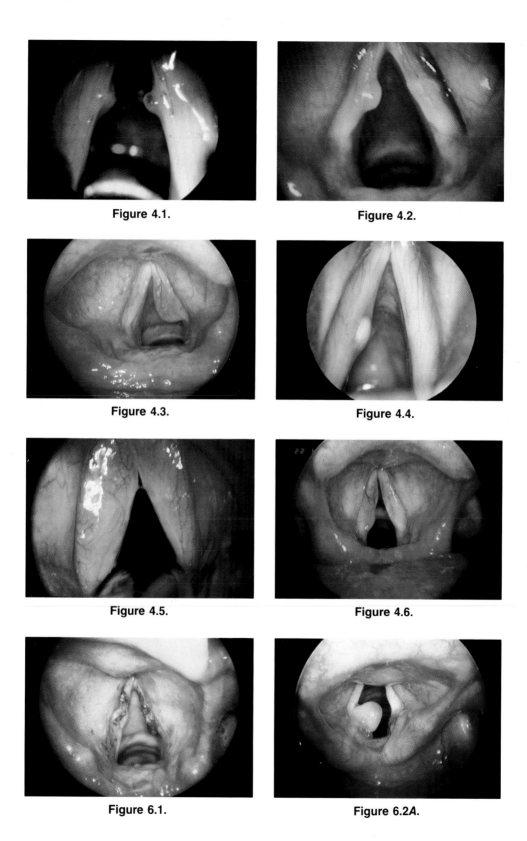

Figure 4.1.

Figure 4.2.

Figure 4.3.

Figure 4.4.

Figure 4.5.

Figure 4.6.

Figure 6.1.

Figure 6.2*A*.

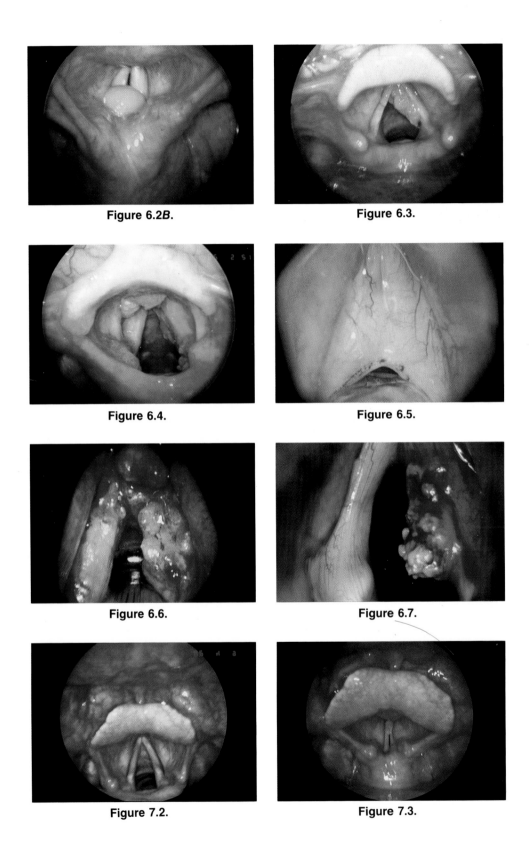

Figure 6.2*B*.

Figure 6.3.

Figure 6.4.

Figure 6.5.

Figure 6.6.

Figure 6.7.

Figure 7.2.

Figure 7.3.

# Understanding
# Voice Problems

## *A Physiological Perspective for Diagnosis and Treatment*

SECOND EDITION

# Understanding Voice Problems

## *A Physiological Perspective for Diagnosis and Treatment*

## SECOND EDITION

*Raymond H. Colton, Ph.D.*
Professor of Otolaryngology and Communication Sciences
Department of Otolaryngology and Communication Sciences
SUNY Health Science Center at Syracuse
Syracuse, New York

*Janina K. Casper, Ph.D.*
Associate Professor of Otolaryngology and Communication Sciences
Department of Otolaryngology and Communication Sciences
SUNY Health Science Center at Syracuse
Syracuse, New York

*With Contributions from*
*Minoru Hirano, M.D.*
Professor and Chairman
Department of Otolaryngology—Head and Neck Surgery
Kurume University School of Medicine
Kurume, Japan

Color photography by Eijii Yanagisawa, M.D.

LIPPINCOTT WILLIAMS & WILKINS
A **Wolters Kluwer** Company
Philadelphia · Baltimore · New York · London
Buenos Aires · Hong Kong · Sydney · Tokyo

*Editor:* John P. Butler
*Managing Editor:* Linda S. Napora
*Production Coordinator:* Linda Carlson
*Copy Editor:* Bonnie Montgomery, M.A., CCC-SLP
*Designer:* Julie Burris
*Illustration Planner:* Lorraine Wrzosek
*Typesetter:* Peirce Graphic Services
*Printer:* R.R. Donnelley & Sons Co., Crawfordsville, IN

*Printed in the United States of America*

**Library of Congress Cataloging in Publication Data**

Colton, Raymond H.
  Understanding voice problems: a physiological perspective for diagnosis and treatment / Raymond H. Colton, Janina K. Casper; with contributions from Minoru Hirano; color photography by Eijii Yanagisawa.—2nd ed.
     p.     cm.
  Includes bibliographical references and index.
  ISBN 0-683-02059-5
  1. Voice disorders—Pathophysiology.   I. Casper, Janina K. II. Hirano, Minoru, 1932–   .  III.
  Title.
  [DNLM: 1. Voice Disorders—physiopathology. 2. Voice Disorders—therapy.
     3. Voice Disorders—diagnosis. 4. Larynx—physiology. WV 500 C725u 1996]
  RF510.C65 1996
  616.85′5—dc20
  DNLM/DLC
  for Library of Congress                              95-33492
                                                            CIP

*The Publishers have made every effort to trace the copyright holders for borrowed material. If they have inadvertently overlooked any, they will be pleased to make the necessary arrangements at the first opportunity.*

To purchase additional copies of this book, call our customer service department a **(800) 638-3030** or fax orders to **(301) 824-7390.** For other book services, including chapter reprints and large quantity sales, ask for the Special Sales Department. International customers should call **(301) 714-2324.**

***Visit Lippincott Williams & Wilkins on the Internet: http://www.lww.com.*** Lippincott Williams & Wilkins customer service representatives are available from 8:30 am to 6:00 pm, EST.

04 05 06
7 8 9 10

*To David W. Brewer, M.D.*
*our teacher, colleague, friend, and*
*a fine human being*

# Preface

A time when books on the topic of the voice and its disorders were few and far between is easily recalled by those of us who have been working in this area for 15 or more years. In recent years we have been witness to an explosion of interest in the voice by clinicians, scientists, physicians, and singers. This multidisciplinary interest in the voice has led to a remarkable sharing of knowledge through the establishment of voice clinic teams, the publication of dedicated scholarly journals, electronic communication, and an abundance of conferences spanning not only a broad range of topics but also spanning the globe.

We are indebted to those who pioneered and pursued an interest in phonation, in how the larynx works, and in how to alter or correct its function. They persevered despite criticism by some who found these early efforts lacking in scientific stringency. We, our students, and our patients are the beneficiaries of their persistence. Nevertheless, much remains to be done. Although heartened and encouraged by the increasing numbers of scientists and clinicians, teachers and singers interested in study of the larynx and voice production, we are dismayed by its continuing "stepchild" status in training programs for speech-language pathologists and otolaryngologists, and in singing pedagogy programs.

That, in large measure, is the reason for this book. We have been fortunate in being part of an interdisciplinary team that has studied normal and disordered phonation both clinically and experimentally for many years. Through this experience we have evolved a philosophy and framework for the examination of laryngeal function and for clinical management of the voice-disordered patient that we believe differs from others in its emphasis. Over the years we have presented our ideas in many lectures and courses and, if we are to judge by feedback received, have found our approach to be well received and helpful. That approach was our guide, which led to the first edition of this book. We intended it to be used by students and practitioners alike in all of the specialty areas involved in the management of the voice, including otolaryngology, speech-language pathology, and coaching of the singing and dramatic voice. We intended this book to be used as a reference text by other medical specialists, such as pediatricians, family practitioners, and internists, who might be the first to come in contact with the patient with a voice disorder. Indeed, with the burgeoning of managed care, this may be increasingly the case and the primary source of referral for examination and treatment.

The enthusiastic acceptance of the first edition of this book greatly exceeded our hopes. We are gratified by the positive comments and the acceptance of our approach to understanding voice problems from our colleagues from all over the world as well as our students. We are especially pleased that our first edition has now been translated into Portuguese.

We believe that understanding voice disorders must begin with an understanding of normal phonatory physiology and acoustics. Based on such knowledge, the student, speech-language pathologist, or otolaryngologist can better understand the pathophysiology that results from misuse, abuse, pathology, or neurological involvement. Because there is not a one-to-one relationship between physiology and acoustics, it is not always possible to predict specific pathology or alterations in physiology on the basis of acoustics or perception alone. Thus, neither acoustic nor perceptual data are sufficient for the diagnosis and treatment of voice disorders. Knowledge of the pathophysiology together with understanding the acoustic and perceptual factors and individual psychodynamics must all be added to the equation in determining diagnosis and planning treatment.

We are firm advocates of the differential diagnosis model and have attempted to emphasize that throughout the text. A differential diagnosis can only be carried out if it is based on knowledge. Indeed, one of the fascinations of the area of voice is the amalgamation of knowledge from various fields that must be brought to bear on the diagnostic process. The team approach is thus an ideal mechanism to support this need. The approach to management has at its core the normalization of physiology, which we believe will bring with it normalized phonation. When normalization is not a realistic goal due to structural or neuromotor constraints, then the approach builds on making the most of what remains functional. The choice of therapy technique is predicated upon a knowledge-based problem-solving approach, rather than on an uninformed gunshot approach. The "if it works, use it" approach may be occasionally successful but may be totally inappropriate at other times. It is important to know when to use a technique and to be able to at least speculate about why it works or fails to do so. The clinician must understand the nature of the altered physiology, must take into account the psychological dynamics that may be operative, and must then be able to select an appropriate approach to rehabilitation that will address these issues. The intertwined relationship between the voice and the person is an essential component in both diagnosis and management. However, even in the patient with a psychologically based voice disorder, the deviations in the manner of voice production and voice use must be understood.

In writing this book we have presumed that the reader will have been exposed to the study of laryngeal anatomy, physiology, neuroanatomy, and neurophysiology. Therefore, the chapters dealing with these topics appear at the end of the book and are designed to be sources of reference rather than extensive teaching chapters.

There is much written about the voice that has yet to be substantiated by experimental data. We have made note of such gaps in our knowledge base in many parts of the book. We have also chosen to put ourselves out on a limb by raising questions about some long-held beliefs. In doing so, we have brought to bear whatever data are available to support our positions, and, where data have been lacking, we have had to rely on theoretical constructs. Although differences exist in the types of voice problems that occur at various points along the lifespan, we have chosen to embed that information wherever appropriate in the text, rather than to devote entire chapters to specific age groupings. Similarly, we have not set aside a chapter specific to the problems of the professional voice user; there is liberal mention made of matters specific to that group throughout the chapters.

We have confined ourselves to those problems having laryngeal integrity and function at their core. Thus, there is little discussion of the difficulties with voice experienced by the deaf and by those with severe hearing impairment. Although we have come to learn that there may be physiological differences in phonation between the hearing and the (congenitally) deaf, the problem usually lies primarily in the absence of acoustic input, not in abnormality of the larynx. For the same reason we have excluded discussion of the resonance problems of hyper- and hyponasality. The velopharyngeal mechanism and the anatomical structures involved in that mechanism are at the core of most resonance problems, rather than the phonatory mechanism. Another problem area that is absent from this book is that of the patient without a larynx. The phonatory demands of that population require the learning of an alternative mode of sound production that can no longer involve the larynx. Such problems are unique to this group and are well and thoroughly covered in other readily available publications.

The structure and philosophy of this revised edition remain essentially unchanged. However, we have attempted to update material, to include more information in certain areas and to respond to some of the requests of those who have used this book as a primary text.

Chapter 1 introduces the study of the larynx, beginning with its important biological functions. The uniqueness of our human ability to speak is dependent in part on the ability of the larynx to produce the acoustic signal we call voice. The changes in that signal that accompany lifespan changes are reviewed, as is voice production. Various models of the team approach to the diagnosis and management of voice disorders are introduced. Chapter 2 is key to the philosophy of this book. We have approached the process of differential diagnosis in the manner usually experienced in the real world when the patient presents with certain symptoms. We follow the process through the steps that the practitioner must pursue in narrowing the possibilities until a diagnosis and etiology are assigned. Case studies are presented as an aid to understanding the process. Our scheme rests on nine primary symptoms of disorders of voice and expands from there to the various signs—perceptual, acoustic, and physiological—that would be consistent with the symptom.

In Chapter 3 Dr. Minoru Hirano discusses the histology of laryngeal structures and the histopathology of laryngeal lesions. Chapter 4 addresses misuse and abuse of the larynx, with a focus on the physiological effects related to specific behaviors. Expanded information on stroboscopic findings is a feature of this revised text. One of the unique aspects of this book is a lengthy section in this chapter devoted to the effects of drugs on the voice. The use of over-the-counter as well as prescription drugs is extensive. Their effects on the laryngeal mucosa have been largely overlooked. There is still a paucity of experimental evidence about these effects. Voice problems associated with nervous system involvement are discussed in Chapter 5. Although voice problems in this population are extensive, the available data on the acoustic parameters of the voice or the physiological parameters of airflow and laryngeal muscle action potentials are exceedingly limited.

Chapter 6 is devoted to a discussion of voice problems associated with organic disease, trauma, and the geriatric voice. These are areas about which the speech-language pathologist must be knowledgeable. A section on geriatric voice has been added to this edition and the information on stroboscopic findings has been expanded. An extensive section on taking the voice history introduces Chapter 7, and its length emphasizes our concern about the relatively minimal training speech-language pathologists and otolaryngologists usually receive in this critical area of communication between patient and practitioner. The remainder of the chapter is given over to descriptions and discussion of methods of laryngeal examination and testing procedures, both instrumental and noninstrumental. The section on stroboscopy has undergone expansion and updating for this revised edition. Dr. Hirano's discussion of phonosurgery, the surgical management of voice problems, is the topic of Chapter 8.

The focus of Chapter 9 is vocal rehabilitation, the primary method used to alter phonatory behavior. The chapter begins with a discussion of some general concepts, principles, and guidelines that we feel are critical to the undertaking of a vocal rehabilitation program. The role of voice therapy in the treatment of disorders associated with voice misuse or abuse, pathology, neuromotor involvement, and some unusual problems is discussed. A variety of specific treatment techniques are offered. Each is described, and a rationale for its usefulness is provided. This section contains materials that are new to this edition. Some controversial areas related to voice therapy and some unresolved issues are discussed, and the final sections of this chapter briefly address the issues of prevention and malpractice.

Chapters 10–12 were described earlier as reference chapters. They deal with the anatomy, physiology, and neuroanatomy and neurophysiology of the vocal mechanism, in that order. It is our intent that these chapters be referred to frequently as a differential diagnosis is pursued. Chapter 13, the final reference chapter, provides normative data against which patient data can be compared. By placing this material in a separate chapter, we have made it readily accessible for reference use. And finally, the Appendix offers a variety of forms and protocols that we have found to be useful in our assessment and examination procedures.

As much as possible, we have attempted to construct our sentences so as to avoid the use of sex-specific pronouns. When this attempt resulted in convoluted language structure that became an obstacle to understanding, we have chosen to use gender pronouns (i.e., his or her) interchangeably. The reader should be aware that despite the particular pronoun used, we are speaking of both sexes unless it is clearly stated otherwise. Furthermore, because this book is intended for a broad audience, we have adopted the use of the English alphabet rather than phonetic symbols to describe vowel sounds (such as /ee/ for the sound in "see").

We are indebted to Minoru Hirano, M.D., for his valued additions to this book in the chapters on histopathology (Chapter 3) and on surgical intervention (Chapter 8). Dr. Hirano has been a leader and innovator in the study of vocal fold physiology and in many other aspects of the study of the larynx and the voice.

Many others have helped in diverse ways with the preparation of this book. Dr. David W. Brewer has, throughout the years, been a source of constant support and encouragement, and he has been so for this project as well. We thank him for that and for his insightful reading and critique of much of the text. We acknowledge the help of the late Samuel Mallov, Ph.D., Professor Emeritus of Pharmacology, SUNY Health Science Center at Syracuse, who checked the accuracy of our comments about the effects of drugs on the voice. Martha Hefner, medical illustrator at the SUNY Health Science Center, along with Elinor Griep, Brian Harris, and Craig Palmer, provided splendid illustrative material, and always with a smile. We are grateful for the generosity of Eijii Yanagisawa, M.D., in sharing with us his superb photographic skills. Others have read various sections of the manuscript in preparation and have given us valuable direction. We wish to thank Peak Woo, M.D., Fran Lowry, Carol Friedenberg, the late Herbert N. Wright, and Joanne Chilton. And, for this revised edition we want to thank the many colleagues who have offered support and encouragement by adopting this textbook for use with their students and by providing us with such useful and positively reinforcing feedback.

We each have families who have been supportive and patient throughout this process. They have been deprived of attention, of our presence, and of the availability of the computer, but not of our gratitude and love.

# Contents

# Chapter 1

# Introduction and Overview

## BIOLOGICAL IMPORTANCE OF THE LARYNX

The structures that make up the larynx play a role in support of an important life-sustaining function, that of respiration. The vocal folds (both true and false), the aryepiglottic folds, and other structures within the larynx were designed to protect the airway from foreign substances. The chief architect of the human body realized that the respiratory system needed multiple levels of protection from the harmful effects of the environment. There are therefore numerous protective mechanisms in the respiratory tract, but the most vigorous exist in the larynx. Some are mechanical and act to close off the airway; others are expulsive and serve to force foreign substances out of the airway. All are reflexive and operate under involuntary control.

Many sensory endings within the larynx collect information about the state of the larynx and transmit this information via several reflex arcs, as well as directly, to the central nervous system. (See Chapter 12 for more detailed information.) These sensory systems exist to inform the brain about the state of the environment within the respiratory tract. Wyke (1967, 1969) has written extensively about these reflex control mechanisms. The various levels of these reflex mechanisms within the larynx provide an elaborate system of precautions to protect the airway and maintain life. For example, sensory endings in the laryngeal lining respond to mechanical forces such as air pressure, and these sensory endings signal information about the state of these forces to higher centers. Although these reflex mechanisms speak primarily to the biological importance of the larynx, they may also be very important to consider in understanding the physiology of normal human phonation and its disorders.

Speech is an overlaid function; that is, the systems used to produce speech were developed long before man learned to speak. These systems have evolved over eons and reflect the unique place of speech in human existence. Clear evidence of this evolution is seen in the multiplicity of the protective laryngeal reflex mechanisms. It is important to recognize that these protective "natural" acts may sometimes be the cause of a voice disorder. For example, excessive coughing, a protective act, can result in trauma to the vocal folds and cause edema, which in turn will interfere with the vibratory characteristics of the vocal folds. By the same token, rapid, random movements of the vocal folds at rest may interfere with normal vibratory motion. Central neurological dysfunction or disruption in a reflex arc may create abnormal motions, which may interfere with phonation or, indeed, threaten life.

The biological function of the larynx can never be ignored. The examiner who accidentally touches the back wall of the pharynx when performing an indirect mirror examination or rigid endoscopy can attest to the rapid reflexive motions of the pharynx and larynx that result from the "gag" reflex. But the reflex or biological functions of the larynx can be subtle in their effects and may not be apparent to both the untrained observer and the experienced eye. Many reflex endings are sensitive to small changes of movement or air pressure that serve to inform the central nervous system about the normal operation of the airway. The respiratory cycle itself and the activity of the nerve controlling the diaphragm may be affected by these changes. They also affect the discharge pattern of the intrinsic laryngeal muscles. The effects of these subtle changes are important to consider for an understanding of the physiology of normal voice production.

We are still young in our understanding of the physiology of the human body. Our fascination with modern instrumentation has produced a good deal of information about human voice production (Baken, 1987). Nevertheless, the fundamental mechanisms of bodily function and regulation must not be ignored. Reflexes are primitive neural control subsystems. They operate at a very low level in the hierarchy of neural functioning and control large muscle actions. But these mechanisms are always there, waiting in the wings, so to speak, to alter body function. Our awareness and appreciation of their role should be apparent to us and to our patients if we are truly to understand human voice function.

## THE LARYNX AND THE VOICE

The voice is an integral part of that uniquely human attribute known as speech. The larynx and its capabilities are important in two broad areas: biological function and speech. The larynx houses the major source of sound used during speaking. The vocal folds produce a tone that becomes modified by the pharynx, palate, tongue, and lips to produce the individual sounds of speech. Voice is present for most vowels and for many of the consonants. The point in time at which the vocal folds begin to vibrate relative to the movement of the other articulators (i.e., lips, tongue, palate, etc.) is critical if the speaker is to produce the intended sound. The larynx must operate in close synchrony with other parts of the speech production apparatus if intelligible speech is to be produced. Although the voice is not visible to the eye during speech production, its absence or malfunction is obvious.

In addition to its role as a carrier of words, the voice can also produce music and express emotion—it acts as a mirror on the inner self. The singer with superb control of the vocal instrument brings immense pleasure to the listener. Although the singer's words may be conveying a verbal statement, the phrasing, control of pitch, and dynamic range may communicate an even stronger message. In classical singing, for example, it is the rare listener who is not enthralled by the sound of a clear and beautiful high C, sung with ease, power, and majesty. The singing of a choir or the chanting of prayers can lead to a unique religious experience.

The actor's voice, resonant and full of meaning, can add significantly to the message and the intensity of emotion. Indeed, the actor's delivery of the words can sometimes be more engrossing to the listener than the words themselves.

The voice serves as an emotional outlet. Both laughter and crying release emotion and frequently serve important cathartic functions. Shouts of joy and screams of rage or fear convey meanings that are easily recognized.

The voice reveals the inner self. It is a reflection of the personality of the individual. We recognize the stereotypical driving, hard-hitting voice of the salesperson, the nasal singsong of the perpetual whiner, and the monotonous, de-energized voice of the depressed. The voice of an outgoing person may be characterized by variety in the pitch, loudness, or quality. On the other hand, a monotone voice, one with little variety, may characterize the withdrawn individual or the loner who wishes not to be disturbed. Markel and his colleagues (1964, 1973) have shown that the pitch, loudness, and tempo of the voice can be used to reflect the personality of the individual and correlate well with other standardized tests of personality measurement.

The speaker's voice is used to attract as well as to repel people. A soft, soothing voice is more apt to calm an agitated person than a strident and loud voice. On the other hand, a strident, loud voice may be effectively used to repel someone. How many times have we used the loud, "firm" voice to dispense with a pushy salesperson or avert a physically threatening situation?

The voice can reveal a person's physical state, as well as the physical state of the larynx. The weak or tremulous voice identified with illness is easily identified, and the voice altered by laryngeal pathology is identified as abnormal.

Yes, the voice is a powerful tool that not only delivers the message but also adds to its meaning. In learning to understand the voice, it is not enough to understand its mechanical functioning. It is also necessary to recognize the important information the voice conveys about the speaker.

## VOICE CHANGES IN LIFE

The voice changes dynamically, minute by minute. But there are long-term changes that are associated with growth and decline in life. At the major stages of life, the uses of the voice are different, as are the demands placed upon it. The reasons for these differences are many and include biological maturation and the emotional and social changes that occur in the individual's life.

### The Voice in Infancy and Childhood

In the first few weeks of life, the infant voice is used to express pain, pleasure, displeasure, and hunger. Crying, the major avenue of communication for the infant, is rich in its ability to communicate (Lester, 1985).

Crying reflects the beginning ability of the infant to control his or her voice. It is a gross physical act that can be described as ballistic in nature. In other words, crying, once started, runs its course and stops. Little can be done to stop the crying once it has begun. As the infant grows older, he is more responsive to the environment and also gains more control of the physical apparatus used to produce the cry. Consequently, the quality of crying is seen to reflect physical and psychological growth. As the infant gains finer and finer motor control, the cry becomes increasingly controllable and much more purposeful in its use.

The next most obvious voice use change occurs as the child begins to use the voice in the production of speech sounds. Concurrently, the child is learning the sounds of his specific language. Then, the child can use the voice to express ideas and moods. As the child matures, increasingly complex and sophisticated differentiation of acceptable modes of vocal behavior develop. This differentiation begins in infancy. The infant's vocal response to a caretaker's familiar voice differs from that given to an unfamiliar voice. Generally, the child's vocal response differs based on the familiarity of the voice heard. Children learn that the voice of the playground is not the voice of the classroom. Such differentiation continues through life in many subtle ways.

The voice reflects the physical development of the child. The infant possesses a larynx that is pliable and has a low level of neuromuscular coordination. It is also small, with short vocal folds. The small structure means that the pitch of the infant's voice will be high. The infant's ability to control the tension of the vocal folds is limited. Moreover, the limited ability of the infant to control the air pressure required for speech results in short bursts of sound, much of which is rather loud. As the infant grows, the ability to control vocal pitch and loudness increases (Boone, 1987). This development is reflected in the longer cries, which are lower in pitch and vary in loudness depending on the circumstances.

In summary, during infancy and childhood the characteristics of the voice depend on the physical, cognitive, and emotional maturation of the child. The physical size of the vocal folds is a major determinant of the fundamental frequency of the child's voice. The infant, with a small larynx and short vocal folds, exhibits the highest vocal pitch, whereas the older child, whose larynx has grown, possesses a lower vocal pitch. Adult vocal pitch is not attained until puberty, when the larynx reaches its adult size.

Loudness variation is less affected by these growth changes and more affected by the level of motor control exhibited by the child. Quality variation reflects physical growth changes of the vocal folds, changes in the size and shape of the entire vocal tract, and finer control of the neuromuscular system. Differentiation of appropriate voice use characteristics depends not only on physical abilities but also on cognitive and social growth and awareness.

## The Voice of the Adult

By age 18 years or so, the voice reaches its mature or adult stage. The fundamental frequency is where it will remain for several decades. The individual has full control over the dynamic range (loudness) of the voice and can produce many variations of pitch and voice quality. These vocal abilities reflect the maturation of the anatomical and physiological systems for the support of speech (Kahane, 1982).

Although the adult voice has been attained by age 18 years, there is still much refinement that can occur to expand vocal abilities. Indeed, vocal training for the singer or the actor most appropriately begins when this level of maturation has been reached. Pitch range can be extended, vocal control can be increased, and voice quality can be enriched.

The way the voice is used depends on the demands of the situation. These demands may include the teacher's need to instruct and maintain discipline, the minister's need to deliver a forceful sermon or to be consoling, or the salesperson's need to sell a product.

It is easy to take the voice for granted. Often we abuse it with constant use and frequent misuse. We abuse it with smoke and alcohol and expect it to be unaffected. It is only when we experience difficulty talking that we cease taking it for granted and seek help. Often we have difficulty recognizing abusive habits and making the necessary changes, even when our lives are threatened.

## The Aged Voice

After 65 years of age or so, the voice begins its decline, much the same way other body functions begin to decline (Beasley & Davis, 1981; Kahane, 1981). The voice, however, does not always mirror the extreme or rapid changes that may occur in the physical functioning of the body. Aged individuals in good physical condition possess voices that are similar in their characteristics to the voices of those of younger persons (Ramig & Ringel, 1983). Some singers can maintain their voices well into their 70s. The voice may retain the essential elements of beauty, although it may not exhibit the range or degree of vocal control that was present in younger years.

But for others, the voice readily betrays the effects of aging. Voices that show a decline or increase in vocal pitch, decreased control of loudness, or changes in voice quality may be showing signs of diminished physical status. Acoustic changes such as upward or downward frequency shifts, poorly controlled loudness, and quality changes reflect to some degree the physiological changes that occur in the larynx with increasing age.

The vocal demands of the aged adult are different from those of the younger adult. After retirement, the salesperson no longer must use that voice to sell a product. The retired minister no longer has to deliver that forceful sermon. The decline of bodily function is usually accompanied by reduced demand on the system. That is not to say that the voice is no longer important to the elderly. On the contrary, the voice is important, but in a different way. It retains its importance in the communication process. It is used to maintain contact with friends and relatives. For some individuals, verbal communication becomes the only way to maintain human contact and control of the environment.

## *Production of the Voice*

To most lay people, the way in which the voice is produced is a mystery. The term "voice box" is commonly used to refer to the larynx, the voice-generating mechanism. Most people know they have one and that it is somewhere in the throat below the chin. From experience they know that when they have laryngitis, they cannot talk, or their voices sound "funny," but few understand why those changes occur. Some people may be aware that after strenuous voice use, such as yelling at a sports event, their voices may sound hoarse. They surmise that the hoarseness has to do with "straining" the voice. Some people may even realize they can manipulate their voices in many ways, for example, raise or lower pitch, increase or decrease loudness, and change their voice quality. This is such common knowledge that it is taken for granted without thought about the workings of the mechanism that is capable of producing such changes.

Understanding phonatory physiology goes beyond knowing laryngeal anatomy and recognizing various laryngeal pathologies (Aronson, 1990; Kahane, 1982). Treatment of the voice-disordered patient demands such a knowledge base. Disturbed physiology may be a by-product of pathology and may persist after the pathological condition is resolved. On the other hand, disturbed physiology may be the cause of tissue changes. Whatever the treatment modality, restoration of normal function, or the closest possible approximation of it, is the goal.

The basic concepts of phonatory physiology have been understood for many years (Lieberman, 1968; van den Berg, 1958). Recent technological advances have, however, significantly increased our knowledge base (Hirano, 1981a; Kahane, 1981). The inaccessibility of the larynx, especially during the phonatory act, has hindered our ability to understand its functioning more fully. In 1855 Garcia developed the laryngeal mirror (Moore, 1937) and made it possible to visualize the larynx with the naked eye. Since then, greatly improved techniques of laryngeal visualization as well as sophisticated analyses of laryngeal acoustics and improved methods of measuring physiological events related to phonation have resulted in a greater understanding of phonatory physiology (Fritzell & Fant, 1986).

Understanding the physiology of phonation is intimately bound up with an understanding of laryngeal anatomy and neuroanatomy, as well as respiratory function. Changes in the structures, in the tissues, or in motor control, whether the result of neurological insult, trauma, congenital anomaly, lesion, or disease process, will distort normal physiology in some fairly predictable ways. This disturbed physiology will, in turn, have an effect on the acoustic characteristics of the voice. Physiology can also be altered by changes in muscular and skeletal tensions, with concomitant changes in the acoustics. Therefore, there is an interdependence and interaction among anatomy, physiology, neurology, and acoustics. It is necessary to understand this interaction in order to treat the voice problem effectively. It is imperative that teachers of the professional voice increase their working knowledge of the complex phonatory process.

All users of voice, as well as those who treat or train it, can benefit from an understanding of how the voice works. Simple knowledge of the effects of vocal abuse and the need for good vocal hygiene could be potent preventive measures for reducing the incidence of vocal nodules and certain polyps. There are some people who, without the benefit of specific voice training, are able to use their voices in strenuous ways without encountering any vocal problems. They are the exceptions. Most people who use the voice in strenuous ways will develop vocal difficulty.

Most professional voice users have had vocal training, although it is rare for such training to include more than a cursory understanding of phonatory physiology. Typically, voice coaches have been taught by other voice coaches, and techniques are passed on that are believed to produce the desired results. There is little objective evidence that these techniques do what they are purported to do. Although some techniques appear to be spectacularly successful, others have done unwitting damage to voices.

Professional voice users need to understand the workings of their instrument in order to use it most effectively and maintain its health. In addition to professional singers and actors, the category of professional voice users should be expanded to include teachers, coaches, ministers, salespersons, cheerleaders, and others who use their voices extensively and strenuously in the performance of their occupations.

## THE VOICE TEAM

There are many professionals representing numerous disciplines or fields of study who are concerned with the voice. Some are concerned with basic studies of laryngeal function, others are concerned with medical problems affecting the voice, and others are concerned with the evaluation and treatment of voice problems. Still other disciplines are focused on developing the voice to its pinnacle of performance ability. Each discipline brings its particular focus and area of expertise to bear on diagnosis, treatment, or teaching.

The internist, the family practitioner, or the pediatrician may be the first specialist to come in contact with a patient with a voice problem. These primary care physicians must be aware of the voice as a sign of health or illness. For example, persistent hoarseness is recognized among medical personnel and the public as one of the early warning signs of cancer. There are other vocal symptoms that if recognized can be helpful in the early diagnosis of certain disease processes. Recognition and identification of the existence of a problem is only the first step. This must be followed by appropriate treatment or referral for further evaluation and/or treatment.

The otolaryngologist is the most appropriate specialist for the diagnosis and treatment of medical laryngeal problems. Although relatively few otolaryngologists specialize in the treatment of voice problems, most will be expected to treat a variety of laryngeal problems. Laryngitis, vocal fold nodules, polyps, loss of voice, or hoarseness of undetermined etiology are among the problems that affect the voice and are typically seen by otolaryngologists.

As is true for otolaryngologists, there are many speech-language pathologists who are engaged in working with the voice disordered patient, but relatively few have made this an area of specialization. The appropriately trained speech-language pathologist is the specialist who diagnoses and treats problems of phonatory function. The mode of treatment offered by speech-language pathologists focuses on the modification of phonatory behavior. Indeed, the speech-language pathologist's broad-based understanding of behavior, whether it be the result of inappropriate voice usage, disturbed physiology, or a manifestation of underlying psychological problems, uniquely qualifies this professional to aid in the diagnostic process, as well as to provide a primary resource for nonmedical treatment.

Voice scientists have added immeasurably to our understanding of phonatory physiology and acoustics through experimental verification of hypotheses. They are not usually directly involved in either treating or teaching the voice user. However, the information available from laboratory studies of the voice can be helpful in establishing a diagnosis, validating treatment approaches (Verdolini & Titze, 1994), and in documenting change in vocal function as a result of treatment. Furthermore, much can be learned about phonatory physiology from the study of abnormal function.

Neurolaryngology, the specialized neurological approach to laryngeal function, is a fairly new and developing area of knowledge, with far-reaching clinical implications. Many movement disorders have laryngeal components that have not been well documented and are not well understood. Indeed, it is not unusual for a phonatory problem to be the first symptom of a motor disorder. A neurolaryngologist could be a valuable member of any team concerned with voice disorders.

Imaging techniques are powerful tools assisting in the diagnosis of pathologic conditions. Radiologists whose special area of expertise focuses on head and neck problems are frequently involved in initial and subsequent assessments of laryngeal abnormality. The information relative to the size, location, and extent of a lesion, which can be obtained through a variety of imaging techniques, is frequently critical to diagnostic and management decisions, especially those that involve surgery. Imaging techniques such as MRI or CT scan hold promise of providing additional information about the state of the larynx and the vocal tract during speaking and singing.

Patients whose voice problems are an expression of deep-rooted emotional problems may require psychotherapy (Aronson, 1990; Aronson, Peterson, & Litin, 1966; Diehl, 1960). Referral to a psychotherapist is indicated when it has been determined that the vocal problem exhibited by the patient may be an expression or symptom of significant psychiatric disability. Our understanding of the bond between voice and personality has been enhanced by the contributions of the fields of psychiatry and psychology.

Teachers and coaches of the singing and the speaking voice are interested in maximizing the individual potential of each of their students while maintaining the health and structural integrity of the vocal mechanism. Their unique knowledge of the professional voice and their deep interest in its correct use necessitates a good knowledge of vocal anatomy and physiology. This is especially true because the vocal demands on singers and actors are frequently much greater than for the average speaker. Furthermore, even subtle changes in vocal production may be critical to a performance.

The number and variety of disciplines involved in the understanding and management of the voice give testimony to the complexity of the process of phonation. Our experience in the "team approach" to understanding the voice and its disorders has led us to an appreciation of the active involvement of a variety of disciplines working together in the assessment process. The benefits of this interactive interdisciplinary team approach accrue not only to the patient, but also to the professionals involved. Each team member brings a particular perspective and knowledge base to the diagnostic process, extending by far the single examiner expertise. For example, the otolaryngologist is highly skilled in assessment of the health or disease state of the larynx, the speech-language pathologist specializes in the phonatory function of the mechanism and the manner in which that may be disturbed by various conditions, and the singing coach recognizes problems in vocal technique that are specific to the singing voice.

The team approach may take various forms, each with its own set of advantages and disadvantages. A description of several models follows.

## Model A

The patient is seen individually during the course of a few hours by various specialists who are located within the same facility or in close proximity. The team of specialists may subsequently meet to discuss their various findings and agree on a treatment plan or individual reports may be directed to the team leader who incorporates them into a complete report with recommendations for treatment.

### ADVANTAGES

The patient is seen on a single day insuring that all specialists are seeing the patient at the same point in the course of the problem. Each specialist has the necessary time to carry out a complete evaluation. The opportunity for interaction among team members exists if the team meets together to discuss the findings. Although it may take a few hours, this model nonetheless can be a time saver for the patient.

### DISADVANTAGES

The process involves duplication of information that the patient must provide to each specialist. Team members do not have the input from other findings until after they have made their own assessments and arrived at their own plan. Even though the examinations take place within a few hours, patients do fatigue and the voice heard by one examiner may be quite different from that heard by another. The patient is usually not present when the team meets precluding further immediate assessment based on input from any individual specialist. Furthermore, if there is a time lag between the actual examinations and the team meeting, much can be lost through dulling of memory. If individual findings are reported to a single individual, the opportunity for invaluable interaction among specialists is lost.

## Model B

The patient is seen individually by various specialists over the course of several weeks. In this type of model individual reports are typically sent to a single individual who is the manager of the case. That individual blends all of the information and makes recommendations for treatment.

### ADVANTAGES

The only plus for this model is the involvement of various disciplines rather than a single specialist who functions without the benefit of additional information.

### DISADVANTAGES

This process may take some time to complete. Over that course of time, the patient's problem may undergo various changes in type, degree, and severity. Thus, each specialist may be seeing quite a different picture. There is no opportunity for true interdisciplinary interaction. It is time consuming for the patient and may prolong a problem by postponing appropriate intervention. Most of the disadvantages cited for the first model also apply here.

## Model C

The patient is seen either by the laryngologist or the speech-language pathologist and a videolaryngostroboscopic examination is done. The history and tape may then be reviewed jointly by these two specialists and a diagnosis and treatment plan agreed to, or, after the tape is reviewed individually, a consensus is reached regarding diagnosis and treatment. Additional specialists may be consulted as needed.

### ADVANTAGES

This model may be a time saver for all concerned—the patient has one examination and only one specialist's time is involved in the examination. If specialists review the examination together, a degree of interdisciplinary interaction is preserved.

### DISADVANTAGES

The patient is usually not present when the specialists meet thus precluding the possibility of additional examination or data gathering at that time. Acoustic and other laboratory data may not be obtained at the time of the initial examination. If the specialists do not jointly review the examination tape, there is a lack of interaction. If further assessments are needed the time necessary to complete the examination becomes extended and interaction of all involved usually becomes minimal.

## Model D

The model which we find most satisfactory is one wherein a number of specialists are present and interact with the patient and each other at the time of the videolaryngostroboscopic examination with the opportunity for further individual assessments to follow. In our model, laboratory data (acoustic and physiological) are obtained immediately prior to or following the endoscopic examination. The team discusses the findings, presents the diagnosis and treatment plan to the patient with full opportunity for questions to be raised and answered (Figure 1.1).

### ADVANTAGES

An obvious advantage of this model is that all of those involved hear the same sample of voice and observe the larynx at the same time. Each specialist has the opportunity to ask questions during the history taking and to request that a specific phonatory task or nonphonatory gesture be elicited during the examination. For example, the speech-language pathologist may wish to assess laryngeal function through the use of both the rigid and the flexible endoscopes in order to appreciate aspects of phonatory physiology. There is an opportunity for immediate discussion of the case and because the patient is still present, further examination is possible if it seems warranted. Diagnosis and treatment plan are formulated by the team and discussed with the patient. The

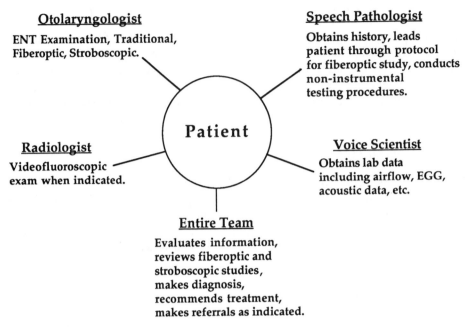

**Figure 1.1.** Team approach.

interdisciplinary interaction is extremely valuable. The history and findings are clearly recalled by all without reliance on memory over time.

## DISADVANTAGES

The number of people present (three or more) can sometimes be overwhelming to patients if they have not been prepared to expect this. The history can only address major areas and may not uncover more subtle or underlying problems which are not appropriately discussed in the presence of the full team. Often such problems, if present, emerge when the patient begins an individual treatment protocol. At that time the individual practitioners attain a better understanding of the patient and can more appropriately explore other issues.

Although we are committed to the team approach, we recognize that it is not a universal mode of operation. Otolaryngologists often see patients with voice problems in their offices and refer to a speech-language pathologist only those patients they feel are appropriate candidates for voice therapy. Those referrals may frequently be based on indirect mirror examinations with minimal information provided to the speech-language pathologist. ASHA guidelines and Preferred Practice Patterns make it clear that all patients with voice disorders must have a laryngological examination prior to the initiation of voice therapy.

When referrals for voice therapy fail to provide adequate information on which to base a therapy approach, it is incumbent on the speech-language pathologist to request additional information. That can be accomplished in a variety of ways. Professional protocol requires that additional information be sought from the referring physician. If the speech-language pathologist is appropriately trained in phonatory function assessment and has access to videostroboscopic equipment, such an examination is appropriately carried out. If neither of these avenues provides the necessary information, patients can be directed to a voice laboratory or other resource where additional information or a second opinion may be obtained.

## SUMMARY

The larynx serves essential reflexive biological functions that protect the airway and maintain life. These basic functions determine the limits of voice and may occasionally affect its function. The larynx also provides the acoustic signal for speech, that uniquely human capability. Singing, dramatic exposition, laughing, and crying fulfill additional human needs through the voice. The voice reflects individual identity, personality, and life stage. An understanding of phonatory physiology, as well as of those factors that may disturb it, is necessary for all professionals involved in the care of the voice and for all professional voice users. Assessment of the voice-disordered patient is enhanced by input from various disciplines through a team approach.

# Chapter 2

# Differential Diagnosis of Voice Problems

In this chapter, and throughout this book, we will be using the term "diagnosis" in two distinct ways. In the first sense, it will refer to the process involved when attempting to determine the nature of a problem. That process involves examination and observation, a problem-solving approach. However, in the second sense, the word "diagnosis" refers to the decision that is the end product of the diagnostic process.

The diagnostic process can be likened to solving a puzzle. Each piece of the puzzle must be examined from many perspectives. Each piece is only a part of the total picture. As a piece is found, it is placed into the puzzle, until the picture is complete. As often happens, one or more pieces may be missing. In those instances, more time is required to search for the missing pieces. In the process of diagnosis of voice disorders, there may also be missing pieces. The solution may not be apparent, and ongoing examination of all relevant information must continue.

Analysis of voice problems involves the examination of many individual components. These components include the statement of the problem, the symptoms, and the history or related information, as well as a set of signs observed or measured by the examiners. The examination of these components may involve a variety of procedures, including the following:

1. interview;
2. examination of medical records;
3. rating of auditory perceptual characteristics;
4. measurement of acoustic, aerodynamic, vibratory, and muscle action events;
5. examination of the laryngeal structures and their function;
6. evaluation of other bodily functions and systems as deemed appropriate; and
7. experimental therapy in which attempts are made to manipulate the patient's vocal behavior.

The successful completion of the diagnostic process requires a solid base of information. Diagnosis of voice disorders requires a thorough understanding of laryngeal anatomy and physiology. A fundamental understanding of phonatory physiology is essential so that rational hypotheses can be formulated about the voice problem and the conditions accompanying it. Moreover, the clinician must be able to formulate hypotheses concerning the expected changes in physiology based on analysis of perceptual and acoustic information. The clinician must be aware of and sensitive to the relationship between personality and voice. Knowledge about the various pathologies and how they affect phonation is, of course, essential.

The diagnostic process is differential. That is, it is necessary to consider all the possible causes of a problem and to proceed through them all as if each is the real cause until proven otherwise. The differential aspect of the diagnostic process involves consideration of the basic question, what specific problem or problems might be comprised of these component parts? The available information relative to the patient is then matched against each of these hypotheses in the search for a match, a good fit.

The process of differential diagnosis begins anew with each patient. In the clinical setting, patients present themselves with a complaint. The challenge for the diagnostician is to track down all the pieces of data essential to an understanding of the physiology, to the making of a diagnosis, and perhaps to knowledge about etiology.

## WHAT IS AN ETIOLOGY?

Etiology is defined by *Webster's Third New International Dictionary* as "a science or doctrine of causation or of the demonstration of causes." Symptoms and signs describe various components of the problem, providing part of the raw data necessary for determination of an etiology. The first step in the treatment of any medical problem is determination of its cause, its etiology. Recognition of the correct etiology is essential for proper treatment. It is not only unwise but also potentially dangerous to treat a problem for which a well-considered etiology has not been established. An incorrect etiology may result in improper treatment, lack of needed treatment, or, at the very worst, may compromise a patient's life. For example, laryngitis is a common cause of hoarseness and is treated not only by otolaryngologists but also by pediatricians, family physicians, and internists. In many cases, laryngitis is caused by an upper respiratory infection and is appropriately treated with medication. However, hoarseness may be a sign of many other laryngeal pathologies, including malignant lesions, and as such should be evaluated with all possible etiologies in mind. In our experience, some patients have followed a protracted and unsuccessful course of medical treatment only to have subsequent examination reveal the presence of a vocal fold lesion as the etiology of the hoarseness.

Assigning an etiology is not always easy. It is possible for a condition to be unobservable and to escape careful and thorough examination. It is also possible for a condition to persist when the original cause of the problem is no longer present. For example, an untrained singer may have developed vocal nodules while engaged in strenuous voice use and abuse for a period of several months. That abusive behavior may no longer be present, but the resultant tissue changes persist. It is important to be aware of antecedent conditions that may be responsible for the present problem.

## SYMPTOMS AND SIGNS

The words "signs and symptoms" are used frequently in medical literature (Brewer, 1975). What do they mean, and how can the distinction between them help the diagnostic process?

### *What Is a Symptom?*

A symptom is a complaint. It is what the patient reports about the problem and its characteristics. Symptoms may be described in various ways. The patient may complain of sensations associated with phonation, such as pain along the side of the neck, or soreness in the throat region after prolonged conversation. Other complaints may refer to perceptual characteristics of the voice, such as hoarseness, scratchiness, or perhaps a wobbly voice. Some symptoms can be verified; some cannot. For example, you cannot "feel" the patient's pain or record it. However, the report of pain is a very important symptom and can be a potent factor in directing the clinician's thinking about a problem. Other feelings (e.g., dry throat, scratchy throat, etc.) may also be difficult to verify. Symptoms, verifiable or not, have reality for the patient and must be given serious consideration by the speech-language pathologist and the otolaryngologist.

## *What Is a Sign?*

Signs are characteristics of the voice that can be observed or tested. For example, hoarseness may be the patient's complaint, but it is also a sign that can be observed and measured independently. Signs represent an inventory of vocal characteristics based upon examination, observation, and measurement.

## *Signs Versus Symptoms: Why the Distinction?*

Despite the fact that patients' symptoms have reality for them, they do not tell the full story. Sometimes they can be misleading, they are frequently underreported, and they may not be the most salient and significant vocal characteristics present in the voice. Thus, symptoms may provide only part of the picture of the patient's vocal difficulty.

Signs provide more objective information. Because each sign is not unique, there may be redundancy in the data. For example, hoarseness may include the following acoustic signs: low fundamental frequency, reduced variability of fundamental frequency, increased frequency perturbation, increased spectral noise, and a large s/z ratio. (See "Acoustic Signs" later in this chapter for a more complete discussion.) Which of these component signs are significant is sometimes difficult to determine, and it is not always possible to record all of them in a single patient. However, knowing how one relates to another and to the underlying pathophysiology will assist the speech-language pathologist and the otolaryngologist in properly interpreting the sign and evaluating its significance.

This section will present the major symptoms and signs of voice problems. In the next three sections, we will discuss perceptual, acoustic, and physiological signs. Finally, each of the symptoms discussed in this section will be presented in greater detail, with listing of the major perceptual, acoustic, and physiological signs, as well as potential etiologies that might produce the symptoms and signs. The emphasis throughout this chapter will be on the process of discovering and interrelating the perceptual, acoustic, and physiological signs to the underlying pathology or pathophysiology and eventually to the etiology of the problem.

## MAJOR SYMPTOMS OF VOICE PROBLEMS

In our experience, patients with voice problems tend to present nine major symptoms. Not included in this list are symptoms reflective of a problem with resonance due to incompetent velopharyngeal closure. These have been traditionally considered voice problems but they are not phonatory problems. There may be some other minor symptoms or different classification schemes, but we believe that these nine primary symptoms are basic. It is important to recognize that symptoms do not usually occur singly but more often appear in combination.

*Table 2.1.* Nine Primary Symptoms of Voice Problems

Hoarseness
Vocal fatigue
Breathy voice
Reduced phonational range
Aphonia
Pitch breaks or inappropriately high pitch
Strain/struggle voice
Tremor
Pain and other physical sensations

The nine symptoms shown in Table 2.1 are as follows:

1. Hoarseness: This symptom reflects aperiodic vibration of the vocal folds. Some patients will use the term "hoarse" to refer to this symptom, whereas others might use terms such as "raspy" or "rough" voice.
2. Vocal fatigue: Patients complain of feeling tired after prolonged talking and often state that continued talking requires a great deal of effort. Moreover, they may report occasional raspiness or hoarseness, which tends to be most apparent at the end of a working day.
3. Breathy voice: Patients sometimes complain that they are unable to say complete sentences without running out of air and needing to replenish the air supply in order to continue talking. They further report having difficulty being heard, especially in noisy situations. We usually label the voice as breathy, although patients will not always use this term.
4. Reduced phonational range: This symptom is usually associated with singers who complain that they are experiencing difficulty producing notes that had previously presented no problem. Typically these are the notes that occur at the upper end of their singing range although some singers have difficulty in the transitional area of their frequency range. They may also complain of tiredness and soreness in the throat area.
5. Aphonia: Aphonia means absence of voice. The patient speaks in a whisper and may sometimes complain of a variety of symptoms, including dryness in the throat, soreness, and a great deal of effort in attempting to speak.
6. Pitch breaks or inappropriately high pitch: A patient may complain of periodic squeakiness and of voice cracks. The voice seems out of control, and the patient reports never knowing what sound will come out. Therefore, we have labeled this symptom as pitch breaks, although it is also possible to describe it as the inappropriate use of high pitch or puberphonia. Often this symptom is reported by a male adolescent who uses an inappropriately high pitch as the habitual voice rather than the more typical lower pitched male voice.
7. Strain/struggle voice: These patients report that it is difficult to talk. This may include inability to get voicing started or to maintain voice. They report that it is a strain to talk; they experience a great deal of tension while speaking and become fatigued due to the effort involved.
8. Tremor: Patients may complain that the voice is wobbly or shaky. They are unable to voluntarily produce a steady sustained sound. This shaky voice is usually very regular and consistent.

9. Pain and other physical sensations: Patient reports about pain vary. Some report pain on both sides of the neck lateral to the larynx; others localize the pain to a specific unilateral area or to mid-larynx, a few report pain radiating into the upper chest. In some patients this may be the only symptom, although that is very rare. Other physical sensations reported by patients include feelings of a lump in the throat, feelings of strain or tension, or the sensation of dryness.

These nine symptoms are the most common in our experience, and the terms used are those patients have used themselves in discussing their problem or are descriptive of their reporting. Patients may report several symptoms, but usually the symptom mentioned first or emphasized should be considered the primary symptom and probably will relate most directly to the eventual etiology of the vocal problem.

## MAJOR SIGNS OF VOICE PROBLEMS

### Perceptual Signs

Perceptual signs of voice problems are the characteristics of an individual's voice that are perceived by the listener/observer. Although they are often considered subjective, they have psychological reality and may be assessed objectively and compared across listeners (see Chapter 7 for methods of scaling perceptions). Clinically, the perceptual signs—the clinician's perception of voice characteristics—paired with the history serve as initial guideposts in the process of differential diagnosis.

Many adjectives have been used to describe voice qualities (Aronson, 1990; Colton & Estill, 1981; Perkins, 1971). The list of perceptual signs to be presented in this chapter encompasses a variety of perceptual characteristics that serve to focus our attention on clinically useful voice characteristics. Some of these characteristics have reasonably clear, well-defined, measurable acoustic correlates and others do not. For example, we are not able to differentiate hoarseness and roughness acoustically. Both hoarseness and roughness have increased perturbation and a noisy spectrum. As another example, tension can be observed by a clinician, but its measurement becomes problematic. Indeed, we would be hard put to specify the exact loci of vocal tension, its acoustic parameters, and how to measure it.

Perceptions by their very nature are hard to describe verbally. They are subjective and individual, being influenced by personal preference, experience, and culture. In the following discussion of perceptual signs of voice (Table 2.2), we have grouped them within the broad areas of pitch, loudness, quality, nonphonatory behavior, and aphonia (absence of phonation). The definitions of the terms are worded so as to provide meaningful guidelines without undue restriction on individual experience.

#### PITCH

Pitch is the perceptual correlate of fundamental frequency.

##### Monopitch

This term refers to a voice that lacks variation of pitch during speech. There is a marked absence of inflectional variation and in some instances an inability to voluntarily vary pitch. Monopitch can be one of many signs characteristic of neurological impairments that may affect the voice. It may also simply be a reflection of an individual's personality or, more significantly, of psychiatric disability.

*Table 2.2.* Perceptual Signs of Voice Problems

---

*Pitch*
 Monopitch (reduced pitch variability)
 Inappropriate pitch
 Pitch breaks
 Reduced pitch range

*Loudness*
 Monoloudness (reduced loudness variability)
 Loudness variation (soft, loud, or uncontrolled)
 Reduced loudness range

*Quality*
 Hoarse or rough
 Breathy
 Tension
 Tremor
 Strain/struggle
 Sudden interruption of voicing
 Diplophonia

*Other Behaviors*
 Stridor
 Excessive throat clearing

*Aphonia*
 Consistent
 Episodic

---

### Inappropriate Pitch

This refers to the voice that is judged to exceed the range of acceptable pitch for age and/or sex, being either too low or too high. Norms for fundamental frequency (the acoustic correlate of pitch) are available for age and sex (see "Acoustic Signs" later in this chapter). The high-pitched voice of a young child is perceived to be inappropriate when produced by an adult, and vice versa. Similarly, the pitch range for an adult female voice does not generally extend as low as might be acceptable in an adult male. The perception of voice pitch and the subsequent judgment of the acceptability of that pitch, based solely on perception, can be fraught with danger. Research has shown (Plomp, 1976; Wolfe & Ratusnik, 1988) that other characteristics of voice quality can affect our perception of pitch. Thus, although the hoarse voice of a person with a vocal lesion may be perceived to be lower than acceptable, actual measurement of the fundamental frequency may fail to corroborate that perception (Shipp & Huntington, 1965). The pitch of a voice is related to the size of the larynx and its structures. A vocal pitch higher than expected may reflect underdevelopment or immaturity of the larynx based on endocrinological factors or perhaps a congenital anomaly. Vocal pitch may also be excessively low due to endocrinological factors such as hypothyroidism or the use of male hormone by women. It is also possible for vocal pitch to be too high or too low based on individual preferences or habit.

### Pitch Breaks

Unexpected and uncontrolled sudden shifts of pitch in either an upward or downward direction are readily perceived even by the untrained and unsophisticated listener.

They are frequently associated with the changing voice of the adolescent male and are usually a temporary stage that resolves with time. Occasionally pitch breaks persist beyond the expected laryngeal growth period. Pitch breaks, however, may also occur as a result of laryngeal pathology or as an accompaniment to conditions that involve some loss of neural control of phonation.

### Reduced Pitch Range

Sometimes, a patient may complain about a reduction in pitch range, usually at the high end of the range and an inability to produce these pitches without excessive strain or at all. Very rarely do patients complain about loss of the low end of their range.

### LOUDNESS

Loudness is the perceptual correlate of intensity.

### Monoloudness

This refers to voice that lacks variation in loudness level. The use of increased loudness for emphasis is absent, and there may be an inability to voluntarily vary loudness. In this category, the perception does not attend to the actual level of loudness being used but rather to the variability of the level during speaking. Monoloudness may be (a) an indication of neurological impairment in which the ability to voluntarily control and vary loudness may be lost, (b) a reflection of psychiatric disability, or (c) a habit associated with personality.

### Loudness Variation

When variations in loudness are extreme, either too soft to be heard easily in average conversational settings or excessively loud for the setting, they are perceived as a sign of a problem. Although norms are available for dynamic range (the softest to the loudest sound a person is able to produce; see "Acoustic Signs" later in this chapter), appropriate loudness levels are dependent upon the specific speaking situation. Unpredictable and uncontrolled variation of loudness level, explosive to fading, constitutes another sign of loudness variability that is beyond accepted norms. Voices that are too soft or too loud may be a reflection of auditory dysfunction, of personality, or of habit. A habitually loud speaker may have grown up in a large and noisy family in which excessive loudness was the norm, or may have had to speak loudly in order to be heard by a hearing-impaired relative. The inability to control vocal loudness may also be due to the loss of neural control of the phonatory mechanism or to problems affecting the respiratory mechanism. It is also possible that variations in vocal loudness, from explosive to almost aphonic, may be a reflection of psychological problems.

### Reduced Loudness Range

As was the case for reduced pitch range, this refers to the reduction in a patient's loudness range, usually a loss of the ability to produce loud sounds. Many times, reduced phonational range and reduced loudness range occur in the same patient.

### QUALITY

### Hoarse or Rough

These words are descriptors of a voice quality that is noticeably aberrant in its lack of clarity, its increased noisiness, and its discordance. Although hoarseness/roughness may be the primary perceptual characteristic of an abnormal voice, its perception may be paired with other characteristics such as breathiness, tension, or strain. The degree of hoarseness/roughness in the voice is related to the acoustic correlates of perturbation (see below under "Perturbation") and to the noisiness of the spectrum (see later under "Signal-to-Noise"). Pathologies that affect the vibratory behavior of the vocal folds will usually result in some degree of perceived hoarseness/roughness.

### Breathy

This designation refers to the perception of audible air escape during phonation. The voice lacks clarity of tone and is usually reduced in loudness. A breathy voice quality is related to the amount of airflow produced. Norms for airflow measures are available (see Chapter 13), and its measurement can verify the perception of breathiness. Excessive airflow through the glottis is usually a reflection of inadequate glottal closure. Inability to fully adduct the vocal folds during phonation may be the result of peripheral neurological problems, of central neurological impairment, of the presence of a lesion that interferes with closure, or of improper use.

### Tension

Tension in the voice suggests to the listener a "hard edge" to the voice, combined with hard glottal attacks and sometimes observable muscular tension in the external neck. Tension is a perception that is difficult to verify through measurement. Assumptions can be made about the dynamics of vocal tension, such as increased tension of certain muscle groups, but we do not have adequate data to determine the most salient muscle groups nor the amount of tension that is acceptable in the normal voice. In many instances tension seems to be related to "hyperfunctional" usage patterns. However, it may also be a reflection of compensatory behavior in the presence of some laryngeal pathology or neurological disability.

### Tremor

This sign may be described as regularly rhythmic variations in pitch and loudness of the voice that are not under voluntary control. The voice is perceived as unsteady, "wobbly," quavering. Tremor is a perception that can be verified through measurement. Indeed, the rate of the tremor can be an important factor in determining the underlying pathology (see "Voice Tremor" later in this chapter). Tremor of any type is usually a reflection of a central nervous system dysfunction that results in some loss of control of the phonatory mechanism.

### Strain/Struggle

The voice perceived to reflect strain/struggle behavior suggests difficulty in initiating phonation and struggle to maintain phonation. As speech is produced, there is the perception of inability to control voicing as it fades in and out. Actual voice stoppages may occur. Physical correlates of these perceptions, such as voice onset time, silence, and variations of fundamental frequency and sound pressure level (SPL), are accessible to objective measurement. However, the perception of the strain and struggle behavior is qualitatively unique and is not well expressed by the various objective measurements. There continues to be considerable controversy (Aronson, 1990; Dedo, Townsend, & Izdebski, 1978) regarding the etiology of this type of vocal behavior. However, it would probably be fair to say that neurological dysfunction of some sort is implicated in most cases. Some experts continue to believe that, in a certain percentage of these patients, the etiology is psychological.

### Sudden Interruption of Voicing

A sudden unexpected drop in loudness and an equally unexpected change in voice quality to breathy voice is a very noticeable perceptual sign. The breathy voice may last only a fraction of a second and may occur repeatedly within an utterance, alternating with essentially normal voicing. This perceptual sign of an abnormal voice may be the result of sudden, unexpected, and involuntary abduction of the vocal folds, or delayed adduction when making the transition from unvoiced to voiced phonemes (Ludlow, 1995), the etiology of which is usually neurological dysfunction. Again, these perceived voice characteristics (e.g., loudness variability, airflow changes) are accessible to objective measurement.

### Diplophonia

This word literally means "double voice." It is said to be present when two distinct pitches are perceived simultaneously during phonation. Theoretically this occurs when the vocal folds are under differing degrees of tension or mass and each vibrates at a different frequency. There does not seem to be a consistent pattern of the perception of diplophonia as a consequence of a given pathology.

## OTHER BEHAVIORS

### Stridor

The term refers to noisy breathing, involuntary sound that accompanies inspiration, expiration, or both and is indicative of a narrowing of the airway at a certain point. Although the pitch or quality of the stridorous sound is taken by some to be diagnostic (Cotton & Richardson, 1981), the judgments of these factors appear to be based entirely on perception. Although the frequency and intensity of stridor could be measured, we know of no such measurements. The presence of stridor is always an abnormal finding and one with potentially serious implications since it is a reflection of blockage of the airway.

### Excessive Throat Clearing

A frequent accompaniment to a variety of voice disorders, excessive throat clearing probably represents an attempt by the patient to clear excess mucus from the vocal folds, or it may be a response to the sensation of "something in the throat." It is a natural behavior but is considered a perceptual sign of disordered voice when it occurs frequently and consistently.

## APHONIA

### Consistent

This is an absence of voicing, usually perceived as whispering, that is constantly present. Aphonia may be the result of bilateral vocal fold paralysis in which the vocal folds are unable to adduct or a result of central nervous system dysfunction, or it may be a psychogenic problem.

### Episodic

Episodic aphonia may take a number of forms. A patient may exhibit unpredictable, involuntary aphonic breaks in voice production that last for only a fraction of a second. Another patient may experience aphonic periods lasting minutes, hours, or even days. Yet another patient may experience a gradual fading of voice to the aphonic state, particularly with increased physical fatigue. Momentary involuntary aphonic breaks are not uncommon during the speech of patients with laryngeal pathology. Episodic aphonia may be observed in patients with central neurological dysfunction of the flaccid type, as noted in myasthenia gravis. However, it is possible that episodic aphonia may be psychologically based.

## Acoustic Signs

Voice is produced by movements of the vocal folds interrupting the egressive airstream. The movements of the folds are controlled by the biomechanical characteristics of the folds themselves, the magnitude of the air pressure beneath the folds, and their neural control. Pathology may affect these movements by interfering with any of these variables.

Vocal fold movement results in periodic interruption of the airstream at rates appropriate for the perception of sound. Acoustics is the study of sound, and voice acoustics can provide important information about vocal fold movement. But acoustics is one stage removed from the movements of the vocal folds. Although acoustic signs are, at best, imperfect mirrors of the underlying vocal fold physiology, there is a great deal of correspondence between the physiology and acoustics, and much can be inferred about the physiology based on acoustic analysis. Moreover, acoustic parameters are probably the easiest to record and to analyze objectively. Many acoustic parameters of the speaking voice can be measured by various instruments, such as the Visi-Pitch (Kay Elemetrics) or one of several computer programs (CSL, CSpeech, Dr Speech Science for Windows, MacSpeech Lab).

There are many acoustic signs that may be associated with any given pathology (Table 2.3). Some are unique and others redundant. For example, jitter (variations of period from one pitch period to the next, also known as frequency perturbation) and noise spectrum may reflect the basic aperiodicity of the vibrating vocal folds. Jitter

---

*Table 2.3.* Acoustic Signs of Voice Problems

| |
|---|
| *Fundamental frequency* |
|     Mean or average speaking fundamental frequency |
|     Frequency variability |
|     Phonational range |
|     Perturbation |
| *Amplitude* |
|     Average overall sound pressure level (SPL) |
|     Amplitude variability |
|     Dynamic range |
|     Perturbation |
| *Signal-to-noise ratio (harmonics-to-noise ratio)* |
| *Vocal rise or fall time* |
| *Voice tremor* |
| *Phonation time* |
| *Voice stoppages* |
| *Frequency breaks* |
| *Normal acoustics* |

may be easier to measure and therefore have greater clinical utility. But all acoustic signs reflect some aspect of the underlying pathology of interest.

## FUNDAMENTAL FREQUENCY

The vibrating frequency of the vocal folds is referred to as fundamental frequency. This acoustic characteristic is usually defined as average fundamental frequency or, in the instance of spontaneous speech or reading, speaking fundamental frequency. Also of interest is the variability of fundamental frequency usually expressed as the standard deviation of frequency and sometimes labeled the pitch sigma. The range of frequencies that can be produced by the voice may also be of interest and is called phonational range. Finally, there is considerable interest in the short-term stability of the vocal folds. This stability (or lack thereof) is reflected in the measure termed frequency perturbation.

### Mean Fundamental Frequency

There are considerable normative data on fundamental frequency during speech for males and females of all ages (Baken, 1987). Males should produce average fundamental frequencies during conversational speech between 100 and 150 Hz, whereas females should produce fundamental frequencies between 180 and 250 Hz (Hollien, Dew, & Phillips, 1971). Figure 2.1 presents an example of fundamental frequency as a function of time for a sentence produced by a normal male speaker. The speaking fundamental frequency was 108.5 Hz. Pathology may affect the vibrating frequency, with the result that males or females will produce either too high a frequency or too low a frequency. By too high or too low, we mean frequencies that lie outside these approximate limits.

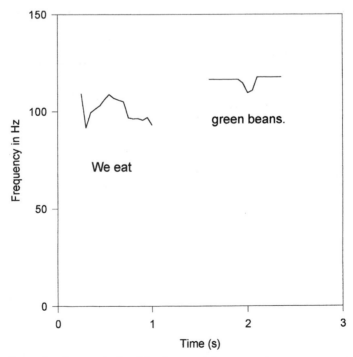

*Figure 2.1.* Example of an analysis of fundamental frequency in a sentence produced by a normal male speaker. The gaps in the plot indicate no measurable fundamental frequency. These gaps correspond to a slight pause between the words "eat" and "green."

Pitch should not be confused with frequency. Pitch is the psychological feature of the voice, whereas frequency is the physical feature. It is possible to perceive a voice as having excessively low pitch without an excessively low fundamental frequency (Wolfe & Ratusnik, 1988).

### Frequency Variability

The standard deviation of fundamental frequency (or pitch sigma) reflects frequency variability for a reasonably large time segment or passage. During speech, both fundamental frequency and intensity vary depending on the sounds, the words uttered, and the intent of the message. Computing the standard deviation of frequency during a sentence or paragraph will provide an estimate of this longer-term variability. In Figure 2.1 the standard deviation of fundamental frequency for the sentence of the normal speaker was 8.9 Hz. In the literature the standard deviation of fundamental frequency is usually expressed in semitones and labeled the pitch sigma. Converting frequency to semitones yields a pitch sigma of 1.9 for this speaker. As a general guideline, normal speakers should be expected to exhibit pitch sigmas between 2 and 4 semitones for both males and females (Baken, 1987; Linville & Fisher, 1985; Mysak & Hanley, 1959; Stoicheff, 1981). Patients are sometimes unable to produce normal variability. This acoustic measure would presumably be related to the perceptual features of monopitch, although little research has been done on these relationships.

### Phonational Range

Phonational range refers to the range of frequencies that a person can produce. Normal young adults should be able to produce a phonational range of about three octaves, with singers slightly higher than nonsingers (Colton & Hollien, 1972; Baken, 1987). Phonational range decreases with age (Linville, 1987).

### Perturbation

Perturbation refers to the irregularity of vibration of the vocal folds that is sometimes called vocal jitter. Such irregularity may be manifested either by irregularities in the time of vibration or in the amplitude of vibration. Variation of glottal period or frequency perturbation refers to the change of frequency from one successive period to the next (Casper, 1983; Horii, 1979, 1980, 1982). Normal speakers have a small amount of perturbation, which may represent variation in vocal fold mass, tension, muscle activity, or neural activity (Baer, 1979; Pinto & Titze, 1990). An example of perturbation in a normal speaker's sustained vowel production is shown in Figure 2.2. The average jitter is expressed as a percentage of the average fundamental frequency and is 0.27 percent. Chapter 13 summarizes some of the data on normal perturbation.

When pathologies affect the vocal folds, their vibrations will show increased aperiodicity (Hecker & Kreul, 1971; Koike, 1967b; Lieberman, 1963). There are many possible pathologies that can affect vibration, including but not limited to growths on the vocal folds, changes in the mucosa, variations in the composition of the vocal folds, variations in muscle function, and variations in the motor control of the muscles controlling the vibration. Thus, perturbation may not be useful for differentiating among etiologies but may reflect the extent of a pathology (Colton, Reed, Sagerman & Chung, 1982).

### AMPLITUDE

There are several acoustic variables that reflect the amplitude or strength of the tone produced by the vocal folds. Many are expressed in decibels. Overall SPL refers to the average sound pressure level of an utterance (sustained vowel, spontaneous sentence,

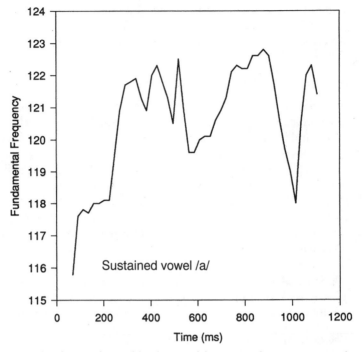

*Figure 2.2.* Example of an analysis of fundamental frequency during a sustained vowel. Note the changes of fundamental frequency, although the speaker was attempting to produce a steady phonation.

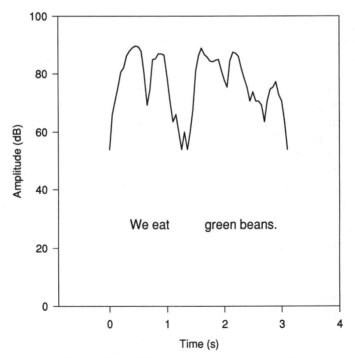

*Figure 2.3.* Example of an analysis of intensity in a sentence produced by a normal male speaker. In general, the humps in the figure correspond to the production of the words in the sentence. The valleys correspond to the gaps between words or very slight pauses.

or paragraph). Amplitude standard deviation is simply a measure of amplitude variability, whereas dynamic range reflects the range of vocal amplitudes an individual can produce. Finally, amplitude perturbation reflects the short-term variation of amplitude from one glottal period to the next.

### Overall SPL

The average overall SPL in decibels provides an indication of the strength of the vocal fold vibration. If a person speaks softly, the overall SPL will be low. Conversely, if a person speaks loudly, the overall SPL will be high. Everyday conversational speech may exhibit SPLs between 70 and 80 dB (Baken, 1987). SPLs as a function of time for a normal male speaker's production of a simple sentence are shown in Figure 2.3. The mean SPL was 76.3 dB.

### Amplitude Variability

During speech or a reading passage, the amplitude of speaking will vary depending on the sounds spoken and the message. Variability of amplitude during speech would be expressed as a standard deviation. The standard deviation of SPL for the normal speaker in Figure 2.3 was 10.28 dB.

### DYNAMIC RANGE

This is the range of vocal intensities that a person can produce. Normal speakers should be able to produce minimum intensities of around 50 dB and maximum intensities of around 115 dB; intensities for males are slightly higher than for females (Coleman, Mabis, & Hinson, 1977). Figure 2.4 presents the mean dynamic ranges as a function of fundamental frequency for the normal subjects in the Coleman, Mabis, and Hinson study. Note how the SPLs at the extremes of the fundamental frequency range are much smaller than the dynamic ranges at the mid frequencies.

### Perturbation

As was the case for fundamental frequency, it is possible that the amplitude of the vocal fold tone will vary from one cycle to the next. This characteristic is called

*Figure 2.4.* The left panel presents the average and range for 10 male subjects, whereas the right panel presents the average and range for 12 female subjects. Each subject produced a sustained vowel at 10% increments of their fundamental frequency ranges and at minimum and maximum SPL.

amplitude perturbation or shimmer. Growths on the vocal folds or poor neural control of the vocal folds would be expected to affect the stability of the vocal folds. Therefore, shimmer should reflect the kind and degree of pathology that a speaker might exhibit. Chapter 13 summarizes some of the available data on shimmer for normal speakers.

### SIGNAL-TO-NOISE RATIO

Noise is random, aperiodic energy in the voice. It may occur throughout the entire frequency range of the voice, or it may be located in certain frequency bands. Normal voices have low levels of noise, whereas abnormal voices show greater noise levels (Emanuel & Sansone, 1969; Fujiu, Hibi, & Hirano, 1988; Hanson & Emanuel, 1979; Isshiki, Kitajima, Kojima, & Harita, 1978; Kitajima, 1981; Newman & Emanuel, 1991; Wolfe & Steinfatt, 1987; Yanagihara, 1967a; Yumoto, Gould, & Baer, 1982; Yumoto, Sasaki, & Okamura, 1984). Two general approaches have been developed for the analysis of noise components in voice.

The first, reported by Yanagihara (1967b), uses spectrograms to classify voices, using the level of noise near the second formants of several vowels. As such, the system is qualitative although based on objective data. It may not provide data that might differentiate subtle differences among patients, differences that might assist in diagnosis.

The second approach analyzes the level of noise directly. An example of this approach is the harmonics-to-noise ratio, a variant of signal-to-noise ratio (Yumoto, 1987; Yumoto, Gould, & Baer, 1982; Yumoto, Sasaki, & Okamura, 1984). Harmonics-to-noise ratios greater than 1 mean that the harmonic energy was greater than the noise energy. Normal speakers are expected to have harmonics-to-noise ratios much greater than 1.

Noise may be generated in two ways. First, there may be a noise source at or near the vocal folds (e.g., air rushing against the open vocal fold). Second, greater aperiodicity of vibration may show up as greater noise in the spectrum (Klingholz & Martin, 1985). Most procedures for the measurement of noise would not be able to distinguish between these two sources. Nevertheless, increased noise levels would be associated with problems that affect the vibrating frequency of the vocal folds or create additional, unwanted sources of sound at the level of the vocal folds.

### VOCAL RISE OR FALL TIME

The ability of the vocal folds to start tone production quickly or to stop phonation quickly may be impaired by pathology. The time it takes to produce a tone of full amplitude is referred to as rise time. The time it takes for the vocal folds to stop producing a tone is called fall time. Rise time is also associated with vocal attack. It has been shown that some pathologies will affect the time it takes the vocal folds to attain their amplitude (Koike, 1967a).

Pathologies affecting the neural control of laryngeal muscles would theoretically be expected to have a pronounced effect on the rise or fall time of glottal amplitude, although little work has been reported on these relationships.

### VOICE TREMOR

Tremor refers to a regular variation in the fundamental frequency or amplitude of the voice (Aronson, Brown, Litin, & Pearson, 1968a; Izdebski & Dedo, 1979; Ludlow, Bassich, Connor, & Coulter, 1986). As a patient attempts to sustain a tone at a constant frequency, there is a slow variation of frequency around the desired constant frequency. Usually, this variation is between 3 and 5 Hz about the mean fundamental frequency, although it could be higher or lower than these limits. Tremor may also be

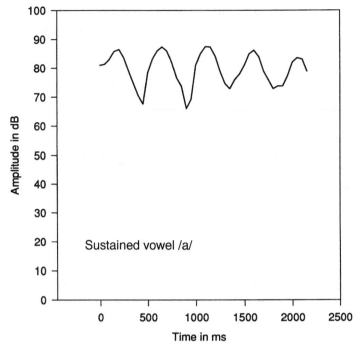

*Figure 2.5.* Voice tremor. A patient with voice tremor was asked to sustain the vowel /a/. The variation of SPL accompanying the tremor during the vowel production is evident in this figure.

exhibited by slow variation in the amplitude of the voice signal. Tremor is usually associated with variations in muscle activity levels or the control of the muscles used in phonation. As such it is usually associated with central nervous system dysfunction and not impaired peripheral motor control or vocal fold pathology.

Figure 2.5 presents an example of tremor on a sustained vowel. Note the slow oscillations of SPL during the production. Measuring the distance between the peaks of the SPL oscillations would yield the tremor rate, which in this example was about 5 Hz.

### PHONATION TIME

Maximum phonation time refers to the maximum time a subject can sustain a tone on one breath. As a rule of thumb, one would expect normal adult male subjects to produce a vowel for about 20 seconds, adult female subjects about 15 seconds, and children about 10 seconds (Kent, Kent, & Rosenbek, 1987). However, these values may vary considerably between people and among age groups. Phonation time may vary as a function of trials. With proper instruction and practice, as few as three trials may be sufficient (Bless & Hirano, 1982; Sawashima, 1966). Short maximum phonation times reflect inefficiency of the phonatory or respiratory system.

Another measure of phonation time is what is referred to as the s/z ratio (Boone & McFarlane, 1988; Eckel & Boone, 1981), or the maximum sustained phonation time of /s/ divided by the maximum sustained phonation time of /z/. A normal speaker would be expected to sustain both the voiceless /s/ and the voiced /z/ for approximately equal durations, resulting in a ratio of 1. However, in the presence of a disturbance of vocal fold vibratory behavior and/or ability to close the glottis, the duration of sustained voicing for /z/ would be expected to suffer. The resulting s/z ratio becomes increasingly larger as the discrepancy between sustained productions of these sounds (z shorter than s) becomes greater. For a group of normal subjects, Eckel and Boone (1981) reported average s/z ratios between 0.4 and 2. Based on the results of their statistical tests between normal and pathological speakers, they suggest that any s/z ratio greater than 1.4 may indicate a vocal pathology. S/z ratios for children were similar (Shearer, 1983; Tait, Michel, & Carpenter, 1980; Weinberg, Bosma, Shanks, & DeMyer, 1968).

### VOICE STOPPAGES

Normal speech consists of phonation, noises, and silences. The latter are usually brief. When silences become longer than normally expected or appear unexpectedly during phonation, they call attention to themselves, disrupt intelligibility, and are considered abnormal. In some disorders, the voice may suddenly stop for a brief period of time and then revert to its previous level. These interruptions would be observable in the spectrum of the sound.

### FREQUENCY BREAKS

Frequency breaks refer to sudden shifts of fundamental frequency either upward or downward. One would expect that these would be related to the perceptual pitch breaks often reported in the literature in the speech of patients with certain vocal pathologies.

### NORMAL ACOUSTICS

Finally, it is possible that a patient with a phonatory problem will exhibit acoustic features typical of a normal voice. In other cases, the differences between a normal and abnormal voice may be so subtle that they are not manifested in these acoustic signs.

## *Measurable Physiological Signs*

The physiological signs that may be affected by pathology include aerodynamic features (airflow and pressure), vibratory behavior (contact area, waveform shape), and muscle activity (as recorded by electromyography). These are summarized in Table 2.4.

*Table 2.4.* Measurable Physiological Signs of Voice Problems

*Aerodynamics*
    airflow (increased, decreased, variable)
    air pressure (increased, decreased, variable)

*Vibratory behaviors*
    aberrant glottal pulse shape
    slowed opening and closing phases of vocal folds
    inadequate or excessive closed times
    irregularity or asymmetry of vocal fold motion
    mucosal wave changes

*Muscle activity*
    absent, reduced, or excessive levels
    involuntary rhythmic variations of level
    sudden, unexpected bursts of activity
    slow rise or fall in amplitude
    diminution of level with sustained phonation
    imbalance of paired muscle activity

## AERODYNAMIC MEASUREMENTS

### *Airflow*

During normal speech, airflow may range between 50 and 200 ml/sec, with males producing higher flows than females (Hirano, 1981b). Usually, the measurement of airflow represents the average flow over several glottal cycles. It is possible to measure the peak flow that occurs during a vibratory cycle. If possible, peak flow measures should be differentiated from the steady airflow rates that occur during speech. The steady airflow rates for speakers with various vocal fold pathologies are greater than those for normal speakers. Normal speakers exhibit a small amount of airflow when the vocal folds adduct, whereas speakers with vocal pathology may produce larger than normal airflows during the closed phase of the vocal folds. If closure of the vocal folds is compromised by a lesion or poor muscular or neural control, airflow rates will be greater than normal.

### *Air Pressure*

The magnitude of air pressure beneath the vocal folds is important in producing vibration and determining the intensity of the sound. Typical pressures beneath the vocal folds (subglottal air pressure, lung pressure, or alveolar pressure) range from about 0.3 to 2.0 kPa[1], depending on the loudness of the sound. Pressures between 0.2 and 0.9 kPa would be expected for conversational speech levels (Brodie, Colton, & Swisher, 1988; Holmberg, Hillman, & Perkell, 1988; Shipp & McGlone, 1971). Higher than normal levels may indicate either excessive lung pressures or inefficient valving of the vocal folds.

Variability of airflow or pressure may be important to measure in persons with vocal pathology. Excessive variation could be associated with poor motor control of the vocal folds or of the respiratory system.

### *Phonation Threshold Pressure*

Phonation threshold pressure is the minimum pressure required to initiate vocal fold vibration (Titze, 1992b). It is dependent on the pitch of the phonation and determined by the degree of opening between the vocal folds, the thickness of the vocal folds, the velocity of the mucosal wave, and the viscosity of the tissue (Titze, 1994). It may be a very important measurement to obtain when describing the pathophysiology of phonation and appears to reflect the level of hydration of the vocal folds (Verdolini-Marston, Titze, & Druker, 1990).

## VIBRATORY BEHAVIOR MEASUREMENTS

Vibratory characteristics of the vocal folds are important in determining the final acoustic output of the vocal folds. Many of these characteristics have been studied using high-speed films. Information about some of the vibratory characteristics can be obtained from stroboscopic examinations or by using indirect techniques for assessing laryngeal function. Some of the more popular systems include (*a*) electroglottography (EGG), (*b*) inverse filtering of the oral airflow waveform (Flowglottogram), and (*c*) photoglottography (PGG).

During normal voice function, the shape of the airflow pulse or the shape of the area pulse is different depending on the mode of vibration[2] (Colton & Estill, 1981;

---

[1]kPa is kiloPascals, a unit of pressure measurement in the MKS (Meter-Kilogram-Second) system. 1 kPa is approximately equal to 10 cm $H_2O$.
[2]The vocal folds may produce different modes of phonation depending on the characteristics of the mucosa, tension in the epithelium and muscle and other inherent physical characteristics of the tissue. See Titze (1994), pp. 97-100 for more information.

Timcke, von Leden, & Moore, 1958). Similarly, the shape of the airflow pulse through the glottis is different (Rothenberg, 1981; Sundberg, 1987). In pathology, the pattern of glottal opening becomes irregular and distorted (von Leden, Moore, & Timcke, 1960), as does the airflow pulse (Colton & Brewer, 1985). Thus, analysis of glottal area from high speed films or airflow waveform shape can help to describe the vibratory characteristics of voice-disordered patients.

## MUSCLE ACTIVITY MEASUREMENTS

Pathology may affect the muscles that control vocal function directly by affecting peripheral function or indirectly by affecting the central nervous system. Clinically, muscle function could be assessed by observing the movements of the structures themselves (i.e., vibration of the vocal folds) or by recording the electrical activity of the muscles (electromyography or EMG). Faaborg-Andersen (1957, 1964; Faaborg-Andersen & Sonninen, 1960; Faaborg-Andersen & Vennard, 1964) was among the first to use EMG in the analysis of muscle function in the larynx. Many studies since that initial work have been concerned with various muscles of the larynx in healthy subjects as well as subjects with voice disorders. EMG is an invasive technique and should be performed only by those skilled in its application. EMG cannot and should not be performed on every patient (Basmajian, 1979). But for a few patients, EMG can be a valuable technique to assess laryngeal function (Faaborg-Andersen, 1957; Lindestad & Persson, 1994; Parnes, 1988; Parnes & Satya-Murti, 1985).

When a muscle is activated for a task, an EMG recording will show a fairly rapid rise in the amplitude of the signal, followed by a consistent level of activity. When muscle activity ceases, the recording will show a fairly rapid fall in amplitude to a low level of baseline activity adequate to maintain the tonus of the muscle (Basmajian, 1979; Kotby & Haugen, 1970). Pathology may severely reduce or increase the background levels as well as the muscle levels during contraction (Kotby & Haugen, 1970; Sawashima, Sato, Funasaka, & Totsuk, 1958). Muscles may be slow to become activated and slow to turn off, or a sudden unexpected burst of muscle activity may be superimposed on steady activity during muscle contraction, or muscles may show normal levels of activity when first contracted but with continued contraction, diminishing levels. There may also be differences of level between pairs of muscles controlling the vocal folds, suggesting a difference of activity between the two muscles (Hiroto, Hirano, & Tomita, 1968). Normal EMG levels, onsets, and offsets will be found in those patients whose laryngeal pathology does not affect muscles or their neural control.

## Observable Physiological Signs

### STROBOSCOPIC OBSERVATIONS

The stroboscope has found increased usage in the diagnosis and treatment of voice problems. Recent models are relatively easy to use and provide sharp imaging (Hirano, 1981b; Hirano, Feder, & Bless, 1983; Kitzing, 1985).

The stroboscope flashes a light at a rate equal to or approximating the vibrating rate of the vocal folds (Alberti, 1978; Kitzing, 1985). If the flash rate is equal to the vibrating rate of the vocal folds, they appear to stand still since they are illuminated at the same phase of their vibratory cycle. If the rate is slightly different from the vibration rate of the vocal folds, they are illuminated at different phases of their vibratory cycle. The effect is a slowing of the vibratory motion of the vocal folds, permitting observation of vibratory details.

*Table 2.5.* Observable Physiological Signs of Voice Problems—Stroboscopic

| |
|---|
| Degree of glottal closure |
| Phase closure |
| Vertical level |
| Amplitude of vibration |
| Mucosal wave |
| Vibratory behavior |
| Phase symmetry |
| Periodicity |

The strobe must measure the fundamental frequency of the vocal folds in order to function. This measure is available to determine the regularity of vocal fold vibration.

The stroboscopic signs of laryngeal pathology are obtained from the recordings of the strobe images (Fex, 1970; Kallen, 1932). Their recognition, like many of the signs previously discussed, depends on the knowledge and skill of the examiner. The signs listed in Table 2.5 are based on those presented by Bless (unpublished technical manual, B&K Stroboscope Course) and Hirano (1981b; Hirano & Bless, 1993).

### Glottal Closure

The extent and configuration of glottal closure can be described based on the stroboscopic images. The terms most commonly used to describe glottal closure include: complete closure, posterior chink, anterior chink, bowed, hourglass configuration, irregular closure, incomplete closure.

### Phase Closure

This parameter refers to the relative amounts of time that vocal folds are open and closed during a phonatory cycle. (Be aware that the stroboscopic image is not a representation of cycle by cycle behavior, but rather a composite of a number of cycles; therefore, the use of the term *phonatory cycle* in discussing stroboscopic observations is not entirely accurate. With that understanding, however, it is convenient to use the term in a stroboscopic context.) In a whisper or in aphonic speech, the vocal folds would be predominantly open, while in vocal hyperfunction the closed phase might predominate. The gauge for normal is an equal distribution of open to closed time.

### Vertical Level

The vocal folds should appear to be on the same vertical level so that as they approximate they appear on a level horizontally. In cases of trauma, paralysis, or other neurological involvement this may not always be true. One fold may appear to lie consistently at a level lower than the other.

### Amplitude of Vibration

This parameter refers to the extent of horizontal excursion of the vocal folds as they open and close during phonation. This parameter is greatly affected by the loudness of phonation, becoming greater as loudness increases. The expected amount of movement from the midline should approximate one third the visible width of the vocal fold. The movement of each vocal fold is rated individually. Differences in movement between the two folds may be diagnostically useful information.

### Mucosal Wave

The mucosal wave is a rippling motion that can be observed as it travels mediolaterally across the superior surface of the vocal folds. It is a reflection of the complex structure and behavior of the vocal folds. Normally the mucosal wave travels smoothly across the visible width of the vocal fold but can be limited by pathology, scarring, or stiffness. In some instances the wave may appear to be larger than normal. This can occur in the presence of highly fluid-filled polypoid degeneration. This parameter is rated separately for each vocal fold.

### Vibratory Behavior

This refers to the presence or the absence of vibratory behavior in the entire vocal fold. The extent of vibratory behavior may vary from normal to partially absent to totally absent. Once again, each vocal fold is rated independently.

### Phase Symmetry

During phonation the vocal folds should appear to move as mirror images of each other. As both folds open in phase they separate in unison and then approach each other and close in unison. That action is referred to as phase symmetry. Variations in this movement can be observed when the voice is disordered. The vocal folds may appear to follow one another with one fold closing (moving toward the midline) as the opposite fold opens (moves away from the midline). This behavior may be constant or it may be intermittently present.

### Periodicity

Periodicity is an estimate of the regularity of vibration of the vocal folds. Judgments of periodicity may be made in a number of ways. Through observation it is possible to subjectively judge whether the movement of the two vocal folds appears to be regular and periodic. Fluctuation and variation of the fundamental frequency can often be observed on screen in the readout of that measure, or it can be observed as slow or rapid variations in the apparent motion of the vocal folds.

### LARYNGOSCOPIC SIGNS

In this section, we will describe those physiological signs that can be observed using a variety of visualization techniques without the stroboscopic feature. These techniques include indirect mirror examination, flexible nasendoscopy, examination with a rigid oral endoscope, direct laryngoscopy under anesthesia, and ultra-high-speed photography. Table 2.6 summarizes the observations that can help to establish a diagnosis. The ability to make these observations may vary with the visualization technique used.

### Vocal Fold Approximation

Variations of vocal fold approximation may include (a) incomplete closure along the length of the one or both vocal folds; (b) bowing of the vocal folds, seen as a central gap; and (c) lack of approximation of the vocal processes, resulting in a posterior chink. These behaviors may be also seen in videolaryngostroboscopic recordings.

### Vocal Fold Movement

Movement of one or both vocal folds may be reduced or absent due to a variety of conditions. The vocal folds may (a) not adduct (move to the midline), (b) not abduct (move away from the midline), or (c) adduct excessively or abduct involuntarily and at inappropriate times during phonation.

*Table 2.6.* Observable Physiological Signs of Voice Problems—Laryngoscopic

Vocal fold approximation
Vocal fold movement
Tissue changes
Pyriform changes
Anteroposterior laryngeal dimensions
Ventricular folds
Anatomical malformations and congenital anomalies
Vocal fold lengthening
Vertical laryngeal position
Involuntary laryngeal activity
Phonatory apraxia
Normal-appearing larynx

### Tissue Changes

There are a host of changes that can affect the vocal fold mucosa. These include edema, inflammation, and benign, malignant, or premalignant lesions. Each has a characteristic appearance and/or site of occurrence (see Chapter 3).

### Pyriform Changes

The opening of the pyriform sinuses usually increases with adductory movement of the vocal folds. Lack of aperture variation of the pyriform sinus cavity is usually a sign of laryngeal paralysis and is a significant sign to note when attempting to differentiate between paralysis and arytenoid ankylosis or dislocation (Brewer & Gould, 1974).

### Anteroposterior Laryngeal Dimensions

During phonation of the sustained /ee/ vowel, the distance between the epiglottis and arytenoids (anteroposterior dimension) is sufficient to allow visualization of the full length of the vocal folds in most normal speakers. However, in some persons, the epiglottis and arytenoids can be seen to approach each other during phonation, thereby shortening this anteroposterior dimension and obscuring visualization of the vocal folds. The extent of the visualization will depend on the phonatory conditions produced by the patient (i.e., pitch, loudness, and vowel).

### Ventricular Folds

The ventricular folds are usually seen superior and lateral to the true vocal folds, and there is variation in the degree of their movement. During phonation they are usually seen to maintain their position relative to the edge of the true vocal folds. However, sometimes they appear to move toward the midline, obscuring all or part of the true vocal folds (Freud, 1962). They may even approximate each other during phonation. Furthermore, their movements may not always be symmetrical.

### Anatomical Malformations and Congenital Anomalies

Structures may be malformed as the result of a congenital anatomical deformity or the result of abnormal growth and development. Laryngomalacia, a softness or abnormal flaccidity of the laryngeal cartilages, is the most common congenital laryngeal anomaly and may resolve by 1 to 2 years of age (Cotton & Richardson, 1981; Hollinger & Brown, 1967). In this condition, there is a characteristic movement pattern of the larynx involving a downward and anterior displacement and a bowing of the aryepiglottic folds during inspiration. Other congenital problems include (*a*) sub-glottal stenosis, a thickening of subglottal tissues that may be sufficient to obstruct the airway; (*b*) vocal fold paralysis, often a temporary condition lasting about 4 weeks (Hollinger & Brown, 1967), and (*c*) laryngeal web, a band of tissue (which may vary in extent) joining the two vocal folds at the anterior commissure.

### Vocal Fold Lengthening

Vocal fold lengthening is usually observed as vocal pitch is raised. This is seen fiberoptically as a lengthening of the distance between the arytenoid cartilages and the epiglottis as the vocal folds elongate. In some persons, the elevation of pitch does not produce this effect.

### Vertical Laryngeal Position

The larynx is able to move in the vertical dimension. This can be visualized in laryngoscopic examination as a rising of the larynx as pitch is raised and a descent below resting level as pitch is lowered. Degree of movement varies among individuals and between trained and untrained singers (Shipp, 1975; Shipp & Izdebski, 1975). For a further discussion on vertical laryngeal position, please see Chapter 4, "High Laryngeal Position."

### Involuntary Laryngeal Activity

Rhythmic involuntary movement of laryngeal structures in the resting state, in the absence of phonation, is often seen accompanying neurologically based disorders (Parnes, Lavarato, & Myers, 1978). Another common observation is the movement of the arytenoids toward the midline. In voluntary effort closure, a medial squeezing and "closing down" of the entire larynx occurs. On occasion, such a movement occurs involuntarily and is described as hyperadduction. The normal larynx, when viewed at rest, maintains a relatively static posture with a fully open glottis. In some individuals, random, arrhythmic movement of various structures may be observed.

### Phonatory Apraxia

Phonatory apraxia is an inability to produce phonation volitionally. Although seemingly normal movement of the vocal folds and other laryngeal structures may be observed during swallow and reflexive activities, it is absent when the person is asked to phonate voluntarily (Aronson, 1990).

### Normal-Appearing Larynx

Despite the perception of a vocal abnormality, the larynx may appear to be normal in structure and function.

## Interrelationships of Perceptual, Acoustic, and Physiological Signs

The signs of voice problems are not independent of one another. That is, there are interrelationships among the physiological, acoustic, and perceptual signs. Simply stated, movements of the vocal folds (physiology) create pressure disturbances in the air (acoustics) that are received by the ear and processed (perception).

A change in the structure of the vocal folds (e.g., a lesion, a tissue change) or a change in their manner of use (e.g., excess tension, inadequate energy) will affect the acoustic signal produced, which in turn will alter the perception of the voice. For example, a mass on the vocal folds may interfere with their closure. Consequently, air will continue to flow during that part of the vibratory cycle in which the vocal folds should be completely closed. This disturbed physiology will create a weak acoustic disturbance. Furthermore, due to the constant flow of air through a small glottal opening, there may be an increase of noise level. The weaker acoustic signal in combination with noise from the air striking the vocal folds will create the perception of breathiness.

As another example, the fundamental vibrating rate of the vocal folds is determined by their mass, length, and tension. If there is a mass on the vocal folds (e.g., a polyp or nodule), the basic vibrating rate will be altered. Vocal folds with a large mass would vibrate at a lower rate, producing a lower fundamental frequency and the perception of a lower pitch (Isshiki, Tanabe, Ishizaka, & Board, 1977). Masses on both vocal folds that are asymmetrical in size will each vibrate at a different rate, producing greater aperiodicity of vibration and increased frequency and amplitude perturbation. Greater perturbation usually is associated with the perception of greater roughness or hoarseness in the voice.

Signs cannot be viewed in a vacuum. Signs interrelate within a domain (physiology, acoustics, or perception) and across these domains. Some are redundant and assist in the confirmation of other signs. Patterns of signs accompany different voice problems and, when considered in combination with laboratory tests, physical examination, and the patient's history, assist in the accurate diagnosis of the voice disorder.

## DIFFERENTIAL DIAGNOSIS OF VOICE PROBLEMS DEMONSTRATED IN NINE CASE STUDIES

In the previous sections we have defined the terminology used to describe the symptoms and signs of voice disorders. In the following sections, each of the nine symptoms will be explored in further detail in the manner of the differential diagnosis process, using case studies. The first case will be presented and followed by a discussion of the process of differential diagnosis as it applies to that case. For each of the other cases, we will present only the case study, with questions designed to guide the reader's thinking. Tables providing those signs that are consistent with each major symptom are also provided throughout the text. Please keep in mind that an individual patient would not necessarily present all of the signs listed in the tables.

### *Hoarseness*

J. H., a 37-year-old woman, was referred for voice therapy by an otolaryngologist who carried out an indirect and endoscopic (not stroboscopic) laryngeal exam and had made a diagnosis of vocal nodules. The history she presented included the following: (*a*) she teaches 7–9 elementary school classes of physical education per day; (*b*) she owns and teaches in a gymnastics school for 3–4 hours per day after the school day and often on weekends; (*c*) this business requires that she spend much time on the phone; (*d*) she is married and has two teenage sons at home; (*e*) she neither smokes nor drinks; and ( *f* ) she describes herself as a very active and vocal person. J. H. reports that she has noticed increased hoarseness for a number of years but that during the past year this hoarseness has worsened in degree and in constancy. She is aware that the hoarseness increases following extended voice use and that she also experiences periods of vocal fatigue, occasional soreness in the throat, and the need to strain to produce voice loud enough to be heard. She sought medical attention at the point when her voice was severely hoarse all the time, her students were unable to hear her, and the fatigue she felt at the end of the day became intolerable.

In the differential diagnosis process, the clinician should now be asking, is this history consistent with a diagnosis of vocal nodules? In view of the gradual onset, increased worsening, and excessive voice usage, a probable cause of her vocal difficulties could be expected to be vocal nodules. However, prior to laryngoscopic examination, the possible diagnoses that could have been entertained, based on the history, include polyps, cancer, keratosis, chronic laryngitis, edema, and intracordal cyst.

At this point, the clinician should be concerned about the compatibility of the perceptual signs and symptoms noted above with the stated history and presenting diagnosis.

Perceptual signs noted at the initial evaluation included hoarse/rough quality, increased breathiness, episodic aphonia, and excessive throat clearing. Increased tension was observed as J. H. worked at producing voice. Acoustic signs included a fundamental frequency of 195 Hz, a phonation range of less than one octave, an s/z ratio of 1.9, and a maximum phonation time of 6 seconds. Her airflow data showed good closure of the vocal folds but with high peak flows.

No additional examinations were recommended at that time, and J. H. began a course of voice therapy. Although it was difficult for her, she began to make significant changes in her voice use habits. A plan was devised whereby she could continue to work but would cease abusing her vocal folds. Throat clearing was eliminated quickly, as were all attempts at loud voice use. J. H. became more dependent on the use of her whistle in place of her voice. She began to demonstrate for her students rather than explain verbally. And her voice improved. Almost immediately she reported that the symptoms of soreness and fatigue abated.

A school vacation allowed J. H. to really "rest her voice" for a week. She talked minimally, without strain and with reduced intensity. At the end of that week, further improvement was noted in her voice. Phonational range was significantly increased, aphonic episodes were no longer present, voicing occurred with minimal effort, and hoarseness was reduced. J. H. returned to her teaching but was extremely careful about voice use. Nevertheless, her voice showed marked deterioration within a week. This rapid vocal worsening raised questions in the clinician's mind.

This rapid vocal worsening was unexpected because J. H. had made significant progress and had engaged in no activities that would be expected to adversely affect the condition of the vocal folds. When such an unexpected change occurs in a patient's condition, the clinician should review the diagnosis and the ensuing therapy. This may lead to the recognition of the need for further examination. In this case, J. H. was scheduled for fiberoptic and stroboscopic examination.

Visualization of the vocal folds utilizing fiberoptic and stroboscopic techniques revealed the presence of a vocal fold cyst. No nodules were apparent. J. H. was scheduled for laryngeal surgery with a recommendation for a course of voice therapy postoperatively.

This case study is an example of the process of differential diagnosis. The questions raised at critical points in the history suggest the thinking process that is essential to the understanding of voice problems and their management. The nature of this particular case also makes it quite clear that the process of differential diagnosis is ongoing throughout the treatment program. A patient's response to treatment (or lack of response) is meaningful information that must become a part of the understanding of the problem. It may, as it did in this case, point to the need for further testing and perhaps a change in diagnosis.

The patient in this case was referred to the speech-language pathologist with a stated diagnosis, vocal nodules, made by an otolaryngologist. The primary symptom expressed by the patient, hoarseness, was consistent with that diagnosis. An examination of Table 2.7 reveals the perceptual signs that may accompany the symptom of hoarseness. A number of these signs were noted in this case during the initial voice evaluation, for example, hoarse voice quality, increased breathiness, episodic aphonia, excessive throat clearing, and increased tension.

*Table 2.7.* Signs That May Be Associated with the Symptom of Hoarse Voice

*Typical complaint: "My voice is hoarse or groggy. People think I have laryngitis."*

*Perceptual signs*
    hoarseness/roughness
    breathiness
    laryngeal tension
    inappropriate pitch
    excessive throat clearing
    episodic aphonia
    pitch breaks

*Acoustic signs*
    restricted phonational range
    restricted dynamic range
    excessive spectral noise
    greater jitter
    greater shimmer
    reduced maximum phonation time and high s/z ratios
    reduced fundamental frequency variability

*Observable physiological signs—laryngoscopic*
    anteroposterior shortening
        functional
    increased ventricular fold activity
        functional
        compensatory
            paralysis
            fixed cord
            inadequate closure
    tissue change
        nodules
        polyps
        carcinoma
        papilloma
        leukoplakia
        edema
        cyst
    color change
        burns
            heat
            chemical
    other vocal fold lesions

*Continued.*

*Table 2.7.* (continued)

---

variations of vocal fold approximation
    posterior chink
        functional
    bowing
        reduced muscle tonus
    keyhole
        aged voice
    incomplete anteroposterior approximation
        paralysis
        functional
        ankylosis
        dislocation
anatomical malformation
    congenital
    malacia
    stenosis
    web
trauma
    blunt
    penetrating
    surgery
normal larynx
    functional
        psychogenic
        misuse
    neurological
    minor or hidden tissue change

*Measurable physiological signs*
    aerodynamics
        increased flow
        increased air pressure
    vibratory
        aberrant glottal pulse shape
        irregularity or asymmetry of vocal fold motion
        muscosal wave changes
    muscle activity
        higher than normal levels
        imbalance of paired muscle activity
        normal activity

---

*"Observable Physiological Signs—Stroboscopic" do not appear in this and Tables 2.8–2.15 because the symptom may be caused by different lesions. Stroboscopic signs associated with specific lesions will be covered in Chapter 4.*

Table 2.7 lists those acoustic signs that would be consistent with the symptom and the perceptual signs. In other words, our ears hear certain vocal characteristics, some of which are accessible to measurement, thereby providing an independent corroboration of our perception. We would therefore expect to find a certain degree of match between the perceptual and the acoustic signs. In this case, we find reduced phonation range, a significant s/z ratio, and reduced phonation time.

Let us examine these factors a little more closely. Remember that hoarseness was given as a perceptual sign. A lesion, such as a nodule, on the vibratory edge of the vocal fold mucosa will disrupt vibratory behavior by adding mass at a specific location on the vocal fold. Addition of the same amount of mass distributed along the entire length of the vocal fold would most likely reduce fundamental frequency. In the case of a nodule, the extra mass loads down the vocal fold and affects its periodicity. Stiffness of the vocal fold cover is also increased due to the biomechanical characteristics of the nodule. This disruption results in a disturbance of the periodicity of the signal, creating a noisy signal that results in a perception of hoarseness. The increased mass and stiffness of the folds will also interfere with their ability to stretch and vibrate at a more rapid rate; therefore, pitch elevation would be affected and phonational range would be decreased.

The s/z ratio is based on the theory that vocal fold vibration sufficient to produce phonation (i.e., /z/) can be maintained for a time period equal to the time that airflow can be maintained without vocal fold activity (i.e., /s/). When a lesion is present on the vocal folds, there is incomplete glottal closure or very brief contact, resulting in a loss of air and a reduction in the ability to sustain phonation. The resulting s/z ratio becomes significantly greater than 1.4, which is reported to be the upper end of the normal range (Eckel & Boone, 1981). Similarly, the maximum time that phonation can be sustained is reduced. When air leakage during phonation is of a sufficient degree, there will be a perception of breathiness.

Excessive throat clearing is a common observation in patients who have vocal nodules or other lesions. These patients report the sensation that something is in the way of their being able to talk and that they must first attempt to dislodge it by clearing the throat, often quite strenuously. Unfortunately, this leads in a cyclical fashion to increased vocal abuse, which results in an exacerbation of the symptoms, which leads to an increased feeling of the need to clear the throat, and so on.

When a vocal fold lesion is present and maximum phonation time is reduced, it is not unexpected to find momentary episodes of absence of voicing. This occurs because the patient is unaccustomed to the reduction in the ability to sustain phonation or because there was insufficient effort, air pressure, or vocal fold approximation to compensate for the extra demands placed on the system by the presence of the lesion.

We would expect that breathiness would be reflected in greater than expected airflow during phonation. Indeed, when this patient was seen for further examination, one of the physiological aerodynamic signs (see Table 2.7) was increased flow. The glottal pulse shape was aberrant, revealing the poor glottal closure. It should be noted, however, that at the time of the reexamination, the amount of breathiness perceived in the voice was considerably reduced from that present at the initial evaluation. This could be due to reduction of general irritation and edema of the vocal folds in response to a marked reduction in abusive and excessive voice use.

Stroboscopic examination, which was helpful in making the diagnosis of a vocal fold cyst, revealed reduced mucosal wave in the area of the cyst (see Table 2.5). The laryngoscopic signs noted on fiberoptic laryngoscopic examination revealed some tissue change, which appeared as a lesion on the superior surface of the vocal fold mucosa at a midway point along its length (see Table 2.6).

During the differential diagnosis process, the pieces must fit together. The process can work from a starting point of the patient's complaint, or it can work backward, as it were, from a previously arrived at diagnosis. It is typical for speech-language pathologists to be in the position of having patients referred with a stated diagnosis. In certain cases, however, the observations and perceptions of the speech-language pathologist and information about the acoustic and physiological signs do not seem to be consistent with the diagnosis. Further examination is often warranted in such cases. On other occasions, as typified by the case of J. H., the symptoms and signs may be consistent with the diagnosis, yet the patient's treatment course suggests the need for further exploration of the case. It is especially important to recognize that in the case of J. H., all the perceptual, acoustic, and physiological signs could have been consistent with the original diagnosis. The stroboscopic and laryngoscopic signs were the determining factors in making the diagnosis, and the suspicion of the speech-language pathologist, based on sudden and unexpected worsening of a condition, was the catalyst for reexamination of the original diagnosis.

Although some case history material was provided in the description of J. H., that part of the diagnostic process has been only briefly considered in this chapter. We do not mean to suggest that it is not an essential part of the process. Indeed, a thorough case history is essential and will be fully covered in Chapter 6.

We will explore the other primary symptoms of voice problems and the differential diagnosis process in the remainder of this chapter. Each will begin with a case study. However, we will not explain each one in the same amount of detail provided for J. H. Consult the tables for listings of all the various signs that we believe to be consistent with the symptom. Following the process should lead the reader to an understanding of the interrelatedness of the various factors, that is, perception, acoustics, and physiology, and the need for complete evaluation. In turn, this understanding should help to eliminate the cookbook approach to voice problems and replace it with the ability to follow the process of differential diagnosis thoughtfully.

## Vocal Fatigue

S. D., a 45-year-old first grade teacher and mother of nine children, complained of feeling vocally tired at the end of each day. She could not identify any recent changes at home, at work, or in her personal health status that might account for the vocal fatigue she was experiencing. However, further discussion revealed that the aide in her classroom had become sick in November and had not been able to return to work. The symptoms had begun in early December, and at the time we saw her, they had persisted for 3 months. When questioned about the specific symptoms of this vocal fatigue, she described a tired feeling in the throat; a feeling of not wanting to talk and, if required to talk, a feeling of having to work to do so; sometimes a feeling of tightness in the throat and chest; and a rough-sounding voice quality that seemed to get worse as the day progressed. She also complained that it was difficult for her to produce a loud voice.

> Q. WHAT ARE THE POSSIBLE DIAGNOSES THAT YOU
> MIGHT BEGIN TO CONSIDER ON THE BASIS OF THIS
> LIMITED INFORMATION?

Although S. D. must use her voice extensively both at work and at home, she reports that she rarely shouts. She does not sing, smoke, or drink. She does not talk on the telephone except when necessary.

Perceptually, we noted a tendency toward a monopitch voice, with little pitch variability during general conversation (Table 2.8). Voice quality was judged to be only mildly to moderately rough, with an apparent increase in the degree of roughness occurring at the end of sentences or breath groups. Voice production seemed unchanged perceptually when S. D. was asked to talk to us as she might to her class or to her children. We also observed what might best be described as a low energy level, as if all systems were working at 50% power.

*Table 2.8.* Signs That May Be Associated with the Symptom of Vocal Fatigue

---

*Typical complaint: "My voice gives out at the end of the day."*

*Perceptual signs*
    monopitch
    tension
    breathiness
    hoarseness

*Acoustic signs*
    restricted phonational range
    reduced variability of fundamental frequency
    normal acoustics

*Observable physiological signs—laryngoscopic*
    variations of vocal fold approximation
        functional
    tissue change
        color
        nodule
    change of laryngeal position
        muscle tension
    normal appearing larynx
        neurological
        myasthenia gravis

*Measurable physiological signs*
    aerodynamic
        increased airflow
    vibratory
        inadequate closed time
    muscle activity
        muscle imbalance
        excessive levels
        variation of level

---

S. D.'s measured speaking fundamental frequency was found to be 205 Hz, and the variability of fundamental frequency around this mean was 3-4 semitones. Phonational range was found to be within normal limits when measured, but it was necessary to work with S. D. first on a pitch-matching task in order to obtain this measure.

Fiberoptic laryngeal examination revealed a structurally normal larynx. Visualization of the vocal folds during speech was often obscured, however, due to approximation of the arytenoid cartilages and the epiglottis. This anteroposterior "squeezing" was marked throughout speaking tasks. When this squeezing is present in a patient, it is not possible to view the vocal folds with a rigid endoscope. With the flexible fiberscope in place, we engaged S. D. in a short period of "diagnostic therapy" in which we asked her to engage in a variety of vocal maneuvers. We began by having S. D. match a very high-pitched vocalization on the vowel /ee/. As we watched her do this, we noted that the vocal folds appeared to lengthen and their full length became visible. The anteroposterior "squeezing" was not visible. We were then able to help S. D. bring the vocal pitch down gradually while maintaining this "open" laryngeal posture.

As she approached speaking fundamental frequency, we became aware of a perceptual difference in vocal quality from what had been heard initially.

Based on the findings of the extended evaluation, a diagnosis of "hyperfunctional voice use" without any laryngeal tissue changes was made, and a period of voice therapy was recommended.

## Breathy

Thirteen-year-old K. B. was referred for voice therapy with the description of a hoarse voice. No diagnosis per se was provided by the referring otolaryngologist. K. B. had been taken to this physician by her mother because of an earache. During the examination the physician had noted the aberrant voice quality and had made the referral for voice therapy. Mrs. B., the mother, reported that she had never been particularly aware of K.'s voice because K. had always sounded this way. Furthermore, none of K.'s doctors, teachers, or other school personnel had ever raised any concern about it.

Despite the mother's lack of awareness of a problem, K. B. was very much aware of her voice being "different." She reported being called derogatory names by other children and being made fun of by them because of the sound of her voice. In addition, she had difficulty in making herself heard in the classroom and was often told to "speak up" by her teachers. Indeed, this had become so distressing to her that she rarely volunteered to speak in class and worried about when she might have to do so.

The rest of the history was essentially negative. K. B. had experienced no serious illnesses, nor had she had any surgery. She had never been involved in an accident, and she had normal hearing and normal intelligence.

### Q. WHAT POSSIBLE DIAGNOSES BEGIN TO BE SUGGESTED?

Perceptual signs included marked breathiness, reduced loudness, and hoarseness and were consistent with the acoustic findings of reduced dynamic range, restricted phonational range, and reduced maximum sustained phonation time (Table 2.9).

### Q. HOW DO THESE FINDINGS AFFECT THE DIAGNOSES YOU ENTERTAINED ABOVE?

Attempts to alter voice quality through a variety of vocal maneuvers were unsuccessful. At no time during the voice evaluation was there any significant change in K. B.'s voice quality. K. B. was then scheduled to be seen in the voice laboratory for physiological and fiberoptic evaluation. Physiological signs included a large amount of airflow leakage and low peak flows. Her electroglottogram showed irregular pulses, suggesting random variations in opening and closing of the vocal folds.

### Q. DOES THIS ADDED INFORMATION NARROW YOUR DIAGNOSTIC CHOICES?

Most revealing, and corroborative of the findings reported thus far, were the stroboscopic and laryngoscopic signs (Table 2.9). K. B.'s larynx was difficult to visualize due to an omega-shaped epiglottis that was oriented in such a way as to frequently obscure the larynx. The larynx was noted to be asymmetric, with the left side appearing to be smaller and less well developed than the right. Left unilateral vocal fold paralysis was observed and glottal closure was never obtained. The stroboscopic examination revealed reduced mucosal wave on the left fold. The diagnosis of congenital vocal fold paralysis was made.

*Table 2.9.* Signs That May Be Associated with the Symptom of Breathy Voice

*Typical complaint: "My voice is weak. I run out of air. People can't hear me."*

*Perceptual signs*
    breathiness
    little loudness variation
    hoarse/rough
    episodic aphonia

*Acoustic signs*
    restricted phonational range
    restricted dynamic range
    reduced sustained phonation time
    increased s/z ratio
    excessive spectral noise
    increased perturbation
    increased shimmer

*Observable physiological signs—laryngoscopic*
    variation of vocal fold approximation
        incomplete a-p approximation (most prevalent)
            paralysis (adductor)
            functional
            ankylosis
            dislocation
            neurological
            ALS
            Parkinson's
            myasthenia gravis
        posterior chink
            functional
        bowing
            aging
            reduced muscle tonus
    lack of movement of one or both vocal folds
        paralysis
        ankylosis
        dislocation
        carcinoma
    lack of change in appearance of pyriform sinuses
        paralysis
    anatomic malformation
        congenital
        laryngomalacia
        trauma
            blunt
            penetrating
            surgery
    tissue change
        burns
            heat
            chemical

*Continued.*

*Table 2.9.* (continued)

---

*Measurable physiological signs*
    aerodynamic
        increased airflow
        increased air pressure
    vibratory
        aberrant glottal pulse shape
        inadequate closed time
        irregularity and asymmetry of vocal fold motion
        mucosal wave changes
    muscle activity
        absent or reduced levels
        imbalance of paired muscle activity

---

### Q. CAN YOU EXPLAIN HOW ALL THE SYMPTOMS AND SIGNS REPORTED IN THIS CASE ARE CONSISTENT WITH THIS DIAGNOSIS?

## Reduced Phonational Range

M. L. is a 39-year-old woman referred to the voice clinic by her choir director for an inability to produce her upper vocal range with clarity. Four months previously she had an upper respiratory infection (URI) during the course of which she had coughed a great deal. She also experienced what she described as acute laryngitis. The symptoms of the URI resolved, including the acute laryngitis, but the coughing persisted for about 2 months. She has continued to note mild hoarseness. Her main concern, however, is that she appears to be unable to produce the top of her range with clarity. Indeed, there have been times when she has been unable to produce the highest notes at all.

### Q. WHAT CONDITIONS ACCOMPANYING AN UPPER RESPIRATORY INFECTION OR PRESENTING AS ITS SEQUELAE WOULD BE IMPORTANT TO CONSIDER?

M. L. has been singing in a choir for many years and has also performed both as a soloist and with another singer for local events such as weddings, funerals, and other social gatherings. She had minimal vocal training many years ago. She neither smokes nor drinks, nor does she perform in loud or smoke-filled settings. She is married and has several grown children. She does not describe herself as either a loud or a constant talker. She is employed at a job that does not require much talking, and all of it is done in a relatively quiet environment. She denies any allergies, takes no medicines, and has no known medical problems.

    Perceptually M. L. presented with an essentially normal-sounding speaking voice (Table 2.10). Although she complained of a mild hoarseness, we found this to be extremely mild and inconsistently present. M. L.'s singing voice was marked by occasional pitch breaks within the upper third of her range. We observed a "reaching" for the high notes with upward and forward tilting of the chin, wrinkling of the forehead, and a generalized body tension, especially the upper body.

### Q. WHAT DO THESE OBSERVATIONS SUGGEST TO YOU?

M. L.'s phonational range was found to be 2.5 octaves at best, which she claims is reduced by at least half an octave from her optimal vocal production. In addition, the

*Table 2.10.* Signs That May Be Associated with the Symptom of Reduced
Phonational Range

---

*Typical complaint: "I am not able to produce the high notes of my range
during singing."*

*Perceptual signs*
   tension
   pitch breaks
   normal-sounding voice

*Acoustic signs*
   restricted phonational range
   restricted dynamic range

*Observable physiological signs—laryngoscopic*
   tissue change of vocal folds
      nodule
      color
   normal appearing larynx
      functional
         misuse
         improper vocal technique
   minor or hidden tissue change

*Measurable Physiological Signs*
   muscle
      excessive levels
      normal physiology

---

highest notes were not produced with what she described as her usual clarity of tone. Her speaking fundamental frequency was 205 Hz. Airflow data revealed elevated peak flows and a small leakage flow but was otherwise normal. Her electroglottogram showed very brief closed times with an unusual break in the closing phase of the signal, suggesting irregular closing patterns.

Fiberoptic examination revealed an essentially normal-appearing larynx. There was the suggestion of some roughness along the edge of the right vocal fold, and a mucus strand formed, broke, and reformed at about the junction of the anterior one third and posterior two thirds of the vocal folds. Her stroboscopic examination was normal.

## Q. WHAT DO THE LARYNGOSCOPIC SIGNS SUGGEST?

A period of diagnostic therapy was provided during which M. L. was instructed to consciously use good breath support, to allow sound to be produced easily without the "reaching" tensions, and to use the type of imagery she recalled from her vocal training in producing the high pitches. The ease of sound production was emphasized, rather than the beauty of the sound. It was gratifying to observe the change in phonatory behavior and to hear the difference in the resulting sound.

The diagnosis in this case seemed to involve a combination of factors. Because some of the precipitating conditions were no longer present, judgments had to be made based on history and current findings. The history of excessive coughing combined with acute laryngitis suggests that the mucosa was sufficiently irritated to begin to show some changes. The slight suggestion of roughness along the vocal fold edge and the presence of the strand of mucus forming and reforming may be evidence of a resolving problem or of an ongoing problem. Although M. L. does not seem to be abusing her voice significantly in speaking, her singing technique is very poor, and there is obvious strain and tension in attempts to produce the upper frequency range. In view of her positive response to diagnostic therapy, at least some of the difficulty she is encountering may be the result of the psychological fear that she has built up concerning her inability to produce those notes. We recommended a resumption of vocal training with periodic monitoring of the condition of the vocal folds.

## Aphonia

P. M., a 32-year-old woman, was referred for voice therapy with a very involved history. She presented for the voice evaluation seated in a wheelchair and with no voice. Indeed, she was so aphonic that she was not even producing a whisper, nor were the voiceless consonants audible.

> Q. CAN YOU EXPLAIN HOW A PERSON COULD
> BE SO APHONIC?

Her history was exceedingly lengthy, often vague, and difficult to follow. Key points seemed to be that she was quite sick for a period of time as a small child and was not expected to survive; she has had frequent upper respiratory problems since then; she had a father who had had tuberculosis; and she claimed to have severe asthma attacks and breathing problems (which had never been observed by anyone else despite numerous hospitalizations). She had been married for a period of time, but the marriage was terminated after she was involved in an automobile accident that left her confined to a wheelchair. This accident resulted in cervical spine nerve root avulsions, but the main reason for use of the wheelchair was her reported "dizziness" and subsequent fear of falling. P. M. lived alone in a trailer. She reported an episode in which a young man broke into her trailer and attempted to strangle her. She denied being raped but stated that he knocked her down and twisted her neck. She began to have some difficulty with her voice following that, but this became worse after she was involved in another automobile accident 3 years later. She did not suffer any injuries in this accident. P. M. wore a hearing aid with a moderate degree of gain for several years. However, a subsequent audiological examination revealed essentially normal hearing sensitivity and showed that she did as well without amplification as she did with it.

   P M. had consulted and been treated by numerous specialists for a variety of problems. She claimed that she was told that her phrenic nerve was damaged and that this was the reason she was unable to speak.

> Q. WHAT DOES THE PHRENIC NERVE INNERVATE, AND
> WHAT EFFECT WOULD DAMAGE TO THIS NERVE HAVE
> ON VOICE PRODUCTION?

During the history taking, P. M. continued to be totally aphonic. Her affect was very pleasant and strangely cheerful given her condition. Some voicing was noted in the voluntary production of a coughing sound, although much support and encouragement were necessary in order to elicit a "fake" cough.

> Q. WHAT DIAGNOSES WOULD YOU CONSIDER AT THIS POINT?

Observation of P. M.'s breathing at rest showed normal abdominal and chest movements. During her attempts at speech, we observed adequate inhalatory behavior, but P. M. seemed to hold her breath while her mouth was moving and expel it at the end of a soundless utterance.

*Table 2.11.* Signs That May Be Associated with the Symptom of Aphonia

---

*Typical complaint: "I lost my voice" or "My voice is gone."*

*Perceptual signs*
    breathiness
    consistent aphonia

*Acoustic signs*
    excessive spectral noise

*Observable physiological signs—laryngoscopic*
    variations in vocal fold approximation
    incomplete vocal fold approximation
    bilateral adductor paralysis
    lack of movement of vocal folds
    phonatory apraxia
    CNS lesion

*Measurable physiological signs*
    aerodynamics
        increased airflow
        increased air pressure
    vibratory
        not applicable
    muscle activity
        unknown

---

### Q. ARE THESE OBSERVATIONS CONSISTENT WITH PHRENIC NERVE DAMAGE?

Because there was no voice production, no acoustic measures could be made (Table 2.11). The airflow trace showed large amounts of airflow unmodulated by the vocal folds. Laryngoscopic examination using the fiberscope revealed a normal-appearing larynx. Vocal fold movement was observed during reflexive behaviors and also during nonphonatory whistling. The movement was noted to be symmetric and quite normal. Since there was no phonation, stroboscopy was not indicated.

A diagnosis of a psychogenic voice disorder was made. P. M. was seen for two sessions of trial voice therapy. During each of these sessions we were able to elicit entirely normal voice quality. Despite the normal sound of the voice and her ability to produce complete sentences naturally and without effort, P. M. was unable to accept return of voicing. She did not acknowledge the presence of voice when she first produced it, and when it was noted by the examiner, she continued to ignore it. P. M. was referred for psychiatric consultation and treatment. She followed up on the consultation but refused treatment. Although she has experienced full return of voice, she continues to have many other problems, both physical and psychosocial.

### *Pitch Breaks or Falsetto*

When S. P., a 20-year-old man, was referred for voice therapy, the referring otolaryngologist reported that examination had revealed a normal larynx but the voice was hoarse. S. P., however, complained that his voice often sounded "squeaky" and that he was aware that his voice was different from that of his friends. He also complained of difficulty in making himself heard at work, where there was often much loud noise.

S. P. was employed as a garage mechanic, had completed high school, shared an apartment with a friend, had never smoked, drank no more than two to three beers a week, and had a steady girlfriend. He had never sustained an injury to his neck, did not believe he had been exposed to any noxious fumes, had experienced no serious illnesses, denied allergies, and was in general quite happy with his life.

Concerning his voice, S. P. reported that he had no memory of ever sounding different. He denied any recent change in his voice and reported that his friends never commented on how he sounded. He believed that they were all simply used to hearing his voice.

## Q. WHAT WOULD BE YOUR NEXT QUESTION?

Our next question was to wonder about the motivation for this consultation, given a situation that seems to have been status quo for a long time and has not had any significantly negative effect on his life. In response, S. P. stated that he just knew that something was wrong and that he had indeed been worried about this for a number of years but did not know what to do about it. The opportunity to do something came about when he sought medical attention for an earache.

## Q. ARE ANY POSSIBLE DIAGNOSES COMING TO MIND?

S. P. presented as a handsome, strong, and muscular young man. Perceptually, however, he had a nonresonant, thin, rather high-pitched voice that sounded somehow out

*Table 2.12.* Signs That May Be Associated with the Symptoms of Pitch Breaks or Inappropriately High Pitch

---

*Typical complaint: "My voice sounds squeaky."*

*Perceptual signs*
  inappropriate pitch level
  pitch breaks

*Acoustic signs*
  higher than expected speaking fundamental frequency
  rapid shifts of fundamental frequency
  restricted phonational range
  restricted dynamic range
  reduced maximum phonation time

*Observable physiological signs—laryngoscopic*
  normal-appearing larynx
    functional
  anatomical malformations
    hormone imbalance
    web

*Measurable physiological signs*
  aerodynamics
    decreased airflow
  vibratory
    inadequate closed times
    mucosal wave changes
  muscle activity
    excessive levels

---

of control (Table 2.12). There were frequent pitch breaks. These were documented acoustically, with rapid shifts of frequency, averaging an octave. Average speaking fundamental frequency was measured at 175 Hz.

### Q. WITH THIS ADDITIONAL INFORMATION, WHAT WOULD YOUR DIFFERENTIAL LIST CONSIST OF?

Additional acoustic signs included a very restricted total phonational range as well as restricted dynamic range (Table 2.12). The referral source had indicated a normal laryngeal examination. The stroboscopic examination revealed small lateral excursions of the vocal folds, and the mucosal wave was suggestive of stiff vocal folds. Such a finding would be expected in falsetto voice phonation due to the high laryngeal tensions and small mass of the vocal folds. Physiological signs included decreased airflow and an inadequate closed phase was seen on the electroglottographic waveform.

The working diagnosis that seemed to be consistent with all of the signs and symptoms was that of puberphonia. With that as a base, it was hypothesized that S. P. should be capable of producing a modal voice of a more appropriate pitch. S. P. was asked whether he had ever produced a different voice even momentarily, and he responded affirmatively. It was found that he could produce a relatively low-pitched (125 Hz) and very resonant voice at will and with ease. Although he had been aware of his ability to do this, he was concerned that this "other voice" sounded very strange and would subject him to ridicule. A short period of using the voice in the clinic setting with reassurance, support, and encouragement was all that was necessary to help S. P. cross that barrier.

### *Strain/Struggle*

R. O., a 45-year-old man who was in a management position with a small industrial firm, was referred for otolaryngological examination by his family physician after a 4-year period of voice difficulty. He had already been seen by several physicians and had also been through a course of voice therapy with no relief of his symptoms. Indeed, he felt that his voice was becoming worse.

R. O. recalls that his initial voice difficulty seemed to be "laryngitis," following which he began to notice "voice breaks." As his symptoms worsened, he found that he began to experience a tightness in his throat as he was speaking, and this did not seem to be related to the length of the utterance. He also reports that he has been unable to detect any pattern related to the severity of his symptoms. Although he thinks that the voice is worse when he is tired or under stress, he can't decide whether the symptoms are actually worse or whether he just becomes more aware of them.

A variety of diagnoses and recommendations for treatment had been made up to this time. These included a bowed vocal fold, requiring teflon injection; overuse of the voice, requiring an extended period of vocal rest; an unexplained problem but one that should be helped by speech therapy; and a psychiatric problem. Voice therapy, as noted, had been tried for a period of 3 months. By his report, the therapy included a variety of relaxation exercises and breathing exercises. R. O. reports that during therapy and during practice, he was occasionally able to produce a very short sentence without difficulty but that otherwise there was no change in his voice.

### Q. WHAT POSSIBLE DIAGNOSES MIGHT BE ENTERTAINED AT THIS POINT AS PART OF THE DIFFERENTIAL DIAGNOSIS?

We found R. O.'s speech difficult to understand (Table 2.13). There was the perception of much vocal tension; sudden interruption of voicing occurred within words,

Table 2.13. Signs That May Be Associated with the Symptom of Strain/Struggle

*Typical complaint: "My voice just stops. I can't get anything out."*

*Perceptual signs*
    strain/struggle voice
    tension
    sudden interruption of voicing
    loudness variation (uncontrolled)
    tremor

*Acoustic signs*
    unexpected voice stoppages
    spectral interruptions
    reduced sustained phonation time

*Observable physiological signs—laryngoscopic*
    effort closure of the larynx
        spasmodic dysphonia
        myoclonus
        hyperkinetic dysarthria
        mixed dysarthria (ALS)
        functional
    anteroposterior shortening of the vocal folds
        spasmodic dysphonia
        functional
    rhythmic movement of laryngeal structures
        spasmodic dysphonia
        ALS
        essential tremor
        myoclonus
    arhythmic movements of laryngeal structures
        spasmodic dysphonia

*Measurable physiological signs*
    aerodynamic
        decreased airflow
        increased air pressure
    vibratory
        excessive closed times
        aberrant glottal pulse shape
    muscle activity
        excessive levels
        sudden, unexpected bursts of activity
        involuntary rhythmic variations of level
        slow rise or fall of signal amplitude

with aphonia extending over a syllable or over several words; initiation of sentences was sometimes louder than the rest of the utterance and seemed somewhat explosive, as if much effort had been required to produce voicing; and there were periods of increasing tightness in the voice as a sentence progressed. Slight tremor was heard only on vowel prolongation.

Acoustic analysis gave evidence of voice stoppages, and maximum sustained phonation time was 8 seconds, a value well below the norm for an adult man. The electroglottographic trace was aberrant, revealing excessively long closed times during the vibratory cycle. Airflow was decreased while air pressures were increased.

### Q. DOES THIS ADDITIONAL INFORMATION SHORTEN THE DIFFERENTIAL DIAGNOSIS LIST, AND IF SO, HOW AND WHY?

This patient was not subjected to electromyography. However, based on the findings from others with similar symptoms and based on other physiological signs, we would expect to find sudden, unexpected bursts of muscle potentials, slow rise or fall of signal amplitude, and excessive levels of muscle activity.

Fiberoptic laryngoscopic examination revealed rhythmic, involuntary laryngeal movement (particularly of the arytenoid cartilages) at rest, effort closure of the larynx at unexpected and unpredictable moments during speech, and occasional apparent anteroposterior shortening of the vocal folds as the epiglottis and arytenoids moved toward each other (Table 2.13). It was not possible to obtain good stroboscopic pictures due to the aperiodicity of phonation.

The working diagnosis made in this case was spasmodic dysphonia. In order to more fully examine this diagnosis, the right recurrent laryngeal nerve was anesthetized by injection of lidocaine. This procedure was carried out in the voice laboratory with the fiberoptic laryngoscope in place. This permitted visualization of the activity of the vocal folds and verified the temporary paralysis of the right vocal fold induced by the injection. The patient was able to speak during this procedure, and it was noted that in the paralyzed condition his voice was produced without strain or sudden voice interruptions but with a breathy quality. R. O. and those present during this procedure found this voice to be a significant improvement.

### Q. WHAT IS THE PURPOSE IN ANESTHETIZING THE RECURRENT LARYNGEAL NERVE? WHY SHOULD PARALYSIS OF ONE CORD HAVE HAD THIS EFFECT ON R. O.'S VOICE?

The results of this procedure were felt to be consistent with the diagnosis of spasmodic dysphonia.

## *Tremor*

We met C. W. in a very interesting way. Her niece had sought assistance for her voice problem and was referred to the voice clinic. During the course of the diagnostic process a family history of voice problems was uncovered. C. W. was the one surviving family member in addition to the niece known to have this problem. She was most interested in coming to the voice clinic for examination.

C. W., 78 years old and in generally good health, states that her voice began to get shaky and wobbly when she was in her early 60s. Although the symptoms were mild at the outset, she reports that they have become gradually worse over the past 18 years. For the past 2-3 years she has found that people often have difficulty understanding her. Her voice has never been free of the wobbliness since it first began, and she reports that stress makes the wobbliness much more pronounced. C. W. recalls that her mother, who lived to be 90, began having a similar problem with her voice when in her 70s. The severity of the problem increased over the span of those years.

Until two years ago, C. W. was never aware of shakiness of any other part of her body. She states that her mother never showed the symptom anywhere but in the voice. However, C. W. now notices that both of her hands become shaky as she engages in an activity, such as bringing food to her mouth. She has no difficulty with activities such as driving her car. Most recently, she has become aware of some slight shakiness in her jaw.

The most prominent perceptual impression is that of vocal tremor (Table 2.14). Beyond that, there is little if any change in pitch to mark for stress or meaning. The vocal tremor is noted in regular and predictable changes in the acoustic signal and occurs about five times per second. Phonational range is restricted to less than one octave. Variations in airflow are found that coincide with the tremor rate, and the glottal pulse shape is aberrant.

The fiberoptic bundle was passed through the nose and was held above the soft palate. Constant rhythmic movement of the palate was observed even though C. W. was not phonating. The fiberscope was advanced, and observation of epiglottis and laryngeal structures revealed similar involuntary movements. While at rest, the arytenoids were observed to rhythmically adduct. During phonation we observed tremor of the larynx. The stroboscope was of no value with this patient because the constantly fluctuating frequency of tremor does not allow tracking of the acoustic signal.

### Q. WHAT DO YOU THINK IS THE NATURE OF THIS PROBLEM, AND HOW DO THE SIGNS AND SYMPTOMS FIT WITH YOUR UNDERSTANDING?

The diagnosis in this case was familial essential tremor. Attempts with experimental therapy were completely unsuccessful in changing any of the characteristics of this speech pattern. C. W. is unable to exert voluntary control over this disorder.

*Table 2.14.* Signs That May Be Associated with the Symptom of Tremor

---

*Typical complaint: "My voice wobbles. My voice is unsteady."*

*Perceptual signs*
    tremor
    monopitch
    monoloudness
    loudness variations/uncontrolled

*Acoustic signs*
    voice tremor
    restricted phonational range
    restricted dynamic range
    less variability of
        fundamental frequency
        intensity
    slow rise or fall in signal amplitude

*Observable physiological signs—laryngoscopic*
    rhythmic movements of laryngeal structures
        essential voice tremor

*Measurable physiological signs*
    aerodynamics
        periodic variations of airflow
    vibratory
        aberrant glottal pulse shape
    muscle activity
        involuntary rhythmic variations of level

---

## *Pain and Other Physical Sensations*

As noted in the initial discussion of these symptoms, they are reported by patients in a variety of ways. Thus, rather than a single case presentation representative of this category, we will present a number of patients who complain of specific types of pain or sensations and relate that sensory information to the underlying pathophysiology.

J. F. reports having a severe cough for several weeks. Following resolution of the cough he noted residual slight hoarseness that did not abate. He also complained of slight soreness and burning type of sensation in a very localized area on the left neck near the posterior aspect of the larynx. He was found to have a contact granuloma over the left vocal process slightly superior to the vocal fold. This was surgically removed but recurred and required two additional surgeries. The granuloma recurred yet again. Each time the soreness recurred and was always localized to the same spot. According to the patient's report, the pain was exacerbated by phonation.

### Q. WHY WOULD PAIN BE PRESENT AND WHAT COULD BE HAPPENING DURING PHONATION TO INCREASE THAT PAIN?

A 24-hour Ph probe study had ruled out gastroesophageal reflux as a contributing factor. J. F. was referred for a course of voice therapy when a videolaryngostroboscopic study revealed a consistent pattern of approximation of the arytenoids occurring prior to closure of the vocal folds. This pattern could be described as a "toeing in" of the arytenoid cartilages.

Voice therapy was directed at changing this closure pattern and reducing the force of the contact. The granuloma reduced in size and the symptom of pain was eliminated.

### Q. WHAT COULD ACCOUNT FOR THE RESISTANCE OF THIS GRANULOMA TO TREATMENT?

That was the question that continued to concern us. A CT scan revealed the probable answer. The left arytenoid was found to be entirely calcified. Thus, the thin mucosal cover overlying a hard and "nongiving" calcified cartilage was unable to absorb the impact forces of arytenoid closure. Although this is not a typical case, it again focuses attention on the need for thorough and ongoing assessment.

L. D. is a 26-year-old woman who has been singing with various local rock groups for approximately ten years. Until this past year she had never experienced more than fleeting hoarseness which never lasted more than two days and such episodes were rare. This year she has noticed increasingly frequent episodes of hoarseness that have now culminated in a constant degree of hoarseness that does not go away. Although this was affecting her singing voice, others seemed not to be aware of it. She was aware that she had to work harder to produce voice, that she was changing musical arrangements to avoid the upper range which was especially difficult, and that she was exhausted by the end of a set. She finally sought medical attention because she began to experience pain and soreness that radiated from the neck down to her upper chest. It was the pain that frightened her into recognizing that she had a problem.

### Q. IN THIS CASE, WHAT SPECIFICALLY DO YOU THINK COULD BE CREATING PAIN OR SORENESS? WHY WOULD THAT SORENESS BE IN THE AREAS DESCRIBED?

L. D. was found to have vocal fold nodules and a course of voice therapy was prescribed. After two sessions of voice therapy directed at eliminating abusive vocal behavior, restricting the amount of talking, and using very soft breathy voice when it was necessary to talk, L. D. reported that the pain was gone. Voice therapy was

Table 2.15. Summary of Perceptual, Acoustic, and Physiological Signs That May Accompany the Nine Major Voice Symptoms

| Perceptual Sign | Hoarse | Vocal Fatigue | Breathy Voice | Reduced Phonational Range | Aphonia | Pitch Breaks, Inappropriately High Pitch | Strain/Struggle Voice | Tremor | Pain and other Physical Sensations |
|---|---|---|---|---|---|---|---|---|---|
| Monopitch | | X | | | | | | | |
| Monoloudness | X | | | | | | | X | |
| Hoarseness | X | X | X | | | | | | X |
| Breathiness | X | X | X | | | | | | X |
| Tension | X | X | | X | | | X | X | X |
| Tremor | | | | | | | X | X | |
| Strain/struggle | | | | | | | X | X | |
| Inappropriate pitch | X | | | | X | | | | |
| Loudness variation | | | X | | | | X | X | |
| Stridor | X | | | | | | | | |
| Throat clearing | X | X | | | | | | X | X |
| Aphonia—constant | X | | X | | X | | | | |
| Aphonia—episodic | X | | X | | | X | X | | |
| Pitch breaks | X | | | X | | X | | | |
| Sudden interruptions | | | | | | | | X | |
| Normal | | | | | X | | | | |

| Acoustic Sign | Hoarse | Vocal Fatigue | Breathy Voice | Reduced Phonational Range | Aphonia | Pitch Breaks, Inappropriately High Pitch | Strain/Struggle Voice | Tremor | Pain and other Physical Sensations |
|---|---|---|---|---|---|---|---|---|---|
| Mean frequency | X | | | | | X | | | |
| variability | X | X | | | | | | X | |
| perturbation | X | X | | | | | | | |
| shifts | | | | X | | | | | |

**Symptom**

| | Hoarse | Vocal Fatigue | Breathy Voice | Reduced Phonational Range | Aphonia | Pitch Breaks, Inappropriately High Pitch | Strain/Struggle Voice | Tremor | Pain and other Physical Sensations |
|---|---|---|---|---|---|---|---|---|---|
| Phonational range | X | X | X | X | | | | X | |
| Mean intensity | X | X | X | | | | | X | |
| variability | X | X | | | | | | X | |
| perturbation | X | X | X | | | | | | |
| dynamic range | X | X | X | X | | X | | X | |
| Spectrum | | | | | | | | | |
| noise | X | | X | | X | | | | |
| harmonic energy | X | X | | | | | | | |
| interruptions | | | | | | | X | | |
| Phonation time | | | | | | | | | |
| maximum | X | X | X | | | | X | X | |
| s/z ratio | X | X | X | | | | | | |
| Unexpected pauses | | | | | | | X | | |
| Tremor | | | | | | | | X | |
| Normal | | | X | | | | | | |
| *Observable Physiologic Sign—Laryngoscopic* | | | | | | | | | |
| Variation of VF approximation | X | | | | X | | | | X |
| Vocal fold movement | | | X | | X | | X | | |
| Tissue changes | X | X | X | X | | | | | |
| Pyriform sinuses | | | X | | | | | | |
| AP laryngeal dimension | X | | | | | | | X | X |
| Ventricular fold activity | X | X | X | | X | | X | | X |
| Anatomical malformation | | | X | | | X | | | |
| Vocal fold length | X | | | | X | | | | |
| Vertical laryngeal position | X | X | | | | | | | |
| Rhythmic movements | | | | | | | X | X | |

*Continued.*

Table 2.15. (continued)

|  | Symptom |  |  |  |  |  |  |  |  |
|---|---|---|---|---|---|---|---|---|---|
| Hoarse | Vocal Fatigue | Breathy Voice | Reduced Phonational Range | Aphonia | Pitch Breaks, Inappropriately High Pitch | Strain/Struggle Voice | Tremor | Pain and other Physical Sensations | Observable Physiologic Sign—Laryngoscopic |
|  |  |  |  |  |  | X | | X | Effort closure |
|  |  |  |  |  |  | X | | | Arrhythmic movements |
|  |  |  |  | X | | | | | Phonatory apraxia |
| X | X | | X | | X | | | | Normal |

|  | Symptom |  |  |  |  |  |  |  |  |
|---|---|---|---|---|---|---|---|---|---|
| Hoarse | Vocal Fatigue | Breathy Voice | Reduced Phonational Range | Aphonia | Pitch Breaks, Inappropriately High Pitch | Strain/Struggle Voice | Tremor | Pain and other Physical Sensations | Measurable Physiological Sign |
| X | X | X | X | X | X | X | X | | Airflow |
| X | X | X | | X | | X | | | Air pressure |
| X | | X | | | | X | X | | Glottal pulse shape |
| | X | | X | | | | | | Open/closed phases |
| X | | X | | | | | | | Vibratory behavior |
| | | | | | | | | | Muscle |
| X | X | X | X | | X | X | | X | levels |
| | X | | | | | X | X | | rate changes |
| | | | | | | X | | | bursts |
| | | | | | | | | | onset/offset |
| | | | | | | X | | | level decay |
| X | X | X | | | | | | | paired muscle activity |
| X | | | X | | | | | | Normal |

continued for another six sessions with eventual resolution of the nodules. L. D. had no further complaint of pain.

### Q. WOULD THIS BE CONSISTENT WITH YOUR RESPONSES TO THE QUESTION ABOVE?

A 35-year-old minister, R. S., complained of vocal fatigue and of soreness on both sides of the neck lateral to the larynx. This soreness was especially intense as he was giving sermons. Laryngovideostroboscopy using a rigid oral endoscope with sustained vowel productions revealed essentially healthy vocal folds with good vibratory behavior, normal mucosal wave, normal amplitude, good closure, and good phase symmetry. Very slight inflammation of the larynx was observed.

### Q. WHAT OTHER TYPE OF EXAMINATION MIGHT YOU WANT AND WHY?

We felt that use of the flexible nasendoscope might allow the patient to provide a sample of the speech he uses when he gives a sermon thereby allowing us to visualize phonatory behavior in that mode. What we observed did not come as a total surprise. Marked anteroposterior squeezing was noted and the entire larynx moved superiorly as he began phonation.

### Q. DO THESE OBSERVATIONS HELP TO EXPLAIN THE NATURE AND LOCATION OF THE PAIN AND VOCAL FATIGUE OF WHICH THE PATIENT COMPLAINED? HOW AND WHY?

### SUMMARY

In this chapter, a basic approach to the diagnosis of voice problems is presented. The approach, based on the medical model of differential diagnosis, carefully considers the patient's symptoms (complaints) and relates them to the signs of the patient's voice problem. There are four categories of signs: perceptual, acoustic, measurable physiological, and observable physiological.

Nine primary symptoms are presented: hoarseness, vocal fatigue, breathiness, loss of range, aphonia, pitch breaks, strain/struggle, tremor, and pain. These are defined and discussed within the context of case studies of individual patients.

Signs can be observed and tested independently of the patient's report. The major perceptual signs associated with voice problems include those related to pitch, loudness, and quality, as well as aphonia and nonphonatory signs. Acoustic signs include reduced phonation and dynamic range, higher or lower fundamental frequency, perturbation, low or high intensity, and spectral noise. Measurable physiological signs include reduced or excessive airflow and pressure, aberrant airflow or electroglottographic waveform, reduced or excessive muscle activity, and unusual muscle activity. Observable physiological signs are those stroboscopic signs that include mucosal wave, level of folds, symmetry of vocal folds, and amplitude of vocal fold motion. Laryngoscopic signs include tissue change, vocal fold approximation, anteroposterior approximation, movement of the vocal folds, and anatomic malformations. Table 2.15 presents a summary of the relationships between symptoms and signs discussed in this chapter.

Case studies have been presented to illustrate the symptoms of a voice problem and the signs associated with each symptom. The process by which the symptoms and signs are considered in the making of the diagnosis of a voice problem is emphasized in this chapter. The diagnosis of a voice problem is an ongoing, dynamic process. It is incumbent on those who work with patients with voice disorders to continue to ask questions about the nature of the problem and the treatment approach.

# Chapter 3

# Laryngeal Histopathology

## HISTOLOGY OF THE NORMAL HUMAN LARYNX: OVERVIEW

Histologically, the larynx consists of cartilages, muscles, and mucous membrane or mucosa.

### Cartilage

There are four major cartilages and two adjunct cartilages. The former are the cricoid, thyroid, arytenoid, and epiglottic cartilages, while the latter are the corniculate and cuneiform cartilages. The arytenoid, corniculate, and cuneiform cartilages are paired, whereas the other three are single structures.

The thyroid and cricoid cartilages are composed of hyaline cartilage; the epiglottic, corniculate, and cuneiform cartilages are made of elastic cartilage. The arytenoid cartilage is composed of both hyaline and elastic cartilaginous material. The main portion of the arytenoid cartilage is composed of hyaline cartilage, while the portion that meets its contralateral counterpart, including the vocal process, is made of elastic cartilage.

Cartilage is made of cells called chondrocytes and an intercellular substance containing mucopolysaccharide sulfate and fibers. Hyaline and elastic cartilage are most markedly differentiated by the type of fibers of which they are made. Hyaline cartilage has very thin, dense collagenous fibers, while elastic cartilage contains dense elastic fibers.

### Muscle

There are five major muscles in the larynx: the cricothyroid, the thyroarytenoid, the lateral cricoarytenoid, the interarytenoid, and the posterior cricoarytenoid. The interarytenoid muscle is a single muscle; the other four are paired. In addition, there are two thin, paired muscles: the thyroepiglottic and aryepiglottic muscles. Part of the thyroarytenoid muscle is located in the vocal fold and is called the vocalis muscle. All these muscles are striated (Fig. 3.1).

### Mucosa

The mucosa of the nearby alimentary canal typically consists of four layers: the epithelium, the lamina propria, the lamina muscularis mucosa, and the tela submucosa. In

*Figure 3.1.* Histological picture of a striated muscle (a part of the vocalis muscle). Note the existence of fine striations.

contrast, the laryngeal mucosa lacks the lamina muscularis mucosa. As a result, the lamina propria and the tela submucosa of the laryngeal mucosa cannot be differentiated. Therefore, the entire mucosa beneath the epithelium is called the lamina propria.

The epithelium in the larynx is basically pseudostratified ciliated epithelium. The exceptions to this include the membranous vocal fold and the inner aspect of the arytenoid cartilage, where stratified squamous epithelium covers the structures. Metaplasia of pseudostratified ciliated epithelium into stratified squamous epithelium occasionally takes place throughout the larynx.

Histological structure of the mucosa, especially that of the lamina propria, varies among the various structures of the larynx. In the following paragraphs, the structure of the mucosa at different areas of the larynx will be described.

### Basement Membrane Zone

The basement membrane zone (BMZ) is an area between the epithelium and the superficial layer of the lamina propria. It is responsible for securing the epithelium to the lamina propria (Figure 3.2a). Gray has described some of the fine anatomy of this region (Figure 3.2b) (Gray, Hirano, & Sato, 1993; Gray, Pignatari, & Harding, 1994). Note how the basal cells of the epidermis are attached by the attachment plaques (AP) to the sub-basal dense plate (DP) to the anchoring filaments (AFL) through the lamina densa of the BMZ to anchoring fibers (AF) to the superficial layer of the lamina propria. Many of the structures are composed of one or more proteins. One such protein, epidermolysis bullosa acquisita (EBA) is involved in the actual attachment of the epithelium to the underlying tissue. The lamina densa area contains proteins that add strength to the BMZ. Type IV collagen is also found in the lamina densa region and perhaps elsewhere.

The BMZ may be very susceptible to injury due to vibration and shearing forces. The fibers that anchor the BMZ loop from the lamina densa into the superficial layer of the lamina propria and then back to the lamina densa (Gray, Pignatari, & Harding,

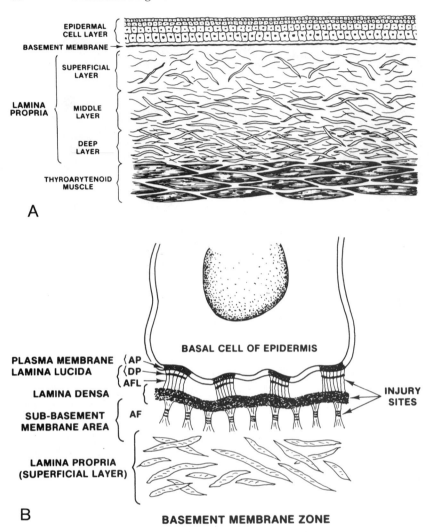

*Figure 3.2.* **A,** Schematic of the basement membrane zone in relation to the epithelium and lamina propria. **B,** Arrangement of structures in the basement membrane zone.

1994). Collagen type III fibers also appear to pass through these loops creating an arrangement that resembles a chain-link fence.

Diseases and injury may damage these fragile connecting links between the epithelium and the BMZ. It is conjectured that some aberrations of or injury to the BMZ may be the cause of nodules and other benign tumors. Fibronectin is a protein implicated in wound healing and is found in the BMZ. Once laid down, it tends to stay and has been implicated in scar formation (Gray, Hirano, & Sato, 1993). It has been found in human vocal nodules. Interestingly, neither fibronectin nor collagen type IV is found in human polyps (Gray, Hirano, & Sato, 1993).

## Epiglottis

Figure 3.3 shows a histological photograph of the laryngeal aspect of the epiglottis. The epithelium is basically pseudostratified ciliated epithelium. The lamina propria is loose and thin. Underneath the mucosa lies the epiglottic cartilage, which consists of elastic cartilage.

*Figure 3.3.* Histological picture of the mucosa of the laryngeal surface of the epiglottis. *E,* epithelium; *LP,* lamina propria; *C,* cartilage.

*Figure 3.4.* Histological picture of the mucosa of the ventricular fold. *E,* epithelium; *LP,* lamina propria; *G,* gland.

## Ventricular Fold (False Vocal Fold)

Figure 3.4 depicts a histological picture of the ventricular fold. The ventricular fold is covered with pseudostratified ciliated epithelium. The lamina propria has many glands and is very thick.

## Posterior Wall of the Glottis

Figure 3.5 shows a histological picture of the mucosa of the posterior wall of the glottis. The mucosa has pseudostratified ciliated epithelium. The tissue of the lamina propria is loose at the thin superficial layer but dense with elastic and collagenous fibers and glands in the thick deep layer. Underneath the mucosa lies the cricoid cartilage.

## Subglottic Region

A histological photograph of the mucosa of the subglottic region is shown in Figure 3.6. The epithelium consists of pseudostratified ciliated epithelium. The lamina propria is loose and contains some glands. The cricoid cartilage underlies the mucosa.

The mucosa of the vocal fold, the sound generator, will be described in detail in the following sections.

## VOCAL FOLD IN ADULTS
### Basic Structure at the Vocal Fold Edge

For the purpose of vocal function, the most important concept about vocal fold structure is that the vocal fold is a multilayered vibrator. A histological frontal section of an adult human vocal fold (Fig 3.7A) and a schematic presentation of the layered

*Figure 3.5.* Histological picture of the mucosa of the posterior wall of the glottis. *E,* epithelium; *LP,* lamina propria; *G,* gland; *PC,* perichondrium; *C,* cartilage.

*Figure 3.6.* Histological picture of the mucosa of the subglottic region. *E,* epithelium; *LP,* lamina propria; *G,* gland; *PC,* perichondrium; *C,* cartilage.

structure (Fig. 3.7B) demonstrate this concept, the most important one to remember about vocal fold structure when considering vocal function.

The vocal fold is composed of mucosa and muscle. The mucosa consists of two parts: the epithelium and the lamina propria. The epithelium is stratified squamous cell epithelium around the vocal fold edge, as described earlier, and, from a mechanical point of view, it can be regarded as a thin capsule of the vibrator. At the vocal fold edge, the lamina propria displays a unique structure. It can be divided into three layers: superficial, intermediate, and deep.

The superficial layer, often referred to as Reinke's space, is loose and pliable and can be likened to a mass of soft gelatin. It is this layer that vibrates most markedly during phonation. If it becomes stiffened by pathologies, including inflammation, tumors, or scar tissue, its vibratory movements are disturbed, resulting in dysphonia. The intermediate layer consists primarily of elastic fibers that are something like soft rubber bands, whereas the deep layer consists chiefly of collagenous fibers that can be likened to cotton thread. The vocal ligament is the name given to the structure that comprises the intermediate and deep layers of the lamina propria. Thus, the tissue in the lamina propria becomes stiffer as the muscle is approached.

The vocalis muscle forms the main body of the vocal fold and, from a mechanical point of view, when contracted it is like a bundle of stiff rubber bands.

The superficial layer of the lamina propria is clearly delineated from the intermediate layer. The border between the intermediate and deep layers, however, is not very clear. In the vocal ligament, elastic fibers decrease while collagenous fibers increase as the muscle is approached. The border between the lamina propria and the muscle is not clearly delineated at the vocal fold edge. Some fibers of the deep layer of the lamina propria insert into the muscle layer.

*Figure 3.7.* **A,** Histological picture of a frontal section of an adult human vocal fold. **B,** Schematic presentation of the layer structure. *E,* epithelium; *LP,* Lamina propria; *LPs,* superficial layer of the lamina propria; *LPi,* intermediate layer of the lamina propria; *LPd,* deep layer of the lamina propria; *VOC,* vocalis muscle; *EC,* elastic conus.

*Figure 3.8.* Blood vessels of the vocal fold. *ANC,* anterior commissure; *PE,* posterior end of membranous vocal fold; *VFE,* vocal fold edge.

From a mechanical point of view, the five layers described above can be reclassified into three sections: the cover, consisting of the epithelium and the superficial layers of the lamina propria; the transition, composed of the intermediate and deep layers of the lamina propria, or the vocal ligament; and the body, composed of the vocalis muscle (Fig. 3.7B).

Around the vocal fold edge, the elastic and collagenous fibers in the lamina propria as well as the muscle fibers of the vocalis muscle run roughly parallel to the edge. This arrangement of fibers facilitates vibratory movements.

Blood vessels in the mucosa of the vocal fold edge come from both the anterior and posterior ends of the membranous vocal fold and run roughly parallel to its edge (Fig. 3.8). All of the blood vessels are very small, and few vessels enter the mucosa directly from the underlying muscle. This blood vessel arrangement is also advantageous to the maintenance of vibration.

No glands that give marked resistance to vibratory movement are found in the mucosa around the vocal fold edge.

## Variation of the Structure along the Length of the Vocal Fold

The layered structure around the vocal fold edge varies along the length of the vocal fold. Figure 3.9A is a schematic drawing of a horizontal section of an adult human vocal fold and Figure 3.9B is a histological section of a vocal fold.

At the anterior end of the vocal fold, the intermediate layer of the lamina propria becomes thick, forming an oval mass called the anterior macula flava, which is composed of a fine mesh of elastic fibers, fibroblasts, and stroma. Anterior to the anterior macula flava lies another mass consisting primarily of collagenous fibers, called the anterior commissure tendon. This tendon is connected to the deep layer of the lamina propria lateroposteriorly, to the anterior macula flava posteriorly, and to the thyroid cartilage anteriorly. Thus, the stiffness of the tissue changes gradually from the pliable membranous vocal fold to the stiff thyroid cartilage.

At the posterior end of the membranous vocal fold, the intermediate layer of the lamina propria forms another oval mass, which is referred to as the posterior macula flava. Its structure is similar to that of the anterior macula flava. It is connected to the vocal process of the arytenoid cartilage with a small intervening transitional area. The transitional area is stiffer than the macula flava but less stiff than the cartilage. The tip of the vocal process is composed of elastic cartilage, which is less stiff than the hyaline cartilage that constitutes the main portion of the arytenoid cartilage. Thus, again, the

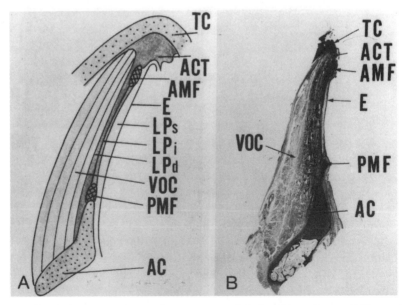

*Figure 3.9.* **A,** Schematic presentation of the structures. *TC,* thyroid cartilage; *ACT,* anterior commissure tendon; *AMF,* anterior macula flava; *PMF,* posterior macula flava; *AC,* arytenoid cartilage; *E,* epithelium; *LPs,* superficial layer of lamina propria; *LPi,* intermediate layer of lamina propria; *LPd,* deep layer of lamina propria; *VOC,* vocalis muscle. **B,** Histological picture of a horizontal section of an adult human vocal fold.

stiffness of tissue changes gradually from the pliable membranous vocal fold to the stiff arytenoid cartilage.

The structures at both ends of the membranous vocal fold appear to have a roll of tissue designed possibly to protect the ends from mechanical injury caused by the vibration of the folds during phonation.

## VOCAL FOLD STRUCTURE IN NEWBORNS

The structure of the vocal fold edge in newborns differs greatly from that in adults, with the most marked differences occurring in the lamina propria of the mucosa. Figures 3.10A and C are histological pictures of the vocal fold of a newborn; Figures 3.10B and D are schematic presentations of the structures.

The epithelium at the vocal fold edge is squamous cell epithelium that does not significantly differ from that in adults. The lamina propria is very thick relative to vocal fold length, and it is rather uniform in structure. There is no ligamentous structure. Almost the entire lamina propria is rather loose and pliable. However, some fibrous tissue, which appears to be the immature maculae flava, is aggregated at the anterior and posterior ends of the membranous vocal fold.

## Development of Vocal Fold Structure

An immature vocal ligament appears between the age of 1 and 4 years. In this stage, however, the ligament is very thin and does not touch the vocalis muscle. There is no differentiation between the layer of elastic fibers and the layer of collagenous fibers. In other words, during this developmental stage the lamina propria does not yet have the three-layer structure. Differentiation of the two layers in the vocal ligament begins sometime between 6 and 12 years of age, and the ligament becomes thicker. After the age of 15 years, a clear three-layer structure of the lamina propria is consistently observed. Maturation of this layered structure of the vocal fold seems to be completed around the end of adolescence.

## CHANGES IN VOCAL FOLD STRUCTURE WITH AGING

There are great individual differences in changes in vocal fold structure as a function of aging. However, certain tendencies have been observed; the epithelium does not show any consistent and significant changes with aging and the superficial layer of the lamina propria tends to become edematous and thicker with age (Fig. 3.11A). The density of fibroblasts, collagenous fibers, and elastic fibers in this layer tends to decrease. These changes tend to be more marked in men than in women.

Age-related changes in the intermediate layer of the lamina propria are noted in men, but occur less frequently in women. These changes include a loosening and atrophy of elastic fibers in the intermediate layer (Fig. 3.11B). As a result, this layer tends to become thinner. Occasionally, deterioration of the contour of this layer occurs, caused chiefly by a fibrotic change in the deep layer of the lamina propria.

Changes in the deep layer of the lamina propria also take place more markedly in aging men than in aging women. Collagenous fibers tend to become thicker and denser with aging, which results in the deep layer becoming thicker. Occasionally, collagenous fibers increase locally and run in various directions, displaying a condition referred to as fibrosis (Fig. 3.11C). The muscle tends to become atrophied with age.

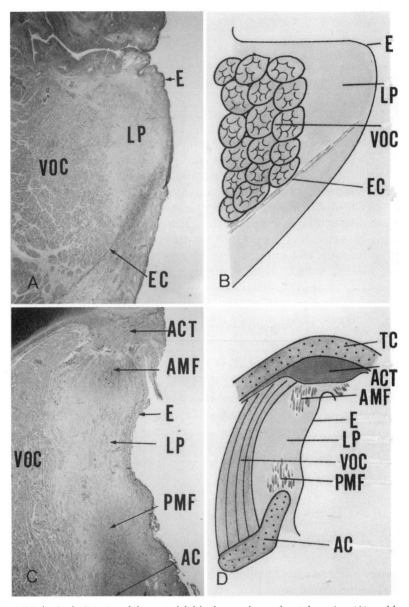

*Figure 3.10.* Histological pictures of the vocal fold of a newborn: frontal section (**A**) and horizontal section (**C**). Schematic presentations of these structures: frontal section (**B**) and horizontal section (**D**). *E,* epithelium; *LP,* lamina propria; *VOC,* vocalis muscle; *EC,* elastic conus; *TC,* thyroid cartilage; *ACT,* anterior commissure tendon; *AMF,* anterior macula flava; *PMF,* posterior macula flava; *AC,* arytenoid cartilage.

## HISTOPATHOLOGY OF NON-NEOPLASTIC DISEASES OF THE MUCOSA

### Epithelial Hyperplasia and Dysplasia

The term "epithelial hyperplasia" implies any kind of pathology in which hyperplastic thickening of the epithelium is the primary lesion (Fig. 3.12A). When the lesion is as-

*Figure 3.11.* Histological pictures demonstrating geriatric changes in the lamina propria of the mucosa of the vocal folds. **A,** Edema (*arrow*) in the superficial layer (a 61-year-old man). **B,** Atrophy of elastic fibers (*EF*) in the intermediate layer (a 47-year-old man, upper figure; the lower figure is a control, a 27-year-old man). **C,** Fibrotic changes (*arrow*) in the deep layer (a 53-year-old man).

sociated with atypical cells, it is called epithelial dysplasia (Fig. 3.12B). Lesions such as leukoplakia, hyperkeratosis, pachydermia, and acanthosis fall into this category.

Lesions of the hyperplastic and dysplastic type are regarded as precancerous conditions. Carcinomas occasionally develop from hyperplastic or dysplastic epithelium. Clinically, differentiating carcinoma in situ or very early invasive carcinomas from epithelial hyperplasia or dysplasia is often difficult.

*Figure 3.12.* **A,** Epithelial hyperplasia. **B,** Dysplasia.

*Figure 3.13.* Histological picture of a vocal fold with epithelial hyperplasia (*arrow*).

*Figure 3.14.* Histological picture of a vocal fold with nodule (*arrow*).

The lesions in this category originate from the epithelium and may enter the superficial layer of the lamina propria (Fig. 3.13). The lesion never invades the vocal ligament unless it becomes malignant. It may be unilateral or bilateral. It is usually asymmetrical and is not uniform within the affected vocal fold. Glottic closure is occasionally disturbed. From a mechanical point of view, the mass and stiffness of the cover increase, whereas the mechanical properties of the transition and the body are

*Figure 3.15.* Histological pictures of vocal fold with polyp (*arrows*). **A,** Whitish polyp in which edema is the dominant pathology. **B,** Reddish polyp in which intratissue bleeding, hyaline degeneration, and thrombosis are the dominant pathologies.

not affected. The lesion occasionally interferes with the vibratory movements of the contralateral vocal fold.

## Vocal Fold Nodules

Vocal fold nodules develop around the vocal fold edge at the middle of the membranous vocal fold. They are whitish, tiny sessile bumps and are usually bilateral although the lesion may be of unequal size. The lesion is in the superficial layer of the lamina propria and consists primarily of edematous tissue and/or collagenous fibers (Fig. 3.14). The lesion may be symmetrical and may prevent the glottis from closing completely during phonation. The mass and stiffness of the cover are slightly increased, whereas the mechanical properties of the transition and body are not affected. The lesion may slightly interfere with vibratory movements of the contralateral vocal fold.

## Vocal Fold Polyp

Vocal fold polyps usually develop around the vocal fold edge at the middle of the membranous vocal fold. They may be reddish or whitish, small or large, sessile or pedunculated, unilateral or bilateral; usually they are asymmetrical. The lesion is in the superficial layer of the lamina propria. The histological features of the lesion are edema (Fig. 3.15A), intratissue bleeding, hyaline degeneration, thrombosis (Fig. 3.15B), proliferation of collagenous fibers, and/or cell infiltration. Glottic closure is impeded. The mass of the cover is increased, but the stiffness of the cover varies depending on the pathology. It is increased when bleeding, hyaline degeneration, thrombosis, proliferation of collagenous fibers, or cell infiltration is the main pathology. When edema is the primary pathology, the stiffness of the cover decreases. The mechanical properties of the transition and the body are not affected. Polyps interfere with vibratory movements of the contralateral vocal fold.

## Reinke's Edema

There are several different terms for Reinke's edema: polypoid degeneration, chronic polypoid corditis, chronic edematous hypertrophy, and polypoid vocal fold. Histologically, one finds primarily edema in the superficial layer of the lamina propria (Fig. 3.16). It is neither degeneration, inflammation (-itis), nor hypertrophy. The membranous vocal fold is edematous and swollen along its entire length. The lesion is usually bilateral and is asymmetrical in most cases. The glottis usually closes completely during phonation. The mass of the cover is increased while the stiffness of the cover is usually decreased. The mechanical properties of the transition and body are not affected. The edematous lesion interferes with vibration of the contralateral counterpart.

## Epidermoid Cyst

Epidermoid cysts are basically in the superficial layer of the lamina propria (Fig. 3.17). Occasionally they have a tiny opening to the laryngeal lumen; they may also insert partly into the vocal ligament (Fig. 3.18). The cystic wall is lined with thin squamous cell epithelium. Cysts contain caseous material and may be compared to a balloon full of fluid. The lesion may be unilateral or bilateral, small or large. The vibrating structures are usually asymmetrical. Glottic closure is often impeded. The mass and stiffness of the cover are increased. The mechanical properties of the transition and the body are usually not affected. The cyst often interferes with vibratory movements of the contralateral vocal fold.

*Figure 3.16.* Histological picture of a vocal fold with Reinke's edema (*arrow*).

*Figure 3.17.* Histological picture of a vocal fold with epidermoid cyst (*arrow*).

## *Nonspecific Granuloma*

There are three types of nonspecific granulomas that develop within the glottic region: intubation granulomas, contact granulomas, and granulomas caused by gastroesophageal reflux. Granulomas are found at the vocal process of the arytenoid cartilage or on the lateral wall of the posterior glottis (Fig. 3.19). The membranous vocal fold is not affected. Histologically, granulomas consist chiefly of proliferated capillaries, fibroblasts, collagenous fibers, and leukocytes (Fig. 3.20). They may or may not be covered with epithelium. The lesion may be unilateral or bilateral. Granulomas impede glottic closure only when they are very large. There is no effect on the mechanical properties of any layer of the membranous vocal fold.

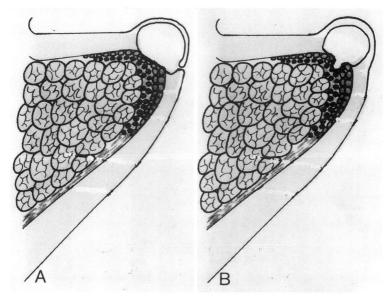

*Figure 3.18.* Variations of epidermoid cyst of the vocal fold. **A,** A tiny opening to the laryngeal lumen. **B,** Partial insertion into the vocal ligament.

*Figure 3.19.* Location of nonspecific granuloma (*dotted area*). *PW,* posterior wall of the glottis; *LW,* lateral wall of the posterior glottis; *PEV,* posterior end of the ventricle; *CVF,* cartilaginous portion of the vocal fold; *TVP,* tip of the vocal process; *MVF,* membranous portion of the vocal fold.

*Figure 3.20.* Histological pictures of a nonspecific granuloma of the glottic area. **A,** Entire view. **B,** Greater magnification.

*Figure 3.21.* Histological picture of a vocal fold with sulcus vocalis (*arrow*).

## Sulcus Vocalis

The term "sulcus vocalis" refers to a furrow along the entire length of the edge of the membranous vocal fold. The vocal fold edge is bowed to a greater or lesser extent. Although the lesion may occasionally be unilateral, in most cases it is bilateral and roughly symmetrical. The glottis does not close completely during phonation. Histologically, the sulcus is located in the superficial layer of the lamina propria (Fig. 3.21). The epithelium in the sulcus is occasionally thickened. Collagenous fibers are frequently increased, and capillaries are decreased in number around the sulcus. From a mechanical point of view, the mass of the cover is reduced whereas the stiffness of the cover is increased. The mechanical properties of the transition and the body are not affected.

## *Vocal Fold Scar*

Scarring can occur any place on the vocal fold as a result of trauma, surgery, burn, or inflammation. Scar tissue consists of dense collagenous fibers and is much stiffer than the normal tissue of the vocal fold mucosa and the muscle. The glottis often does not close completely during phonation. The mass of each layer varies, depending upon the amount of scarring, whereas the stiffness of the layer(s) involved is increased.

## HISTOPATHOLOGY OF NEOPLASTIC DISEASES

### *Carcinomas*

Most carcinomas of the vocal fold are squamous cell carcinomas. They originate from the epithelium and invade the deeper structures, including the lamina propria and the muscle (Fig. 3.22). The lesion is originally unilateral, but it can extend to the contralateral side. The vocal fold tissue is asymmetrical and glottic closure is usually disturbed. Both the mass and the stiffness of the cover are increased. The mass and stiffness of the transition and the body are increased when these structures are involved. The carcinomatous mass interferes with vibration of the contralateral vocal fold.

### *Papilloma*

Papillomas originate from the epithelium and may invade the lamina propria and the muscle. The lesion may be unilateral or bilateral, and it is usually asymmetrical. Histologically, papillomas consist of proliferated neoplastic epithelial cells growing in a papillary shape (Fig. 3.23). The lesion impedes complete glottic closure during phonation. The mass and stiffness of the cover are increased. The mass and stiffness of

*Figure 3.22.* Histological pictures of vocal folds with carcinoma (*arrows*). **A,** Lesion confined to the mucosa. **B,** Lesion involving the muscle. *VOC,* vocalis muscle; *TC,* thyroid cartilage.

the transition and the body are increased when these structures are affected. The papilloma mass interferes with vibratory movements of the contralateral vocal fold.

## HISTOPATHOLOGY OF NEUROMUSCULAR DISEASES

The most frequent neuromuscular disease of the vocal fold is paralysis caused by recurrent laryngeal nerve (RLN) lesions.

From a neuropathological point of view, there are three types of paralysis: neuropraxia, axonotmesis, and neurotmesis (Fig. 3.24). In neuropraxia, conduction of nerve impulses is temporarily blocked. It is caused, for example, by injection of local anesthetics. It does not cause muscle atrophy, and the neuromuscular system recovers to its normal state. Axonotmesis is a condition in which the axons of the nerve are sectioned, and neurotmesis refers to a condition in which the nerve fibers are entirely cut. In

*Figure 3.23.* Histological picture of vocal fold with papilloma (*arrow*).

*Figure 3.24.* Three types of paralysis. **A,** Neuropraxia. **B,** Axonotmesis. **C,** Neurotmesis. *Dotted area:* Conduction of neural impulses is temporarily blocked. *Solid area:* Axon is degenerated.

*Figure 3.25.* Histological picture of a horizontal section of a vocal fold with RLN paralysis, demonstrating muscular atrophy. *E,* epithelium; *LPs,* superficial layer of lamina propria; *VL,* vocal ligament; *m,* atrophic muscle.

both conditions, the portion of the nerve peripheral to the site of lesion degenerates, and the muscle becomes denervated. The nerve may or may not regenerate, and the muscle may or may not be reinnervated accordingly. When the muscle is not reinnervated, it becomes atrophied. In many clinical cases, the RLN is only partly affected, meaning that some motor units are affected while others are not.

Vocal fold paralysis is unilateral in most cases. Glottic closure is usually disturbed because of lack of adduction of the affected vocal fold. Figure 3.25 shows a histological picture of a vocal fold in which marked atrophy of the vocalis muscle has resulted. In cases of vocal fold paralysis associated with muscle atrophy, the mass and stiffness of the body are decreased. Paralysis without muscle atrophy results in decreased stiffness of the body, and the mass of the body may be slightly decreased. In any case, the mechanical properties of the cover and the transition are basically not affected.

## SUMMARY OF IMPLICATIONS FOR VOCAL PHYSIOLOGY

In understanding the effect of various pathological conditions on the sound generation properties and the vibratory behavior of the vocal folds, it is important to consider the following parameters:

1. Localization of the pathology
2. Symmetry of both vocal folds
3. Uniformity within each vocal fold
4. Glottic closure
5. Layered structure
6. Mass and stiffness of each layer
7. Interference with vibratory movements of the contralateral vocal fold

Table 3.1 summarizes these aspects for varying pathological conditions. Since each parameter can vary from case to case for a given pathology, the table describes the most typical states for each pathology.

Table 3.1. Summary of Various Pathological Conditions

| Pathology | Location of Pathology | Symmetry | Uniformity | Glottic Incompetence | Layer Structure | Cover | | Transition | | Body | | Interference |
|---|---|---|---|---|---|---|---|---|---|---|---|---|
| | | | | | | Mass | Stiffness | Mass | Stiffness | Mass | Stiffness | |
| Epithelial hyperplasia and dysplasia | Epithelium → Superf. layer of lamina propria (Cover) | Deteriorated | Deteriorated | Occasionally | Frequently deteriorated | Increased | Increased | Normal | Normal | Normal | Normal | Varying |
| Nodule | Superf. layer of lamina propria (Cover) | Maintained | Deteriorated | Partly | Maintained | Increased (slightly) | Increased (slightly) | Normal | Normal | Normal | Normal | Slight |
| Polyp | Superf. layer of lamina propria (Cover) | Deteriorated | Deteriorated | Partly | Maintained | Increased | Varying | Normal | Normal | Normal | Normal | Marked |
| Reinke's edema | Superf. layer of lamina propria (Cover) | Deteriorated | Usually maintained | None | Maintained | Increased | Decreased | Normal | Normal | Normal | Normal | Marked |
| Epidermoid cyst | Superf. layer of lamina propria (Cover) | Deteriorated | Deteriorated | Partly | Partly deteriorated | Increased | Increased | Normal | Normal | Normal | Normal | Marked |
| Granuloma | Posterior glottis | Maintained | Maintained | None | Maintained | Normal | Normal | Normal | Normal | Normal | Normal | None |

| | | | | | | | | | | | |
|---|---|---|---|---|---|---|---|---|---|---|---|
| Sulcus vocalis | Superf. layer of lamina propria (Cover) | Maintained | Maintained | Entire length (slight) | Partly deteriorated | Decreased | Increased | Normal | Normal | Normal | Normal | Normal | None |
| Scar | Varying | Deteriorated | Deteriorated or maintained | In varying degree | Deteriorated | Varying | Increased | Varying | Normal or increased | Varying | Normal or increased | None |
| Carcinoma | Epithelium → Superf. layer of lamina propria → Vocal ligament → Muscle (Cover → Body) | Deteriorated | Deteriorated | Partly | Deteriorated | Increased | Increased | Increased | Increased | Increased | Increased | Marked |
| Papilloma | Epithelium → Superf. layer of lamina propria → Vocal ligament → Muscle (Cover → Body) | Deteriorated | Deteriorated | Partly | Frequently deteriorated | Increased | Increased | Occasionally increased | Occasionally increased | Ocassionally increased | Occasionally increased | Marked |
| Vocal fold paralysis | Muscle | Deteriorated | Maintained | Entire length (marked) | Deteriorated | Normal | Normal | Normal | Normal | Decreased | Decreased | None |

# Chapter 4

# Voice Misuse and Abuse: Effects on Laryngeal Physiology

Vocal misuse and abuse are frequently claimed to be the causes of voice problems. Furthermore, they are thought to contribute to the laryngeal tissue changes that result in the formation of such lesions as nodules, polyps, and contact ulcers. What does misuse and abuse mean? What kinds of vocal activities can be properly deemed to be abusive or somehow improper or unhealthy? When does misuse become abuse? How much abuse or misuse can laryngeal tissues tolerate? How do patterns of misuse evolve, and what maintains them? How do misuse and abuse create voice problems? These questions must be asked, and surprisingly few answers are available. In this chapter we will discuss the current state of knowledge about vocal misuse and abuse.

## MISUSE

Misuse suggests voice production behaviors that distort the normal propensity of the phonatory mechanism to work effectively and efficiently. An efficient system produces its best results with a minimum of effort. A car engine whose various components are in top working condition so that its operation is smooth and uses the least energy to perform its work is said to be operating efficiently. Similarly, a phonatory system in which the individual components are healthy and the coordination and interaction with all of its supporting parts and systems is in tune produces voice in an efficient manner.

There are a number of ways in which that smooth operation of the voice may be altered. Each of us can voluntarily produce voice in a variety of different ways, some of them efficient, some inefficient. Those who work with disordered voices should be able to produce inefficient as well as efficient voice in order to better understand how various changes in voice production can be made. For example, take a breath, and as you begin to speak tighten your chest to the point of almost holding your breath. How does it feel to talk like that? Where do you feel the tensions? How did it change the sound of your voice? As another example, try to squeeze your larynx tightly and speak in a hoarse voice. Think about how that feels and what you have done to change the sound of your voice. As a final experiment, pick a pitch about two tones above your present pitch level and try to converse, and then do this at a pitch about two tones lower than your comfort level. Has your larynx height changed? What does it feel like to try to do this? What does it do to your breathing, your degree of tension, your inflection patterns?

All of these activities could be categorized as vocal misuse, yet all are within the ability of each of us to produce. In Table 4.1 we have identified some of the behaviors that when used habitually constitute misuse. Each of these will be discussed in the following sections.

## *Increased Tension or Strain*

Descriptions of what is meant by increased vocal tension abound but frequently lack specificity. The judgment of vocal tension is most frequently made on a subjective basis. The subjectivity may be the reporting by the patient of the sensation of tension, or sometimes even pain, accompanying speaking, or it may be the judgment of the voice clinician based on auditory and visual observations. There are few objective methods of documenting tension, and there are none that can be put to routine clinical use to provide measurement of specific muscle tensions. Biofeedback using externally placed electrodes has been attempted, but it is not at all clear what specific muscles are being tapped, nor is there sufficient information available to identify which muscles are the most significant in assessment of vocal tension.

In cases of vocal misuse, the laryngological examination may be negative, with perhaps a suggestion of increased redness or slight swelling of the vocal folds. In some cases it is noted that a strand of mucus forms and reforms between the vocal folds at the nodal point, a sign thought by some to be an early indication of or tendency toward nodule formation. We have found flexible fiberoptic examinations to be of significant help in identifying patterns of excessive laryngeal tension in some patients. The specific, observable signs of that tension are hard glottal attack, high laryngeal position, anteroposterior laryngeal squeezing, and excessive medial compression.

### HARD GLOTTAL ATTACK

The hard glottal attack or glottal coup describes a manner of initiating vowels, usually characterized by rapid and complete adduction of the vocal folds prior to the initiation of phonation. This adducted state, which may be accompanied by considerable muscle tension, requires that subglottal pressure be increased in order to overcome vocal fold resistance and initiate phonation. The characteristic sound of a hard glottal attack is an abrupt, explosive, and hard-edged onset of phonation. This form of voice initiation is often visible fiberoptically, especially when subjects are asked to produce isolated vowel sounds (Casper, Colton, Brewer, & Woo, 1989). It appears to be produced in at least two ways. In one method, medial compression of the vocal folds is observed

---

*Table 4.1.* Characteristics of Vocal Behaviors Categorized as Misuse

A. Increased tension or strain
   1. Hard glottal attack
   2. High laryngeal position
   3. Anteroposterior laryngeal squeezing

B. Inappropriate pitch level
   1. Puberphonia
   2. Persistent glottal fry
   3. Lack of pitch variability

C. Excessive talking

D. Ventricular phonation

E. Aphonia and dysphonia of psychological origin

almost simultaneously with the onset of phonation. The second variation is characterized by prephonatory laryngeal constriction in which the ventricular folds approach each other, as do the arytenoids and the epiglottis, obscuring visualization of the true vocal folds. As phonation is initiated, there is a reduction in the forced adduction and a sudden springing open of the larynx as the true vocal folds become visible. It is important to add a note of caution. We have observed occasional evidence of this hard glottal attack in speakers who were judged to have normal voices and who were experiencing no voice problems. It is a behavior that may occur on occasion in most speakers. In some instances the behavior may be a reaction to the examination procedure and the tensions associated with it. Whether or not this particular behavior is identified as evidence of misuse must depend in part on the degree of its presence and the circumstances under which it is observed. In general, when the hard glottal attack is present to a significant degree, it is but one of several behaviors that give evidence of increased tension and strain.

## HIGH LARYNGEAL POSITION

Vertical laryngeal height has been the subject of some study and controversy. It has been reported that untrained singers show greater laryngeal elevation with increased pitch level than do trained singers (Shipp, 1987; Shipp & Izdebski, 1975). There are different schools of thought among singers, singing coaches, and voice scientists relative to the benefits of maintaining a low laryngeal position. Many believe that raising laryngeal height with elevation of pitch is improper singing technique and detrimental to the voice (Sundberg & Askenfelt, 1983). However, more recently, Sundberg reported that an X-ray study of two well-trained female singers revealed an increase in vertical laryngeal height with an increase in pitch, in what he described as a "very elegant" and "well-trained" behavior (Shipp, Guinn, Sundberg, & Titze, 1987). It was suggested that varying laryngeal position may be useful and that raising the larynx during singing may not be abusive.

There are many differences between singing and speaking that make it difficult to suggest that a particular behavior in one activity is the same or has the same effect in the other activity. Raising the larynx results in (*a*) a shortening of the vocal tract, with a subsequent raising of all formant frequencies; (*b*) a stiffening of vocal fold tissues that alters the vibratory pattern and increases fundamental frequency; and (*c*) an increased tendency for tight vocal fold closure. This tight adduction is a desirable and essential part of the swallowing process wherein the larynx elevates and a tight valving maneuver ensues, thereby protecting the lower airway. In speaking, it is not variability of laryngeal height that is suggestive of excessive tension but rather a speaker's tendency to consistently speak with the larynx in an elevated position. Titze states (Shipp, Guinn, Sundberg, & Titze, 1987) that the human body seems naturally to do that which is easiest to do, and it seems to optimize itself for a given task. Further, he suggests that the speaker who constantly maintains a low laryngeal posture may be using more energy in doing so than the speaker who allows the mechanism to move freely.

Vocal tension is characterized by increased tension in both the intrinsic and extrinsic laryngeal muscles. However, we are not yet able to isolate the contributions of each muscle group to voice problems associated with misuse. Indeed, the system as a whole is so interactive that when excessive tensions exist in one muscle, they will probably occur also in some other muscles. Thus, although laryngeal height is primarily controlled by extrinsic laryngeal muscle activity, we cannot attribute a voice disorder to that condition alone and must recognize the total physiological disturbance. A high laryngeal position may be related to excessive tension in both extrinsic and intrinsic muscle groups. Sundberg and Askenfelt (1983) stated that "the muscles used for raising the larynx also may affect the way in which the vocal folds vibrate" (p. 307), which underscores the relationship between larynx height and the voice source. Shipp (1987) also addresses this relationship and reports that increased stiffening of the vocal fold margin results from the upward stretch of tissues created by laryngeal height elevation.

It is not unusual for patients with this particular pattern of hyperfunction to report sensations of pain or soreness in the neck lateral to the larynx, sometimes radiating upward or downward. These patients also report that their voices tend to become worse with increased use and that by the end of the workday they feel it takes too much effort to talk.

### ANTEROPOSTERIOR LARYNGEAL SQUEEZING

In the endoscopic laryngeal examination of voice-disordered patients, we have often observed (usually in the absence of observable pathology) a "squeezing" of the larynx in which the epiglottis and the arytenoids approach each other during phonation. A similar but not identical movement is typical in the production of the low back vowels (e.g., /ah/), when the tongue position dictates a posterior movement of the epiglottis. That movement is a natural one in which none of the "squeezing" elements are present. During production of the vowels /ee/ and /oo/, the epiglottis is normally expected to be pulled somewhat anteriorly and superiorly, making the vocal folds fully visible. This does not occur in patients with a "squeezed" larynx. These patients, even in the production of the /ee/ and /oo/ vowels, as well as other stimulus materials heavily loaded with these vowels, demonstrate anteroposterior "squeezing" behavior to the extent that visualization of the true vocal folds along their full length is often obscured.

Another vocal maneuver that is normally expected to "open" the larynx when it is being viewed endoscopically is pitch elevation. However, persons who tend to habitually use very tight laryngeal posture with anteroposterior shortening do so even as they raise pitch. In fact, they often encounter difficulty in raising pitch and may exhibit a reduced phonational range. We believe that this vocal behavior is an indication of disturbed phonatory physiology, probably due to excess strain and tension.

## *Inappropriate Pitch Level*

A common concept in the voice literature is that of optimum pitch. Clinicians are instructed that the use of a too high or a too low habitual pitch level is a frequent cause of voice disorders. Much therapy time is spent in identifying what is purported to be an individual's optimum pitch, and therapy is then directed toward teaching the patient to use that pitch. We have difficulty with this approach for a number of reasons.

If the fundamental frequency of a person's voice is altered by pathology, for example, it seems to us that attempts to "measure" an optimum pitch are immediately flawed. The most common methodology espoused for obtaining the so-called optimum pitch is described by Fairbanks (1960) and involves obtaining a measure of phonational range. Recall, however, that phonational range is often reduced in the presence of certain laryngeal pathologies and voice disorders. It is important to recognize that despite the apparently widespread use of the concept of optimum pitch, there are no data to demonstrate or document its validity nor its therapeutic efficacy. (See Chapter 9 for further discussion of this topic.)

The physiological approach to voice disorders, based on an understanding of vocal fold physiology and acoustics, suggests that a disturbance of physiology due to mass lesions, manner of use, or abnormal motor control will result in acoustic changes.

Thus, an inappropriate pitch level, if indeed it is present, may well be a sign of a problem rather than the cause of the problem. Attention needs to be paid to the underlying cause of the problem, and when the physiology is normalized or improved, then the pitch level of the voice will also improve or normalize. Indeed, it is quite possible for a person to speak at a totally appropriate pitch level and yet do so in an abusive way.

Judgments of the pitch of a voice can be made subjectively but those perceptions should always be checked against objective measurement of fundamental frequency. Perception of pitch levels can be quite erroneous, especially in the presence of hoarseness or excess noise energy in the voice. Objective measurement of fundamental frequency rather than casual judgments of pitch may be made easily using methods described in Chapter 7 and should always be done before any judgments about the acceptability of this parameter are considered. However, in a very rough voice even measurements of fundamental frequency should be suspect because of the difficulty in obtaining reliable and accurate estimates of the period of vibration.

Inappropriate pitch is typically the hallmark of puberphonia, persistent glottal fry, and lack of pitch variability. It is necessary to recognize, however, that inappropriate pitch may be only one sign of an underlying problem.

### PUBERPHONIA

This category is referred to in the literature by a number of names: adolescent falsetto, pubescent falsetto, incomplete mutation, and mutational falsetto, to name a few. We have chosen to use the term *puberphonia* (not as the most desirable, but as the least objectionable) since it suggests the developmental stage at which this problem is encountered (puberty) and tells us that it involves the voice (*phone*). Rather than add yet another term, we prefer to describe the nature of the problem.

Puberphonia refers most simply to the persistence of a high-pitched voice beyond the age at which voice change is expected to have occurred. This is primarily a male problem. Although some women continue to have very high pitched and childlike voices into their adult years, there is little stigma attached to this situation for two reasons: First, the lowering of the fundamental frequency in women (3–4 semitones) as a result of laryngeal growth is not as marked as for men (one octave); second, women are expected to have higher pitched voices. Thus, the presence of a high-pitched voice in a woman is not always perceived to be as unusual or inappropriate as in a man. That is not to deny, however, that a childlike voice can be inappropriate, can jeopardize a woman's employment status, and can negatively affect how she is perceived.

In cases of puberphonia it is important that a determination be made first as to whether an organic abnormality is present. The adequacy of laryngeal growth must be assessed, and potential endocrinological problems must be ruled out. The laryngeal examination and the history may provide sufficient information regarding these concerns. The vocal symptoms include not only the inappropriately high-pitched voice but also often hoarseness and some degree of breathiness. The voice tends to sound unstable and uncertain, and the patient's reporting often confirms that perception: "It sounds funny, and I never know what it is going to sound like." Pitch breaks may also be heard. Although the onset of the problem is, by definition, during the adolescent growth spurt and the emergence of secondary sex characteristics, it may persist for a considerable length of time before any treatment is sought.

Psychosocial factors, such as difficulty with male identification or with the acceptance of emerging adulthood, are most often cited as the primary etiological factors. Our experience, however, suggests that, if present, these factors are not overwhelming in their expression. It seems quite logical to us that a certain percentage of young boys may have fairly traumatic voice change experiences not only in the psychological sense but also in the physical sense. Pitch breaks may be frequent and extreme, and the lack of control over the voice may be pronounced. Feelings of embarrassment result and are aggravated by a lack of understanding of what is happening. An understandable reaction to such feelings might be an attempt to hold on to the voice that is known (the child voice) and to attain control of what otherwise seems to be an uncontrollable behavior. In many cases, when asked if they have another voice, young men with this problem will answer in the affirmative. In some we have observed a profound sense of relief when this admission has been made and reassurance has been provided about the normalcy of the "hidden" voice. Indeed, for many, little additional treatment has been necessary beyond providing a period of practice in using the new voice, coupled with encouragement and guidance. In others, the process of "releasing" the adult voice (see Chapter 9) is usually very effective in producing a more typical adult voice within a short time period. We are not aware, either through personal experience or perusal of the literature, of posttherapy failures wherein there is a regression to the high-pitched voice. We also have not been impressed that the young men who have presented with this problem in our clinic have had difficulty with male identification. Indeed, we would not describe the sound of their voices as ever having been effeminate. The characteristics of an effeminate voice are comprised of speech mannerisms and suprasegmental differences that go well beyond just the presence of a higher than expected pitch level. We believe that the theory of the domineering mother figure and the weak father figure as the primary underlying cause for the maintenance of the inappropriately high pitch level has not been validated.

We have recently become aware of several cases of "falsetto-like" voice in the female. These voices exhibit instability similar to that described for the puberphonic male with frequent pitch breaks and elevated fundamental frequency. The underlying etiology and the pathophysiology in these cases has not been well explored, but they differ from other psychogenically based voice problems in that the voice has not undergone a recent change. It has been present for many years with no recall of it ever having sounded different. In the cases we have encountered, eliciting and establishing a more appropriate pitch level and vocal stability has been accomplished through voice therapy..

## PERSISTENT GLOTTAL FRY

Glottal fry, or pulse register, is described as one of the three normal voice registers, the other two being loft (falsetto) and modal. These registers are characterized by a change in the mechanical mode of vibration (Fairbanks, 1960), and there is usually a little overlap in the frequency of phonation between adjacent registers. Daniloff, Shuckers, and Feth (1980) state that the physiologically complex larynx "can vibrate in three (or more) relatively different ways, giving rise to airflow modulation that yields acoustically and perceptually distinct vocal quality" (p. 209). Glottal fry is the register lowest in fundamental frequency and the least flexible. The vocal folds are noted to close quickly, and the closed phase of the vibratory cycle is very long relative to the length of the entire period. Moore and von Leden (1958) described the occasional occurrence of two open phases during one vibratory cycle. Zemlin (1988) reported that the closed phase occupies about 90% of the cycle. In describing the characteristics of glottal fry as seen in high-speed motion pictures, he observed tightly approximated vocal folds whose free edges, however, appeared flaccid. Zemlin further noted that air seemed to "bubble up" between the folds near the junction of the anterior two-thirds of the glottis. Glottal fry is produced with much lower airflows than the other registers (Murry, 1971), and air is released in irregularly timed bursts. Pulsated voice, according to Perkins (1983), allows the production of only very low fundamental frequencies, with a decay of energy in every glottal cycle.

Glottal fry has a very characteristic sound, which has been described variously as similar to the popping of corn, the imitated sound of a motor boat engine, or a creaky voice. The vibratory pattern is so slow that individual vibrations of the vocal folds are heard. The amplitude of vocal fry sound is very low.

Although glottal fry is a normal mode of vibration, its consistent and habitual use is atypical and may be considered misuse of the voice. It is difficult to produce glottal fry with adequate volume for many speaking situations. A person using this mode of phonation will show increased tension when attempting to increase vocal loudness. The lack of flexibility of pulse register makes it difficult to achieve variation of fundamental frequency and results in monotonic voice. Complaint of a sense of vocal fatigue and a constant awareness of vibration even below the larynx are typically heard from speakers who habitually use glottal fry.

## LACK OF PITCH VARIABILITY

There are some individuals who speak in a monotone with barely perceptible variations in fundamental frequency, as corroborated by acoustic analysis. A monotonic voice may be a sign of neurological dysfunction affecting the ability to control pitch, a reflection of psychological depression, or it may be an habitual pattern that is a sign of misuse. We have been impressed with the presence of this problem in untrained speakers who lecture or frequently address large groups. They do not know how to modulate their pitch level for maximum communication effectiveness. In this type of pattern, the phonatory mechanism establishes a "set" that rarely varies. This set includes a certain configuration of the vocal folds, with the adductory and contact forces occurring with the same strength and in the same area over and over again. This behavior fails to take advantage of the flexibility of the phonatory mechanism and tends to become fatiguing. It is not unusual to find that persons with this pattern allow their voices to drift into vocal fry at the end of utterances. The delivery usually is perceived as lacking in energy, vitality, and interest.

## *Excessive Talking*

Each larynx has a physiological limit that varies not only from person to person but also intraindividually, as influenced by numerous factors. A healthy, well-rested, well-nourished, emotionally stable individual may encounter no vocal difficulties despite heavy voice use demands. However, should that same person be physically exhausted, eating poorly, and perhaps taking some medication, the same amount of demand on the larynx, or even less, may result in phonatory problems. Factors of individual selectivity are involved in determining the physical tolerance limits of body structures and systems. Therefore, it is not possible to predict whether excessive talking per se will result in a problem or, if a problem does result, how severe the impairment will be.

Excessive talking may result in vocal fatigue. The voice quality may be reported to become slightly rough or hoarse, the voice may sound weak, and the person may report that talking requires effort. Frequently, those who have such complaints in the presence of a chronic pattern of excessive voice use report that a night's rest or a weekend with fewer vocal demands may temporarily restore the voice to normal but that the symptoms recur with the next period of excessive voice use. It is also important not to lose sight of the fact that patterns of misuse do not always occur as single, isolated behaviors. It is, of course, quite possible that the excessive talker is also engaging in other patterns of vocal misuse or abuse. Thus, a distinction should be made between amount of talking and manner of talking (i.e., is it just a lot of talking or is it a lot of talking in an excessively loud or tense voice).

## *Ventricular Phonation*

The diagnosis of ventricular phonation is usually made when laryngological examination reveals greater than expected movement of the ventricular folds toward the midline. Visualization of the true vocal folds is often largely obscured by the compression of the ventricular folds, particularly in indirect mirror examination. Use of the flexible fiberoptic laryngoscope often permits visualization of some part of the true vocal folds or of their adductory and abductory movements. Stroboscopic examination can document whether or not there is actual ventricular fold vibration present.

Ventricular fold phonation has been described as being low in pitch, very hoarse in quality, rattling, rumbling, cracking, reduced in intensity, diplophonic (Aronson, 1990; Case, 1984). However, acoustic data to support these perceptual descriptors are not available. The pathophysiology of ventricular phonation is not well understood (see Chapter 9 for further discussion). We have observed it as a manifestation of a psychogenic dysphonia (Brewer & McCall, 1974), as a compensatory behavior in the absence of adequate vocal fold movement (Woo, Casper, Brewer, & Colton, in press) as one component in a pattern of hyperfunction, and as an unexplained phenomenon. Furthermore, in a study of normal nonsymptomatic speakers, Casper, Brewer, and Colton (1987a) observed much variability in the degree of medial movement of the ventricular folds accompanying adduction of the true vocal folds.

Therapeutically we have found ventricular phonation to be reversible when its etiology is psychological or when it is a manifestation of hyperfunction. Its use as compensatory behavior may well be very functional allowing the individual to produce the best voice of which he is capable. In such instances, it is an appropriate behavior requiring neither change nor elimination unless improved function of the vocal folds can be restored. When the etiology is unclear, or when it is a true compensatory behavior, we have found this increased ventricular fold activity to be very resistant to change through behavioral therapy.

When excess medial compression of the ventricular folds is present in the absence of laryngeal pathology, and when a voice problem seemingly related to this ventricular fold activity is present, ventricular phonation may be considered vocal misuse.

## *Aphonia and Dysphonia of Psychological Origin*

There is no single way to characterize the patterns of misuse of the phonatory mechanism exhibited by persons whose voice problems are psychogenically based. In our experience, we have encountered a wide diversity of patterns, including (*a*) total aphonia in which even the voiceless consonants were inaudible and the vocal folds were maintained in an abducted posture; (*b*) dysphonia in which the laryngeal mechanism was held in a tension equal to that of very forceful effort closure, with episodic bursts of explosive vocalization alternating with extreme hoarseness; (*c*) dysphonia in which the ventricular folds appeared to adduct; and (*d*) dysphonia so variable that it encompassed normal voicing, aphonia, hoarseness, and very strained phonation, all within two or three sentences. In all of these instances, when the physiology was normalized, so too was the voice. Therapeutic approaches to achieve normalization are discussed in Chapter 9.

## DIFFERENTIATING MISUSE FROM ABUSE

Prior to discussing vocal abuse, it is appropriate to return to some of the questions posed in the first paragraph of this chapter. We have thus far discussed the vocal behaviors that we believe constitute misuse. However, the line between misuse and abuse is a very thin one, and perhaps rather than there being a division between the two, the behaviors might be thought of as existing along a continuum. Bear in mind, however, that a continuum is only a scale. It is usually thought to represent lesser or greater degrees of a behavior (in this case), but it does not necessarily imply progression of a behavior or disorder along the continuum. Thus, a pattern of misuse such as puberphonia can remain misuse and may not necessarily develop into a problem of greater severity. We are unable to predict if or when misuse may become abuse and lead to tissue change. It is logical to assume that excessive talking, for example, might at some point result in actual tissue changes. Indeed, many patients with lesions such as nodules or polyps admit to being incessant talkers. However, we all know non-stop talkers who never develop a voice problem. Certainly there are individual selectivity factors operating about which we know little.

How patterns of misuse evolve is often difficult to determine or track down. One of the most frequently asked questions we have encountered clinically, and often a difficult one to answer, is the patient's incredulous wonderment about how it is possible, after several decades of presumably talking correctly, to no longer be doing so. We have no prospective information about this and can therefore only theorize retrospectively, using the information provided by patient recall. There are inherent dangers in doing this because most people are usually unaware of their speaking patterns until they encounter difficulty. To speak, to produce voice, is so innately human that very little conscious effort or thought is involved. Furthermore, memory is often flawed. The tendency to date the onset of a problem to a coincident event or one closely related in time is sometimes very useful, but it may also be totally misleading.

The most common antecedents to vocal misuse that seem to have validity include periods of increased personal tension or of greater than usual demands on the voice. Patients frequently report an episode of what they describe as laryngitis as the precipitating event. This laryngitis is reported to have been but one symptom of a more extensive upper respiratory infection, or it may have been an isolated symptom. Some patients recall periods of voice difficulty in the past that they ascribed to laryngitis and that had always resolved spontaneously within a short period of time. On occasion they may report that these episodes had become increasingly frequent and that each one had taken longer to resolve. Because producing voice is such a "natural" phenomenon, and because sensory feedback from the larynx is so limited, it is possible to change phonatory behavior with little awareness of having done so. In the presence of

*Table 4.2.* Abusive Behaviors

A. Excessive, prolonged loudness

B. Strained and excessive use during period of swelling, inflammation, or other tissue changes

C. Excessive coughing and throat clearing

D. The screamer and noise maker

E. Sports and exercise enthusiast

   1. Observer

   2. Participant

laryngitis, whether due to infection or to vocal fold edema resulting from misuse, adjustments in phonatory behavior need to be made in order to produce any voice. It is conceivable that these changes may go unrecognized and persist after the precipitating condition has resolved, or may contribute to maintaining the condition. One other factor that is often neglected must be considered. That is, we are not the same person from moment to moment or day to day. Our bodies are constantly changing and reacting to nutritional status, to drug intake, to effects of age, to environmental factors, to emotional state. A behavior that may have been present for many years and tolerated by the body may, due to some of the above factors, become intolerable and create what appears to be a sudden change in body function. It is also possible that the body reaches a threshold of tolerance for a certain behavior, the effects of which may have been minimal but cumulative. The changes may have been so gradual as to have gone unnoticed until the cumulative effect surpassed threshold level.

## ABUSE

Recognizing the fine distinction between misuse and abuse and the possibility of misuse becoming abuse, behaviors that we categorize as abuse tend to be harsher than those previously described, with a greater likelihood of causing trauma to the laryngeal mucosa. Table 4.2 presents vocal behaviors that we categorize as outright abuse of the mechanism.

### *Excessive, Prolonged Loudness*

In this category we would include persons who have habituated patterns of excessively loud voice use, those who spend much time talking above high levels of environmental noise, teachers who have come to depend on loudness as a means of capturing and maintaining attention and discipline, cheerleaders, aerobics instructors, some ministers, sports coaches, and untrained or poorly trained singers, speakers, or actors whose activity requires loud voice usage, often in environments not conducive to good voice production.

The mechanism for loudness requires the creation of increased resistance of the laryngeal valve until an appropriate level of air pressure is produced and released. The vocal folds must be adducted strongly to create the increased medial compression required for this valving capability. Awareness of this mechanism results in an understanding of the abusive nature of excessive or prolonged loudness. The laryngeal mucosa, especially along the glottal edge, may become irritated, inflamed, and swollen. This may result in altered mass and affect the stiffness of the cover of the vocal folds. Vibratory behavior is changed and reflected in the sound of the voice. Continued use of the voice in this abusive manner may lead to further tissue changes, resulting in organized local lesions at the point of the greatest force of contact of the vocal folds, that is, the midpoint of the vibratory portion of the vocal folds. (In more generalized pathology, a greater extent of the vocal folds may be affected.) The ability to fully adduct the vocal folds may be altered by mass lesions, and this will change the sound of the voice. Leakage of air through an incompletely closed glottis is heard as noise and adds a breathy component to the voice. As changes in phonatory function occur, there is a natural tendency on the part of the speaker to make compensatory adjustments. However, these attempts often constitute further abuse and can result in greater tissue damage.

Daniloff et al. (1980) have pointed out that untrained speakers and singers have difficulty changing vocal parameters (e.g., pitch, loudness) independently of one another.

Thus, as loudness is increased, the increased air pressure produces faster vocal fold vibration, resulting in an elevation of pitch. This may put additional strain on the mechanism.

## Strained and Excessive Use during Periods of Swelling, Inflammation, or Other Tissue Changes

In the previous section we mentioned the negative effect of continued use of excessive and prolonged loudness after such behavior had already resulted in irritation of the vocal fold mucosa. There are other times when similar caveats must be recognized. Edema of the vocal folds may result from infection, allergic reaction, or noxious environmental agents. Other conditions, such as chronic sinusitis with purulent drainage and gastroesophageal reflux, may serve to irritate and inflame the mucosa. Excessive drying of the tissues, resulting from the use of certain drugs (discussed later in this chapter), extreme dryness of heated buildings (due to inadequate humidification or the use of woodburning stoves for heating), excessive use of alcohol, or reduced function of mucus glands can also increase the vulnerability of the mucosa. The chances of creating further damage to the vocal folds are increased if abusive vocal behaviors occur in the presence of any of these conditions. Tissues that are not in their healthiest and strongest condition are unable to withstand added stress.

It is not at all unusual for a patient to report that a voice problem seemed to begin with an episode of laryngitis, but that normal voice did not return after the infection had cleared. Persons who rely heavily on voice use are often the most likely to engage in abusive behavior by continuing to use their voices during periods of laryngeal irritation. They tend to strain and exert greater than usual effort in order to produce as much voice as possible, and in so doing increase the abuse. They may also produce other tissue changes that persist after the infection has cleared.

## Excessive Coughing and Throat Clearing

It is a normal occurrence for all of us to cough and clear our throats. Coughing may be in response to a local irritation or to infection and serves a life-sustaining purpose in guarding the airway against the entry of foreign objects. The cough reflex evokes a blast of air at high pressure as a mechanism for expelling anything that has attempted to pass through the larynx. It is also the reaction to irritation of the mucosa of the vocal fold edge. The sensation of needing to clear the throat may result from momentary collection of mucus on the vocal folds that interferes with phonation. For some people, certain foods may create a reaction of increased mucus secretions (dairy foods seem to be the most common culprits) and an increased need to clear the throat. An allergic reaction of irritation and swelling of the vocal fold mucosa can also result in the need to cough or clear the throat. During upper respiratory infections or other illnesses, or as a reaction to drugs or treatment such as radiation therapy, the mucus tends to thicken and become tenacious. The sensation aroused seems to make clearing the throat necessary. Inadequate laryngeal lubrication may result from drug effects, from emotional reactions such as stage fright, from excessive smoking or drinking, or from poorly functioning mucus glands.

Chronic cough, usually dry and unproductive, can result from irritation of the mucosa secondary to reflux of stomach contents in patients with gastroesophageal reflux disease (GERD) (Deveney, Benner, & Cohen, 1993; Gaynor, 1991; Koufman, 1991;

Olson, 1991; Wilson, Pryde, Cecilia, & Macintyre, 1989). See Chapter 6 for more complete discussion of this topic.

Occasional coughing and throat clearing are not of concern. It is when these behaviors become excessive or habitual that they can be abusive. The entire larynx and supraglottal structures are involved in a cough. High-speed films of coughing behavior reveal wide glottal opening first, followed by firm and protracted glottal closure during which large lung pressures build up, and ending in a complex expulsive phase (von Leden & Isshiki, 1965). The vocal folds and supraglottal structures, including the posterior pharyngeal wall, are all involved in that final vibratory phase and show periodic undulations of a violent nature. Very vigorous laryngeal activity has also been described during throat clearing (Timcke, von Leden, & Moore, 1959). An understanding of the "violent" nature of these behaviors makes it clear that both excessive coughing and habitual throat clearing can be damaging to the sensitive laryngeal mucosa.

An inventory of abusive behaviors frequently reveals habitual throat clearing as one such behavior. It is not uncommon to find the pattern so habituated that it is almost at an involuntary level and the patient's general level of awareness of it is limited. Most patients who exhibit this behavior report sensations of something in the throat that they feel they must dislodge in order to begin to speak. A habitual, hacking cough and frequent throat clearing are recognized hallmarks of the cigarette smoker and occur in response to the mucosal irritation caused by the noxious agents and the heat of the inhaled substances. They may also be symptomatic of an allergic reaction or other laryngeal irritation.

## *The Screamer and Noise Maker*

Some young children are the prime exhibitors of these behaviors. They tend to be aggressive youngsters who talk a lot, habitually using loud voice in most situations and engaging in much yelling and screaming in interactions with family and friends, be it in anger or in play (Barker & Wilson, 1967; Toohill, 1975; Wilson & Lamb, 1973). Parents frequently report that a child has been a "screamer" since infancy, being perhaps the only one in the family to be so categorized. On other occasions the report implicates other family members who also tend to be "loud" in their vocal behavior. Because of factors of individual selectivity coupled with amount and degree of excessive screaming, a child may begin to exhibit a voice problem. Vocal nodules are often referred to as "screamer's nodes" due to their frequent occurrence in association with excessive screaming and yelling behavior.

Another manifestation of abuse of the voice most frequently noted in young children is that of using the voice to make a variety of sound effects. Not all such behavior need be abusive; however, many of the sounds typically produced by these children tend to involve strained vocalizations. Some children take special delight in producing the most unusual sounds they can devise. Others tend to supply all of the sound effects during play, not only for themselves but also for their friends.

There are many more boys implicated in screaming and noise making than girls. The incidence of vocal nodules is similarly greater for boys than girls (Moore, 1986; Senturia & Wilson, 1968). Aronson (1990) assigns the "abnormal speaking behavior" of these youngsters to personality or emotional factors. Barker and Wilson (1967) studied the amount and type of voice use in the classroom of children with hoarse voices and compared them to a group of children with normal voices. They noted that those with hoarseness produced almost three times as many vocalizations within a

2-hour period than did those with normal voices. These dysphonic children were also observed to be more behaviorally active during unstructured classroom time than the control group of children. A further finding of interest was that 65% of the hoarse children came from families in which there was much intrafamily conflict, while only 35% of the nondysphonic children had such a family background.

## Sports and Exercise Enthusiast

### OBSERVER

Prime demonstrations of vocal abuse may be seen at many sporting or political events. The roar of the crowd is made up of many individual roars. In concert with the crowd noise, it becomes difficult to monitor the loudness of an individual voice. In the heat of the moment, and in keeping with socially accepted behavior, the louder the scream or yell, the better. These loud yells are usually produced with great tension and with elevated pitch, which adds to the degree of tension under which the laryngeal mechanism is held. This behavior and its results are so commonly known that lay people talk about screaming till the voice is gone. Indeed, even Shakespeare commented on this phenomenon in *Henry IV* with the exclamation, "For my voice, I have lost it with halloing and singing of anthems."

The delicate vocal fold mucosa becomes edematous and irritated in response to this abuse, thereby increasing the mass of the folds and interfering with their vibratory behavior. The severity of the vocal symptoms will be related to the extent of this irritation and the tissue reaction to it. However, return to normal or slightly reduced vocal use plus a good night's rest will usually suffice to restore the vocal folds to their normal condition. But should the person continue to use the voice abusively, or place greater demands on it than the weakened mucosa can withstand, further deterioration of both the condition of the mucosa and the dysphonia may occur.

### PARTICIPANT

A number of sports or fitness exercises by their very nature may set the stage for vocal abuse. Whenever it becomes necessary to build intrathoracic pressure, the laryngeal valve is involved, and effort closure of the glottis often results. Producing voice under this condition is very stressful. When lifting weights, for example, it is necessary for the person to build and maintain lung pressure as a ballast against which the weight may be lifted. This is a reflexive behavior when attempting to lift any heavy weight. Weightlifters often produce grunting sounds during the actual lift. It is not difficult to recognize the abusive nature of phonation produced with the larynx and vocal folds in tight adduction and with increased subglottal pressure present. Similar effort closure of the glottis occurs accompanying a tennis serve or a golf drive.

In other types of sports, it is often necessary for team members to yell to one another above the noise of the spectators. Aerobics instructors who not only participate in the routine but also verbally cue the class above the sound level of the music are a new group of voice abusers to encounter problems. Persons who use motorized sports equipment such as snowmobiles and talk above the noise of the engines may also find themselves having repeated episodes of dysphonia.

When dealing with vocal misuse or vocal abuse, it is essential to pursue an exhaustive history of voice use. Patients do not readily identify behaviors other than the obvious ones, such as screaming, excessive talking, and loud singing. It is necessary for the clinician to explore the full range of potentially abusive vocal behaviors. Although we have attempted to highlight many such behaviors, our listing is probably not all inclusive. Each voice clinician will be able to add to it from personal experience.

## DAMAGING EFFECTS OF DRUGS ON THE VOICE

This section of the chapter will deal with the known and potential effects of drugs on the voice. Although the taking of drugs does not come under the category of a vocal behavior, the effects of drugs can be potentially damaging to the mucosa and disruptive to phonation. For these reasons, we have chosen to place this material in this chapter.

Research on the effects of various drugs on the laryngeal mucosa and laryngeal physiology is almost nonexistent. Therefore, in discussing the effects of drugs on voice, we are talking about expected effects based on an understanding of drug action and laryngeal anatomy and physiology. The following summary is based on the work of pharmacologist F. Gene Martin (1983, 1984, 1988), who presents five basic pharmacological principles to keep in mind when discussing the general effects of drugs:

1. Biological response variability: There is wide biological variability in individual response to drugs, based on a large variety of factors including age, body composition, kidney function, genetic inheritance, biochemistry, stress level, disease, drug/drug interaction, and nutritional status. Responses may differ both quantitatively and qualitatively.

2. The placebo effect: The expectation of an effect may influence the type and degree of effect obtained. This is a poorly understood but generally accepted phenomenon.

3. Dose-response relationship: The intensity of the effect of a drug is usually expected to be proportional to the dose administered or taken; that is, the larger the dose, the greater the effect, proportionally. However, the dose-response relationships of most drugs form sigmoid-shaped curves rather than straight lines when their effects are plotted against dosage. Such curves indicate that the intensity of a drug increases gradually at first, then rapidly, and then gradually again, eventually reaching a ceiling or plateau level as the dose is increased incrementally (stepwise). Increasing the dose after the ceiling effect has been obtained produces no further enhancement of effect and may only produce undesirable toxic side effects. Allergic reactions to drugs may appear with any dose, no matter how small, and the intensity of allergic effects is not related to the magnitude of the dose.

4. Multiple effects of a single drug: Drugs may have a multiplicity of effects. Those that are not the specifically intended effect are usually referred to as side effects. These are the effects that most frequently have ramifications for voice production.

5. Drug efficacy versus drug dosage: The efficacy of a drug is of more concern than its potency. Thus, if drug A produces a desired level of response at a lower dose than drug B does, it does not necessarily mean that drug A is better than B. Drug A may, in fact, be worse, if even at its lower dose it produces more undesirable side effects than drug B. It matters little to the patient whether the pill swallowed contains 5 mg or 200 mg of a drug. What matters is the production of an adequate therapeutic effect and the absence of unacceptable side effects with a given reasonable dose.

To those basic principles an additional caution should be included concerning the geriatric population. Elderly people may respond differently, quantitatively or qualitatively, than younger persons do to the same dose of the same drug. This difference in response is due to the loss, reduction, or alteration of certain body structures and functions with aging, as, for example, a reduced ability to metabolize or absorb certain drugs. Furthermore, many drugs are combinations of several agents, each of which may have an effect on the voice. It is important for the consumer to be aware of these combinations and their possible effects.

The voice-related effects of drugs may be classified in the following seven categories: (*a*) coordination and proprioception, (*b*) airflow, (*c*) fluid balance, (*d*) secretions of the upper respiratory tract, (*e*) structure of the vocal folds, (*f*) irritation of vocal fold mucosa, and (*i*) miscellaneous. The various classes of drugs and their effects are shown in Table 4.3.

## *Coordination and Proprioception*

Any agent that is stimulating or depressing to the central nervous system has the potential to affect coordination, including the fine motor control of phonatory behavior. Central nervous system stimulants include amphetamines, dextroamphetamine sulfate (Dexedrine), cocaine, caffeine, and phenylpropanolamine (PPA), the active agent in over-the-counter diet aids. Stimulants are used primarily as recreational drugs and appetite depressants. Their adverse effects may include nervousness and tremor and difficulty in performing acts requiring well-controlled coordination. For example, the shaky or tremorous voice of a person who is highly agitated results from a breakdown of the ability to control fine aspects of voice production.

Central nervous system depressants include alcohol, barbiturates, tranquilizers such as diazepam (Valium) and chlordiazepoxide hydrochloride (Librium), and chloral hydrate. They are used primarily as antianxiety agents and produce a sedating effect that in high enough doses may have a negative influence on muscle coordination. For example, slurred and slowed speech are well-recognized hallmarks of the person who has had too much to drink.

Diazepam (Valium) is often prescribed for patients with a variety of voice disorders. However, administration of diazepam is usually unproductive of any beneficial change in voice production or in the alleviation of voice symptoms. In a study of the effect of diazepam on respiratory and laryngeal muscle activation, Ludlow, Schulz, and Naunton (1988) report strong interindividual respiratory and phonatory effects, which may be age related. Laryngeal activation decreased in their older subjects, while it increased in their younger subjects. The authors caution that use of diazepam as a treatment for spastic dysphonia or other movement disorders affecting the voice may, in some individuals, result in a worsening of symptoms. Furthermore, they call attention to the not uncommon administration of diazepam or other such medications to subjects in studies of laryngeal muscle activity during speech, suggesting that this practice may significantly alter the results of such studies.

Another group of drugs that affect the central nervous system are those that produce an anesthetic effect. Local anesthetics such as benzocaine (Americaine), lidocaine (Xylocaine), procaine hydrochloride (Novocain), or phenol may be the primary ingredients in over-the-counter lozenges and sprays used to treat a sore throat. These agents are capable of blocking nerve impulse conduction and reducing pain sensation. Pain serves as an alarm system, indicating the presence of a problem somewhere in the body. The usual response to throat or laryngeal pain is to reduce voice usage. Reduction of pain by the use of these analgesic agents masks the presence of the problem, and the individual may then be prone to overstressing voice use. Leonard and Ringel (1979) reported some changes in laryngeal behavior following the dripping of a local anesthetic onto the vocal folds.

Table 4.3. Drug Classes and Their Laryngeal Effects

| Drug Type | Coordination and Proprioception | Airflow | Fluid Balance | Secretions of the Upper Tract | Structure of the Vocal Folds | Irritation of the Vocal Fold Mucosa |
|---|---|---|---|---|---|---|
| CNS Stimulants | X | | | | | |
| CNS Depressants | X | | | | | |
| Anesthetics | X | | | | | |
| Bronchial Dilators and Constrictors | | X | | | | |
| Diuretics and Decongestants | | | X | | | |
| Corticosteroids | | | X | | | |
| Drying agents | | | | X | | |
| Wetting agents | | | | X | | |
| Androgens | | | | | X | |
| Lower esophageal sphincter effects | | | | | | X |

## Airflow

Drugs that either dilate or constrict the bronchioles will affect the movement of pulmonary air through the larynx. Bronchodilators, such as albuterol (Proventil, Ventolin), metaproterenol sulfate (Alupent), and others are used primarily as antiasthma agents. Negative side effects may be nervousness and tremor. Bronchoconstrictors potentially have a more adverse effect on voice production. The mechanism most often used to cause bronchoconstriction pharmacologically is an allergic reaction. The effects may vary from very mild discomfort and wheezing to a significant, even lifethreatening effect on respiratory function. Many environmental irritants, such as dust, pollen, and molds, produce similar effects in individuals with sensitivity to these environmental factors.

## Fluid Balance

Fluid balance in the mucosa of the vocal folds may have a very significant and direct effect on voice production. There are many drugs that, either as a consequence of their primary intended effect or as their side effect, work in such a way as to reduce edema. Diuretics, which reduce the formation of edema, are commonly used in the treatment of high blood pressure and heart or kidney failure. Perhaps the most widely used group of agents with the effect of reducing edema are the decongestants, many of which are sold as over-the-counter preparations in tablet, capsule, or liquid form or as topical sprays (e.g., oxymetazoline hydrochloride [Afrin], pseudoephedrine hydrochloride [Sudafed, etc.]). These are used in the treatment of the symptoms of cold, cough, allergy, or sinus problems.

Vocal fold edema, under most circumstances, is the result of protein-bound water (Lawrence, 1987; Sataloff, 1987a) and will not be responsive to diuretic agents. Corticosteroids, often used as drying agents in the treatment of vocal fold edema in performers following vocally abusive episodes, affect protein-bound water directly. Although they are often effective, they offer only a palliative, not a curative, effect. A patient may be using a diuretic agent for a number of reasons not directly related to vocal fold edema. In such instances, the danger of reducing the normally desirable fluid level in the laryngeal mucosa must be kept in mind. Long-term use of decongestants may cause a rebound effect wherein, as the vasoconstrictive effects of the drug wear off, there is a return of the edema and congestion to a greater degree than was previously present. As a result, a vicious cycle may be established in which the patient must continue to take the decongestant in an attempt to counteract the side effect that is being caused by the drug itself. The long-term effects of vasoconstriction and the adverse effects from the loss of adequate fluid balance include a reduction in blood flow to the mucosa; loss of electrolytes with concomitant decrease of potassium level, leading to a decrease in energy and a sedating effect; increased nervousness and tremor; and potential damage to the mucous membranes. Edema formation in reaction to drugs occurs primarily in the form of an allergic response. Agents that cause an allergic reaction in a patient may have more than a single effect. While bronchoconstriction may be one effect, edema of the mucosa may occur simultaneously. Edema of the laryngeal mucosa may also occur in response to vocal abuse, trauma, infection, and environmental allergens.

Corticosteroid inhalants are used in the treatment of asthma. Their effect on voice is not entirely clear. Williams, Baghat, DeStableforth, Shenoi, and Skinner (1983) reported dysphonia and bilateral vocal fold bowing in patients using an inhaled corticosteroid. The vocal fold bowing appeared to be related to the dose and potency of the drug used and was believed to represent a local steroid myopathy. The bowing and concomitant dysphonia were reversed in all patients after cessation of use of the steroid inhalant. Watkin and Ewanowski (1979) reported that prolonged administration of aerosol-delivered triamcinolone acetonide (Kenalog), a drug used by chronic asthmatics, results in significantly altered vocal tract functioning and an elevation of fundamental frequency of approximately 20 Hz. They reported that changes were evident after 1 year of use, with a cumulative effect described after 2 years.

## Secretions of the Upper Respiratory Tract

According to Martin (1983, 1984, 1988), exposure to agents that affect upper respiratory tract secretions occurs with great frequency. Many drugs act as drying agents by causing a reduction in secretions of the salivary and mucus glands. Furthermore, Martin states, a major portion of our lives "is spent in buildings with very low humidity, and we are continuously breathing air with moisture levels similar to that of the Sahara" (Martin, 1988; McClean, 1987; Stoicheff, Giampi, Passi, & Fredrickson, 1983). A vicious cycle ensues in which breathing dry air results in dryness and irritation of the mucosa, which leads to coughing, which serves to further irritate and dry the mucosa.

Among the drugs creating a drying effect, the most common are the antihistamines used in the treatment of allergy, cold, cough, sinus, motion sickness, and insomnia. Drugs functioning as antispasmodic agents ( e.g., atropine, scopolamine, diphenoxylate hydrochloride [Lomotil], etc.) used in the treatment of diarrhea also create a reduction in glandular secretions. The action of antitussive drugs such as codeine and dextromethorphan hydrobromide (Benylin DM), used in cough remedies, is drying, and a side effect is sedation. Antipsychotic agents such as chlorpromazine hydrochloride (Thorazine) and haloperidol (Haldol) and antidepressant agents such as amitriptyline (Elavil) and lithium carbonate (Lithane, Lithobid) cause drying and sedation. The last group of drying agents is the antihypertensive drugs used in the treatment of high blood pressure, such as methyldopa (Aldomet), reserpine (Sandril, Serpasil), and captopril (Capoten).

The most effective wetting agent is water, abundantly available and easily consumed. Ambient humidity may be voluntarily controlled, as may the amount of water consumed. Expectorants, used in the treatment of cough, are agents that increase secretions. However, many of these products contain other drugs that have the opposite effect. Guaifenesin (Robitussin, Glycotuss) is the most commonly used expectorant drug and can be obtained as the only drug in a product. Saliva substitutes (e.g., dibasic sodium phosphate [Moi-stir], sodium carboxymethylcellulose [Salivart], etc.) have recently become available and appear to be very helpful as wetting agents. They are used primarily by persons who have salivary gland pathology but can be effectively used to combat the dry mouth caused by the use of drying agents and also by preperformance anxiety. Thompson (1995) has suggested that the efficacy of wetting agents has not been proved and perhaps the most beneficial effect may be the increased water intake required while taking this medication.

## Changes in Structure of the Vocal Folds

The androgens, which are structurally related to the male hormone testosterone, change the actual structure of the vocal folds. They are used in the treatment of hormonal imbalance (frequently in postmenopausal women) and by body builders seeking to increase muscle mass. Androgens cause an increase in the mass of the vocal folds, which, of course, results in a change in the voice, referred to as the virilization of the voice. Once this change has occurred, it is irreversible (Damste, 1967). A synthetic androgen, danazol androgen (Danocrine), is commonly used in the treatment of benign fibrocystic breast disease, although a side effect of voice change occurs in about 10% of the patients treated. It is not yet clear whether these voice changes are reversible (Martin, 1988). These agents can be used effectively to lower fundamental frequency of the voice in individuals who have undertaken sexual reassignment from female to male.

## Irritation of Vocal Fold Mucosa

Laryngeal tissue (as well as esophageal and pharyngeal) is susceptible to irritation and damage caused by the acidic contents of gastric juices that reflux into the hypopharynx in gastroesophageal reflux disease (GERD). Lower esophageal sphincter (LES) pressure has been reported to be decreased by the following drugs: atropine, dopamine, smoking, calcium blockers, sedatives/tranquilizers, nitrates, theophylline and adrenergic (Gaynor, 1991). Because decrease in the tightness of the LES is implicated in the pathophysiology of GERD it is logical to assume that use of any of these drugs may predispose an individual to GERD. Caffeine, fat, alcohol, and highly spiced foods are also believed to reduce LES pressures. (See Chapter 6 for more information on GERD.)

## Miscellaneous

Martin (1983, 1984, 1988) notes additional agents that are thought by some to have an effect on voice production and on performance, although they do not specifically fit any of the previous categories. These include ototoxic drugs, herbal teas, aspirin, beta blockers, and tobacco and other smoked or inhaled drugs.

### HEARING

A number of drug groups are known to be potentially ototoxic. Some of these are aminoglycoside antibiotics, such as amikacin sulfate (Amikin) and tobramycin sulfate (Nebcin), which are used intravenously in life-threatening disease states. Certain diuretics, referred to as "loop" or "high ceiling" diuretics, such as furosemide (Lasix) or bumetanide (Bumex), used in the treatment of heart failure and high blood pressure, also have the potential to create hearing loss. Some drugs used in chemotherapy for cancer are also suspected to have ototoxic side effects, and their use should be monitored closely. Obviously the loss of hearing will not have a direct effect on laryngeal anatomy, and perhaps not an immediate effect on laryngeal physiology. Indirectly, however, loss of hearing may affect vocal production, and it is likely that vocal physiology may be altered over time. When vocal loudness considerations are a component of a voice disorder, auditory acuity must be taken into account.

### HERBAL TEAS

Certain varieties of herbal mixtures are anecdotally reported to have a soothing effect on the respiratory tract mucosa. They have not been shown to have any medicinal value. In general, it is well to exercise care in the use of any herbal mixtures and to know exactly what they contain.

## ASPIRIN

Aspirin has anticoagulant properties that are not usually of consequence to the average voice user unless that individual has a bleeding disorder or is taking other anticoagulant medication. Because the professional voice user is called upon to use the voice strenuously, the risk of vocal fold hemorrhage may be somewhat increased, and particularly so if that person is taking aspirin or any preparations containing acetylsalicylic acid.

## BETA BLOCKERS

During times of stress and fear, the adrenal glands release the chemicals epinephrine and norepinephrine. It is the increased level of these chemicals that results in rapid heartbeat, tremor, elevated blood pressure, sweaty palms, dry mouth, respiratory tension, nausea, and an urge to urinate. These are also the well-known symptoms of the phenomenon known as stage fright. Beta blockers, of which propranolol (Inderal) is the most common, act to block the effect of epinephrine on glands, smooth muscles, and the heart, thereby reducing the symptoms described above. Whether or not the reduction of symptoms produces enhanced performance has not been determined. Instrument musicians have been reported to demonstrate improved performance and a lessening of subjective stage fright symptoms with the use of beta blockers (Brantigan, Brantigan, & Joseph, 1982; James, Pearson, Griffith, & Newburg, 1977; Liden & Gottfries, 1974). Evidence of their effectiveness in singers is less conclusive. Gates and Montalbo (1987)suggest that low-dose (20 mg) beta blockade had no significant effect on singers' performance. In an earlier study, Gates, Saegert, Wilson, Johnson, Shepard, and Hearne (1985) reported a deleterious effect on singing quality with the administration of beta blocker in high doses (40–80 mg). There does not appear to be strong evidence that beta blockers significantly enhance performance. Indeed, it has been suggested by some that heightened preperformance anxiety serves a useful purpose in that it lends a degree of intensity and excitement to the performance that might be lost if beta blockers were used. Data to support this contention or its corollary are not yet available.

## TOBACCO AND OTHER SMOKED OR INHALED DRUGS

We should not leave this section on the effect of drugs on the voice without some direct mention of tobacco, marijuana, and other drugs that are smoked or inhaled. There is very convincing evidence (Burch, 1981; Hammond, 1966; Kahn, 1966; Wynder, Covey, Mabuchi, & Muchinski, 1976; Wynder & Stellman, 1977) that smoking cigarettes is closely related to laryngeal cancer. The vast majority of individuals who present with laryngeal carcinoma have a history of heavy smoking. Precancerous conditions such as leukoplakia and hyperkeratosis are also closely linked to smoking. Some smokers present with very boggy, polypoid vocal folds (Reinke's edema), a condition that is benign but usually results in significant dysphonia and can be severe enough to compromise the airway. Redness and generalized irritation of the mucosa of the upper respiratory tract and the larynx are often present in persons who use tobacco, marijuana, and other inhaled substances. The harmful effects of inhaling environmental smoke has been documented (U.S. Department of Health and Human Services, 1986). Lung cancer and emphysema are also known to be directly related to smoking. When the respiratory system is compromised, there is a direct effect on voice production. Thus, even in the absence of actual laryngeal pathology, the effects of smoking on lung function are sufficient to produce a broad effect on phonation.

## VOCAL PATHOLOGIES SECONDARY TO VOCAL ABUSE AND MISUSE

### *Nodules*

#### PRIMARY VOICE SYMPTOM: HOARSENESS

#### DESCRIPTION AND ETIOLOGY

Nodules are localized benign growths on the vocal folds that are usually thought to be the result of vocal abuse. They are a reaction of the tissue to the constant stress induced by frequent, hard oppositional movement of the vocal folds. In the initial stages of the formation of a nodule, the trauma causes localized edema on the vocal fold edge. Early or acute nodules are fairly soft and pliable; they may be reddish in appearance and are mostly vascular and edematous. The remainder of the vocal fold may also be edematous, and the entire larynx may be slightly inflamed. In this early stage, the nodule may be evident only on one side and may easily be mistaken for a polyp. With continued trauma, the tissue undergoes hyalinization and fibrosis and becomes firm. Chronic nodules are usually hard, white, thick, and fibrosed. Arnold (1962, 1980) reported that at this chronic stage of nodule development, the epithelium may show hypertrophy, horny or very rough surfaces, and a change in the type of cells present. Chronic nodules are usually bilateral and not always symmetrical in size. Figure 4.1 is an illustration of a pair of vocal nodules.

There is some controversy about the distinction between nodules and polyps. A polyp is a projecting mass with a central core of fibrous tissue of greater density than the lamina propria and covered by a normal or slightly hyperplastic epithelium. Clinically, there are times when the distinction is very clear and other times when the difference is minimal. Histologically, the situation is not much clearer. Fitz-Hugh, Smith, and Chiong (1958) reviewed the histological findings of 300 consecutive cases of benign tumors of the vocal folds. They commented on the difficulty of distinguishing among

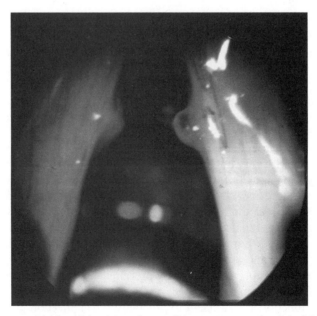

*Figure 4.1.* Vocal fold nodules. Note the small hematoma on the right fold. See color plate.

nodules, polyps, and polypoid degeneration. Many nodules were classified as polyps and vice versa, on review. They eventually concluded that a nodule was a trauma-related lesion consisting of a local nodular or polypoid degeneration of the lamina propria. They state that a polyp has its origin in the subepithelial (or Reinke's) space.

Luchsinger and Arnold (1965) consider general physical constitution, personality, and local laryngeal signs to be important predisposing conditions for nodules (or polyps). Allergies or thyroid imbalances may contribute to precipitating factors; tobacco and alcohol use may be aggravating factors. In adults, nodules occur most frequently in women between the ages of 20 and 50 years.

Nodules may be found in children who are prone to excessive loud talking or screaming. They usually occur in children who have a history of loud, constant voice usage in conversation, in school, at home, and at play. In this age group, they occur most frequently in boys.

### PERCEPTUAL SIGNS AND SYMPTOMS

Hoarseness and breathiness are the major perceptual signs of nodules. Some individuals complain of soreness or pain in the neck lateral to the larynx that may radiate upward to the ear or downward to the upper chest. Some have the sensation of something in the "throat" that they need to try to clear. Difficulty in producing pitches in the upper third of the range is a complaint especially true for singers. The degree of hoarseness or breathiness present may be related to the size and firmness of the nodules and may vary from slight to moderately severe.

### ACOUSTIC SIGNS

Acoustically, a patient with nodules will exhibit increased frequency and amplitude perturbation (jitter and shimmer) with a fundamental frequency within the normal range. Davis (1981) reported pitch perturbation quotient (PPQ) values of 2.61% and 1.87% for two patients with nodules, compared to a PPQ of 0.42% for normal speakers. Others have reported similar greater than normal frequency perturbation measurements in the presence of nodules. Takahashi and Koike (1975) reported a mean relative average perturbation (RAP, see section in Chapter 2 on frequency perturbation) of 0.0084, whereas Ludlow, Coulter, and Gentges (1983) reported a mean jitter of 9.26 microseconds, compared to a normal value of 5 microseconds. Davis also reported an amplitude perturbation quotient (APQ) of 9.07% and 15.33% for the nodule cases, compared to a normal APQ of 6.14%.

Phonational range may be markedly reduced, especially at the upper end. The patient may also show reduced dynamic range, with an inability to produce high sound pressure levels. Eckel and Boone (1981) reported an average s/z ratio of 1.65 for their group of 28 patients with nodules and polyps. Normal subjects produced an s/z ratio of 0.99.

Spectrum analysis of a patient's phonation will show evidence of noise in the spectrum (Arnold & Emanuel, 1979; Yanagihara, 1967b), the degree of which depends on the severity of hoarseness and lesion size. Interestingly, nodules seem to produce little effect on fundamental frequency of phonation (Murry, 1978).

### MEASURABLE PHYSIOLOGICAL SIGNS

Airflows in a patient with nodules may be equal to or slightly higher than normal (Iwata, Esaki, Iwami, & Mimura, 1976; Iwata, von Leden, & Williams, 1972). Tanaka and Gould (1985) reported a mean value of 275 ml/sec for their two patients with nodules. Normal male subjects produce flows of about 125 ml/sec. Woo, Colton, and Shangold (1987) reported a mean flow rate of 265 ml/sec for their combined polyp and nodule group, collapsed across 14 male and 18 female subjects. In their study, normal speakers produced a mean flow rate of 144 ml/sec. The magnitude of the increase of airflow rates appears to depend on the severity of the lesion (Shigemori, 1977). Lung pressures may also be high because of the tendency for an individual to increase the driving force to overcome incomplete glottal closure (Tanaka & Gould, 1985). However, in our sample of 36 females with nodules, we found some elevation of pressure (6.45 cmH2O) versus normal (Colton & Casper, unpublished data). It has also been our experience that patients with nodules may show marked offset flow, but normal and slightly increased peak flow measures. Electroglottograms will show decreased closing times of the vocal folds and an irregular pattern. Normal electromyogram levels would be expected, although it is possible for these to be elevated if the patient shows excessive laryngeal tension.

## OBSERVABLE PHYSIOLOGICAL SIGNS

### Laryngoscopy

Nodules have typically been described as benign lesions located at the junction of the anterior third and posterior two thirds of the vocal folds. It is there that the forces encountered during vibration are the largest (Luchsinger & Arnold, 1965). It must be remembered that the posterior one third of the vocal fold (i.e., the vocal process), is composed of stiff cartilage that does not vibrate. The remaining two-thirds of the vocal folds vibrate, and it is at the midpoint of this vibrating portion that the contact forces will be the greatest. However, in a recent study of 24 patients with vocal nodules, Casper, Colton, Brewer, Kelley, Woo, and Griffin (1995) reported that one third of those patients were found to have nodules located at mid-cord. Laryngoscopically, there may be evidence of incomplete closure of the vocal folds, especially in the area surrounding the nodules or a large posterior chink. Some edema of the folds is not uncommon, and there is increased vascularity.

### Stroboscopy

According to Kitzing (1985), the vocal folds will show normal symmetry and periodicity but reduced amplitudes and mucosal waves at the nodule site and reduced glottal closure. In view of the greater frequency perturbation found in patients with vocal nodules (as reported in "Acoustic Signs," above), Kitzing's finding of normal periodicity is questionable. It is possible that a small nodule may have a minimal effect on the vibratory frequency of the vocal folds. Hirano and Bless (1993) report absence of the mucosal wave in the nodule area when the mass is firm, but find it present and unchanged when the nodule is edematous. In our study of stroboscopic signs in a group of 30 female patients with nodules (Colton, Woo, Brewer, Griffin, & Casper, 1995), the amplitude of the vocal fold movement was slightly reduced. Glottal closure had traditionally been described as having an hourglass appearance. Using frame-by-frame analysis procedures in which even a single frame of vocal fold closure result in a "complete closure" rating (Casper et al., 1995), slightly more than 50% of patients (13 of 24) exhibited an hourglass closure pattern. Only 2 of 24 showed a posterior chink pattern. When viewed as a gestalt (rather than frame-by-frame) the "appearance" of both hourglass closure and posterior chink ratings would be more predominant. Furthermore, half of the nodules were described as being pinpoint in shape with the other 50% described as broad based.

## PATHOPHYSIOLOGY

A nodule will increase the mass of the cover of the vocal fold. The stiffness of the cover will be increased by a hard and firm nodule and decreased or unchanged by a soft and pliable one (Hirano, 1981a; Hirano & Bless, 1993). It has been theorized that the mechanical properties of the transition layers and the muscle will not be affected by the nodule. However, Gray's recent work on the Basement Membrane Zone (Gray, 1991; Gray, Hirano, & Sato, 1993; Gray, Pignatari, & Harding, 1994) suggests that area as the possible site of some damage. Because the mechanical properties of the cover are very important in determining the vibratory characteristics of the vocal folds, a nodule may have a pronounced effect on the mechanics of vibration. The extra mass along the medial edge of the vibrating vocal folds results in increased aperiodicity of vibration, greater frequency perturbation, and greater hoarseness. Depending on the size of the nodule, glottal closure will also be affected. Incomplete closure (such as occurs in the hourglass configuration) will permit increased air escape, resulting in the perception of breathiness.

## Polyps

### PRIMARY VOICE SYMPTOM: HOARSENESS

### DESCRIPTION AND ETIOLOGY

There are a number of forms a polyp may take, and the subsequent effects and treatment may also vary. If the polyp is localized, it may show up as pedunculated (attached only by a slim stalk) or sessile (closely adhering to mucosa). Another variant is that of hemorrhagic polyp, which has the appearance of a blood blister. If the lesion is diffuse, it may cover one-half to two-thirds of the entire length of the vocal fold and is usually referred to as polypoid degeneration or Reinke's edema. The distinction between polyp and polypoid degeneration is sometimes confusing. According to Lowenthal (1958), they are very similar in that they are localized or diffuse inflammatory tumors involving the space of Reinke. Histologically, both types are very similar.

Polyps are thought to result from a period of vocal abuse, although they can occur as the result of a single traumatic incident, as for example, yelling at a basketball game. Luchsinger and Arnold (1965) consider that polyps and nodules have the same etiology and differ only in degree. According to Jackson (1941), a polyp is larger and more vascular, edematous, and inflammatory than a nodule, which is described as an organized mass of tissue (Fig. 4.2).

*Figure 4.2.* A single vocal fold polyp. See color plate.

Polyps are usually unilateral, although sometimes a small polyp can be found on the contralateral side. Although polyps usually occur on the free margin of the vocal folds, they may also be found on the superior surface of the folds as well as subglottally. In the latter case, there may be little or no alteration in the voice. They may also involve almost the entire length of the vocal fold (Fig. 4.3).

It is easy to see how acute nodules can be mistaken for polyps. Polyps usually occur in Reinke's space (the superficial layer of the lamina propria) and may consist of dilated blood vessels, fibrotic tissue, and small hemorrhages.

### PERCEPTUAL SIGNS AND SYMPTOMS

Typical perceptual signs of a polyp include hoarseness, roughness, or breathiness. In addition, the patient may report the sensation of something in the throat.

### ACOUSTIC SIGNS

The acoustic features created by a polyp are very similar to those of a nodule. Increased jitter and shimmer would be expected depending on the location of the polyp. Davis (1981) reported a PPQ of 0.60% and an APQ of 11.68% for his one patient with a polyp. Normal PPQ is 0.42% and APQ is 6.14%. Reduced phonational and dynamic ranges, as well as increased spectral noise, would also be anticipated acoustic characteristics. Unfortunately, data to support these expectations about the magnitude of phonational ranges and spectral noise in patients with polyps are not available.

### MEASURABLE PHYSIOLOGICAL SIGNS

Increased airflow may be present if the polyp interferes with complete glottal closure. In one report, 18 patients with polyps had an average airflow rate of 162 ml/sec (Iwata, von Leden, & Williams, 1972), whereas in another report (Iwata, Esaki, Iwami, & Mimura, 1976) an average airflow rate of 253 ml/sec was reported for 29 male patients and 247 ml/sec for 19 female patients with unilateral polyps. Patients with bilateral polyps had airflow rates of 256 ml/sec (8 males) and 359 ml/sec (8 females). For their 7 patients with polyps, Tanaka and Gould (1985) reported a mean flow rate of 223.71 ml/sec. Woo et al. (1987) reported a mean flow rate of 265 ml/sec for their combined

*Figure 4.3.* Large sessile polyp, involving the entire length of the vocal fold. See color plate.

polyp and nodule group, collapsed across 14 male and 18 female subjects. In their study, normal speakers produced a mean flow rate of 144 ml/sec. Subglottal or lung pressure also appears to show an increase due to attempts to produce phonation in the presence of a leaky glottis (Tanaka & Gould, 1985). We have observed that patients with polyps tend to have greater than normal vibratory flows. Electroglottograms tend to show decreased closing times of the vocal folds and irregular patterns. Muscle action potentials would be expected to be normal, unless the patient showed excessive laryngeal tension.

## OBSERVABLE PHYSIOLOGICAL SIGNS

### Laryngoscopy

Polyps often can be visualized with standard laryngoscopy. They appear as rather large masses on one vocal fold, sometimes with a very broad base, sometimes attached to a stalk. Most times they appear somewhat translucent, although on occasion they may be filled with blood and therefore appear reddish in appearance.

### Stroboscopy

Stroboscopically, asymmetry of motion of the vocal folds and increased aperiodicity are noted. Polyps tend to show distinct phase differences between the two folds, especially if the lesions are grossly different in size or if the lesion is unilateral. The amplitude of the vocal folds is reduced, but the effect of the polyp on mucosal waves, especially in the vicinity of the polyp, may vary from being decreased or absent (as in the case of a hemorrhagic polyp), to being increased (as in large sessile polyps) to being normal (as in a pedunculated polyp). Glottal closure may also be affected (Hirano, Feder, & Bless, 1983; Kitzing, 1985). In our study of 24 patients with polyps (Colton, Woo, Brewer, Griffin, & Casper, 1995), the most common closure pattern was irregular. Aperiodicity of vocal fold movement may be increased although in our study (Colton et al., 1995) the most frequent periodicity category rating was regular. In some instances, the polyp lags in movement behind the vocal fold proper and thus appears as a "coupled" movement. Also in our study, the amplitude of vocal fold movement was moderately decreased, especially for the affected fold. Vibration of the affected vocal fold was also altered by presence of the lesion (Colton, Woo, Brewer, Griffin, & Casper, 1995); i.e., there was little or no mucosal wave, especially over the site of the lesion.

## PATHOPHYSIOLOGY

A polyp will increase the mass of the cover of the vocal folds. If the polyp is soft, edematous, and pliable, the stiffness of the cover will be decreased (Hirano, 1981a). However, if bleeding, hyaline degeneration, or other histological changes are present, stiffness of the cover may be increased (see Chapter 3). The mechanical properties of the transition layers and the muscle will not be affected. As described in the case of nodules, the mechanical properties of the cover will determine the vibratory characteristics of the vocal folds. The extra mass at the midpoint of the vibrating vocal folds results in increased aperiodicity of vibration, greater frequency perturbation, and greater hoarseness. However, if the polyp is pedunculated, there will probably be little effect on vibration because the mass of the polyp does not affect the cover directly. Depending on the size of the polyp, glottal closure may be affected. If excessive air can escape through the closed glottis, breathiness will be perceived.

## *Intracordal Cysts*

### PRIMARY VOICE SYMPTOM: HOARSENESS

### DESCRIPTION AND ETIOLOGY

Intracordal cysts appear as small spheres on the margins of the vocal folds (Fig. 4.4) and sometimes on the superior surface. They may be mistaken for early nodules because small nodule-like growths may appear on one cord but not the other. Cysts are predominantly unilateral. Cysts may also occur in association with vocal nodules (Monday, 1983).

Intracordal cysts may be caused by blockage of a glandular duct in which there is retention of mucus (Monday, 1983). Because there is no way for the mucus to escape, a cyst may, with time, grow larger. Another type of cyst, usually smaller than a retention cyst, is the epidermoid cyst. Epidermoid cysts of the vocal folds have a strong similarity to epidermal cysts of the skin.

Most patients with intracordal cysts are young adult women (Bouchayer, Cornut, Witzig, Loire, Roch, & Bastian, 1985; Monday, 1983). Cysts often occur in professional voice users.

### PERCEPTUAL SIGNS AND SYMPTOMS

Typical signs of a cyst include hoarseness and a lowered pitch. The patient may report a "tired" voice.

### ACOUSTIC SIGNS

Data are not available on the acoustic characteristics of the voices of patients with cysts. We might expect data similar to those for nodules, since the effect on the vocal folds appears to be similar.

### MEASURABLE PHYSIOLOGICAL SIGNS

Again, there are few physiological data available on patients with cysts. However, higher than normal average airflows might be expected as a result of elevated offset

*Figure 4.4.* Intracordal cyst. See color plate.

flows and higher than normal peak flows. The closing phase of the vocal folds, as seen in an electroglottogram, may also be slower than normal.

## OBSERVABLE PHYSIOLOGICAL SIGNS

### Laryngoscopy

Identification of a cyst can be very difficult. Bouchayer et al. (1985) report that in only 10% of their cases was a cyst obvious on initial examination. However, the appearance of fullness of the vocal fold and dilated capillaries raised the suspicion of a cyst in 55% of cases. Endoscopically, cysts are sometimes highlighted by a persistent light reflection from the slightly raised area of the cyst.

### Stroboscopy

Stroboscopy has been found to be very helpful in the diagnosis of a cyst because there is an absence of mucosal wave in the area over the cyst. Other signs include greater aperiodicity and reduced glottal closure (Kitzing, 1985). We have found that the vibration of the two folds is often asymmetric, especially over the area of the cyst (Colton, Woo, Brewer, Griffin, & Casper, 1995). Amplitude of the affected side, in particular, will be reduced.

## PATHOPHYSIOLOGY

A cyst originates in the superficial layer of the lamina propria (Hirano, 1981a). As it grows, it increases the distance between the cover and the lamina propria but usually does not extend into the layers. A cyst increases the mass and stiffness of the cover, whereas the transition layers and the body are unaffected.

## Edema

### PRIMARY VOICE SYMPTOM: HOARSENESS

### DESCRIPTION AND ETIOLOGY

Edema refers to the buildup of fluid that occurs primarily in the superficial layers. When it occurs in the first layer of the lamina propria, it is referred to as Reinke's edema since Reinke's space occurs in this layer (Fig. 4.5). Other names used to refer to

*Figure 4.5.* Reinke's edema. See color plate.

this problem are diffuse polyposis or polypoid degeneration. Some apparent swelling of the vocal folds, especially when localized, may also be a sign of a cyst. The lesions are seen bilaterally but are usually asymmetric in size.

Edema is a natural reaction of tissue to trauma and misuse. In addition to vocal abuse, chronic Reinke's edema is most often associated with smoking. It appears to occur more frequently in females, especially if they are long-term smokers (Bastian, 1986; Nielsen, Hojslet, & Karlsmose, 1986).

## PERCEPTUAL SIGNS AND SYMPTOMS

Typical symptoms of edema include a lower than normal pitch level and hoarseness. If the condition is particularly severe, the patient may complain of shortness of breath because the edematous vocal folds may partially block the airway. In some cases of edema (not polypoid) patients complain of loss of pitch range and increased effort required to produce voice.

## ACOUSTIC SIGNS

The fundamental frequency of phonation is lower than that expected for the sex and age of the patient. Bennett, Bishop, and Lumpkin (1987) reported a mean fundamental frequency of 108 Hz for their group of 29 females with Reinke's edema, and 91 Hz for their 6 male patients. There may be increased frequency and amplitude perturbation, as well as the presence of spectral noise due to the hoarseness. There are, however, few experimental data available to support these hypotheses.

## MEASURABLE PHYSIOLOGICAL SIGNS

Electromyographic recordings may also show no abnormalities. Flow glottograms may show greater aperiodicity of phonation and greater than normal mean and peak airflows. Pressures and vocal efficiency measures may be within normal limits.

## OBSERVABLE PHYSIOLOGICAL SIGNS

### Laryngoscopy

In Reinke's edema the vocal folds have the appearance of enlarged fluid-filled boggy structures. They do not appear firm or solid. The edema usually involves the full length of the vocal folds bilaterally. In some respects, Reinke's edema gives the appearance of a broad-based polyp occupying the full length of the vocal fold. Vocal folds may also be seen to be edematous, but without the boggy appearance of Reinke's. In such cases, they have a firmer, rounded appearance, rather than a flat, superior surface.

### Stroboscopy

Stroboscopic features of Reinke's edema are expected to show greater than normal excursion of the mucosal wave and complete glottal closure. In our study of four patients with Reinke's edema (Colton, Woo, Brewer, Griffin, & Casper, 1995), the mucosal wave was slightly decreased but glottal closure was complete. We have found that the vibration of the two folds is often symmetrical. In superior surface edema, the stroboscopic appearance may be quite different. Both amplitude of vibration and mucosal wave may be decreased.

## PATHOPHYSIOLOGY

Edema affects the superficial layer of the lamina propria. The mass of the cover is increased. However stiffness may depend on the specific nature of the lesion. Bennett,

Bishop, and Lumpkin (1987) suggested that Reinke's edema disturbs the elasticity of the cover, resulting in decreased stiffness. Such a reduction in stiffness would allow for greater amplitudes of vibration. The transition layers and body are not affected in Reinke's edema. The increase in bulk and reduction of stiffness would contribute to a lowered fundamental frequency of vibration.

## *Laryngitis*

### PRIMARY VOICE SYMPTOM: HOARSENESS

### DESCRIPTION AND ETIOLOGY

Laryngitis is an inflammation of the vocal folds and larynx. It may result from exposure to noxious agents (tobacco, alcohol, drugs), acidic gastric contents (GERD), environmental agents (allergens, dust), or vocal abuse. Laryngitis may also be the result of upper respiratory infections, which have a generalized effect on the mucosa of the respiratory tract, including the larynx (Fig. 4.6). The problem may be acute or chronic. Acute laryngitis resulting from bacterial infection is not directly related to vocal abuse. However, it does affect voice production and indirectly may be aggravated by abuse, as will be described later. Chronic abuse can lead to chronic laryngitis with persistent inflammation and perhaps a thickening of the vocal folds. Laryngitis may lead to tissue changes, such as nodules, polyps, or hypertrophy of the laryngeal epithelium.

### PERCEPTUAL SIGNS AND SYMPTOMS

The symptoms of laryngitis include marked roughness or hoarseness of the voice with accompanying sensations of discomfort and dryness in the throat. When secondary to infection, the hoarseness may persist for some time after the infection has been controlled. Continued heavy use of the voice during this time may contribute to the laryngitis and the continued hoarseness. The pitch level of the voice may appear to be either higher or lower than normal, and it will be difficult to speak in a loud voice.

*Figure 4.6.* Chronic laryngitis, with polypoid change. See color plate.

## ACOUSTIC SIGNS

Greater than normal frequency and amplitude perturbation would be expected. Taka-hashi and Koike (1975) found a mean RAP of 0.0069 and 0.0078 in their two female patients with chronic laryngitis. Their nine normal subjects had a mean RAP of 0.00582. Takahashi and Koike (1975) reported a mean fundamental frequency level of 103 Hz for one of their female patients with chronic laryngitis, and 284 Hz for the other. Thus, it appears that fundamental frequency may be either elevated or reduced. This may be related to the severity of the cordal involvement. One would also expect that phonational range would be reduced (Shipp & Huntington, 1965). Maximum sustainable intensities may be much lower than normal. Finally, there should be greater than normal spectral noise in the voice.

## MEASURABLE PHYSIOLOGICAL SIGNS

When laryngitis is present, airflow and air pressures may be elevated, especially if there is incomplete glottal closure. However, average airflows appear to be within normal limits (Hirano, 1981b; Hollien, 1975; McGlone, Richmond, & Bosma, 1966). Based on our experience, vibratory airflows show increased variability from one cycle to the next, and there may be greater than normal offset and peak airflows. Woo et al. (1987) reported a mean flow rate of 222 ml/sec for their combined acute, chronic, and radia-tion laryngitis group, collapsed across 7 male and 11 female subjects. (Normal speakers produced a mean flow rate of 144 ml/sec.) The electroglottographic signal may show marked variability from one cycle to the next, although closure times may be normal. Electromyographic levels would be expected to be normal or slightly elevated.

## OBSERVABLE PHYSIOLOGICAL SIGNS

### Laryngoscopy

Laryngitic larynges in the acute stage show a marked redness; small, dilated blood ves-sels may be visible on the inflamed folds. Chronic laryngitis may not be marked by in-flammation, but rather by thickened epithelium.

### Stroboscopy

The vocal folds may show increased asymmetry and aperiodicity, with reduced mu-cosal waves and reduced amplitude. We have noted a jerk-like movement of the mu-cosal wave, in which the wave appears to travel along part of the surface at one speed, then changes its speed for the remainder of its travel. The movement may also be called biphasic (Woo, personal communication, 1988). There is a stiff, jerky quality to this movement.

## PATHOPHYSIOLOGY

Laryngitis affects the cover of the vocal folds by increasing its stiffness, with little ef-fect on the mass of the vocal folds.

## OTHER COMMENTS

Chronic laryngitis, if allowed to continue untreated, may result in serious complica-tions, including laryngitis sicca, which is characterized by marked atrophy of the mu-cosa of the larynx. The major abnormality is the lack of vocal fold lubrication due to the reduction or absence of glandular secretions. The vocal folds will become dry and sticky, and a chronic cough may be present as the system attempts to remove the thick secretions on the vocal folds. On occasion, laryngeal crusting may result, requiring surgical removal.

Other forms of laryngitis result from diphtheria, tuberculosis, and syphilis, all of which are extremely rare. Another special form of laryngitis is acute epiglottitis, in which the inflammatory changes affect the mucosa of the epiglottis. Epiglottitis may be life threatening if the epiglottis becomes sufficiently enlarged to result in airway obstruction. Emergency treatment may be required. Antibiotics may be used to control the infection or steroids may be used to reduce the inflammation (Sataloff, 1987a).

## *Sulcus Vocalis*

### PRIMARY VOICE SYMPTOM: HOARSENESS

### DESCRIPTION AND ETIOLOGY

Sulcus vocalis refers to a condition in which a furrow along the upper medial edge of the vocal folds is observed. Bastian (1986) describes it as an "epithelial-lined furrow or pocket whose lips parallel the free edge of the cords" (p. 1974). In a cross-section of the vocal folds, the furrow appears as a pocketed ledge on the medial surface of the vocal folds (Fig. 4.7). The longitudinal extent of the furrow is variable, as is its depth. If very deep, it seems to divide the cord in half. According to Arnold (1980), sulcus vocalis may be associated with other laryngeal or oral asymmetries.

The etiology of sulcus vocalis is uncertain, although Bastian (1986) attributes it to vocal misuse and abuse. Luchsinger and Arnold (1965) in their review of the literature summarized the possible etiological factors as being congenital, developmental, or traumatic. Bouchayer et al. (1985) argued for a congenital etiology. The disorder is rather rare, at least in Europe and the United States (Luchsinger & Arnold, 1965); it may be more prevalent in Japan (Hirano, 1981b). According to Hirano and Bless (1993), sulcus vocalis is either congenital or the result of repeated chronic inflammatory processes.

### PERCEPTUAL SIGNS AND SYMPTOMS

Symptoms include a breathy, hoarse voice quality that apparently is due to incomplete closure of the vocal folds and disturbed vibratory behavior. The pitch of the voice may be lower than normal, and the loudness may be reduced.

### ACOUSTIC SIGNS

Phonational and intensity ranges would be expected to be reduced, although there are no data available to support this expectation. There may be elevated levels of spectral

*Figure 4.7.* Schematic of a coronal cross-section of the vocal fold with a sulcus vocalis: a, the mucosal cover; b, the vocal ligament; c, muscle; d, sulcus entrance.

noise in the voice. We might also find greater than normal frequency and amplitude perturbation, although of small magnitude.

## MEASURABLE PHYSIOLOGICAL SIGNS

Airflows may be slightly elevated (Shigemori, 1977). We would expect vibratory flows to show greater than normal perturbation and slightly greater than normal airflow leakage (offset flow). Electroglottographic recordings should show increased perturbation with the possibility of short closed times.

## OBSERVABLE PHYSIOLOGICAL SIGNS

### Laryngoscopy

Laryngoscopically, a sulcus will be seen as a depression or line along the upper medial edge of the vocal fold. The depression may extend the entire length of the vocal fold and may vary in depth from shallow to very deep.

### STROBOSCOPY

We have found diminished amplitudes of vocal fold movement with little continuity of the mucosal wave across the sulcus. A mucosal wave can usually be seen across the uninvolved superior surface of the vocal fold. A narrow, spindle-shaped glottal chink closure configuration with bowed vocal fold edges is described by Hirano and Bless (1993).

### PATHOPHYSIOLOGY

The sulcus is located in the superficial layer of the lamina propria, which decreases the mass of the cover but may increase its stiffness. The body and the transition layers are normal.

*Figure 4.8.* Vocal abuse.

## SUMMARY

Misuse and abuse of the voice have been defined, and the specific ways in which they occur have been discussed. The goal of this chapter is to sensitize the practitioner to the many forms that misuse and abuse of the phonatory mechanism may take. The primary misuses of the voice include hard glottal attack, elevated laryngeal posture, anteroposterior squeezing, and inappropriate pitch level. Abusive behaviors include excessive coughing and throat clearing, yelling, shouting, cheerleading, and prolonged loud talking. Abusive behaviors result in mechanical trauma to the vocal folds or vocal processes. Continued trauma may result in tissue change that will alter the vibratory characteristics of the vocal folds, which in turn results in hoarseness or roughness in the voice. In some cases, the tissue alteration will prevent complete glottal closure and result in the production of breathy phonation. An understanding of these behaviors will allow the clinician to help patients make a thorough inventory of their own behaviors.

The goal of this chapter's section on drugs is to increase awareness of the potential phonatory effect of a vast array of pharmaceuticals, many of which are frequently considered to be quite benign, especially if they are of the over-the-counter variety. There are certainly many overriding reasons why drugs must be used in the treatment of various conditions, even if some degree of voice change may occur. However, the practitioner who works with the voice patient must be aware of the effects various drugs may have on voice and/or on mucosal tissues. This can be critical for the professional voice user.

In the last section, a variety of specific tissue changes associated with vocal misuse and abuse have been reviewed, including vocal nodules, polyps, cysts, edema, laryngitis, and sulcus vocalis. Although some of these conditions may be caused by infection, viral agents, external trauma, congenital disposition, or disease, vocal abuse is often considered to be involved. Recognition of the contribution of abusive behaviors to these conditions is necessary in order to arrive at a treatment protocol that will be effective in reducing and/or eliminating these vocal problems, with the least trauma and expense to the patient (Fig. 4.8).

# Chapter 5

# Voice Problems Associated with Nervous System Involvement

## ROLE OF THE NERVOUS SYSTEM

The nervous system is that portion of the body concerned with the control of other body functions. Viewed as a unit, it is responsible for the total control of all systems in the body, even self-regulating systems that are capable of carrying out their own functions. The smaller units of the body's organizational system (cells, tissues, and organs) function only within their own little world and in an environment that must be controlled. It is the responsibility of the nervous system to create this environment by regulating systems that provide for the proper nourishment, temperature regulation, gas exchange, and by-product disposal necessary for all the component parts to work effectively.

Coordination of function is another aspect of the control exerted by the nervous system. One system must work at the proper time if another system is to function properly. Within a system, the various parts must perform their tasks at the proper times for the final output of the system to be meaningful and productive. The necessity for coordination is even more apparent in the production of skilled motor acts involving the various striated muscles of the body. Simple walking is an example of a highly skilled motor act involving the proper contraction and relaxation of different muscles for its action.

The nervous system is divided into two major parts: the central nervous system and the peripheral nervous system. The central nervous system (CNS) is that portion residing within the cranial cavity or skull and vertebral column. The peripheral nervous system (PNS) resides throughout the body outside of the cranium. The central nervous system is responsible for the initiation and coordination of function, whereas the peripheral nervous system carries the instructions of the central nervous system to the various organs and muscles of the body.

The nervous system may also be divided into two components, according to whether information is conducted to the central nervous system (afferent) or from the central nervous system (efferent). Indeed, information from muscles, organs, and tissues is needed by the central nervous system for proper control to be maintained. Information from the outside world via the several senses is also used by the central nervous system to make it possible for the body to exist in the hostile world. Without the nervous system, the body cannot live. With a damaged nervous system, the body cannot function "normally" in its environment.

## GENERAL CHARACTERISTICS OF NERVOUS SYSTEM DYSFUNCTION

The nervous system may malfunction due to disease, abnormal growths, accidents, or trauma. The nature of the malfunction will depend on where the problem occurs. In some cases there will be difficulty in initiating an action or activity, while in others the activity will begin without difficulty but control of it may be impaired. In still other cases, incoming information will be distorted or nonexistent, so that the nervous system will not have the proper information for the control of motor or organ activity appropriate for the task at hand.

The central nervous system is responsible for initiating skilled motor acts that involve the starting and stopping of motor activity. Walking is a good example of an activity that must be initiated and terminated. Most internal body functions are ongoing; that is, once started, they continue or else the body will to cease to function (e.g., blood flow, respiration, temperature regulation). Other internal body functions are episodic and may be stopped and started (e.g., digestion, hormone production). Speech itself is a very good example of an act that is constantly started and stopped even during its execution. There are centers and cells within the central nervous system that have this function of starting an act. If damaged, the initiation of the act may not take place or will be delayed, uncertain, or otherwise impaired.

The central nervous system also coordinates function. There are many examples of the need for coordination of body systems, the act of walking being just one. Speech is also a highly coordinated event involving coordination within bodily systems (e.g., phonation, respiration, articulation) and among these systems. Damage to the central nervous system may affect control of coordinated function.

Lower brain centers, including the spinal cord, maintain a measure of control, albeit local, on muscles and systems. For example, muscles must be maintained in a state of readiness for action. Muscle tone reflects this state of readiness. Muscles show steady levels of electrical activity even when they are not being used for a motor act. This state of readiness is often regulated and maintained by lower neuron systems. The central nervous system exerts its control by inhibiting the activity of the lower centers, so that they do not get out of control. Damage to the central nervous system can result in the disruption of this inhibition and the production of unnecessary or unwanted movements.

Finally, incoming sensory information is critical for the control process. The central nervous system must know when the right foot has touched the floor in order to command the left leg to rise and move the left foot forward. Otherwise the walker will fall flat on his face or cease moving. The central nervous system relies on visual information in order to properly control the hand and arm in reaching for the glass of water on the kitchen table. Deprived of sensory information, the organism will not know about the environment and its potential effects. Incoming sensory information need not be entirely external. Internal sensory information is also critical for neural control. Examples of internal sensory information include joint kinesthetics, position sense, pain, pressure and temperature. Kinesthetic feedback from joints and muscles must be available if skilled movements are to be possible. The job of the central nervous system is to receive and integrate information and prepare a proper plan for dealing with it.

## ROLE OF THE NERVOUS SYSTEM IN PHONATION AND SPEECH

Speech is a complex, fine motor act that involves several diverse systems or parts of systems for its execution. The respiratory system, basically designed for the exchange of gases for use by the tissues of the body, is also used for speech, with contributions from the digestive system, primarily the mouth, jaw, and teeth. Speech requires the use of the respiratory system mechanically, that is, for the generation and control of the airflows and pressures needed for speaking. Thus, the control of the respiratory system for life support and the control of the respiratory system for speaking are quite different. The nervous system must provide the control appropriate to the task at hand. Furthermore, during speech, there must be a high level of coordination among the chest wall, the abdominal mechanical system, the larynx and pharynx, and the lips, tongue, teeth, and mandible so that all function at the proper time and for the length of time necessary for the production of the individual sounds. During the act of speaking, the system receives information about the state of its structures and muscles via both kinesthetic and acoustic feedback. Thus, the auditory system is yet another important system that must enter into the control exercised by the nervous system.

Disease, malformation, or injury will affect the control capabilities of the nervous system. The manifestation of nervous system damage will vary depending on where the lesion occurs. If the lesion occurs at the cortex, many components of speech may be affected, including the ability to use language, to initiate speech, to produce muscle movements necessary to produce intelligible speech or control muscle movements, or to receive information from the body systems about where they are and what they have done. The symptoms and signs that the patient presents are critical to the proper diagnosis of the problem and identification of the source of the problem.

In this book, we are interested in the effects of nervous system damage on the control of phonation. Although the system remains complex, there is a finite set of brain sites and pathways that have been shown to be important for the control of phonation. Lesions will produce specific symptoms that will help the diagnostician identify the site of lesion. Some of the possible problems affecting phonation and their possible locations in the nervous system are discussed by Barlow, Netsell, and Hunker (1986). They note that in the lateral precentral cortex, there appears to be a convergence of pathways from other parts of the brain that may be the site of the final common pathway through the brain to the periphery. Lesions at this site would be expected to result in complete loss of phonation because input from the higher control centers will have been lost. Furthermore, lesions in this area and other adjacent areas would also be expected to produce loss of function in other muscles concerned with speech. Consequently, such lesions will be expected to produce aphonia or dysphonia, dysarthria, and perhaps even aphasia. Lesions in the anterior cingulate cortex are also reported to produce akinetic mutism in humans (Barlow, Netsell, & Hunker, 1986). In monkeys this area seems to be critical for the control of conditional, learned vocalization. Lesions in other areas of the brain (e.g., basal ganglia, periaqueductal gray) produce a disruption in phonation characterized by breathiness, roughness, tremor, or complete disruption of vocalization. Lesions in the cerebellum result in ataxic dysarthria and changes in the velocity of lip and jaw movements and would presumably affect the speed of movements of structures in the larynx. Larson, Sutton, and Lindeman (1978) concluded that the cerebellum is very important in the control of pitch and loudness of phonation but is not required for the initiation of phonation.

An effective and convenient organizational scheme for the consideration of the neurological problems that affect phonation would recognize the levels of organization within the nervous system, as discussed above. The following is such a scheme, proposed by Ward, Hanson, and Berci (1981). It is both simple and effective as an aid in understanding how a specific lesion or syndrome may affect phonation.

1. Afferent sensory, autonomic
2. Efferent motor

> Upper motor neuron (cortex and pyramidal tracts)
> Extrapyramidal (reticular substance)
> Cerebellar
> Nuclear (lower motor neurons)

We have adopted this scheme, with slight modifications, as the organizational framework for consideration of neurological problems that affect voice. It is most effective in emphasizing the role of a specific area of the nervous system in the control of phonation and in the ultimate determination of the pathophysiology of a voice problem.

## ORGANIZATION OF THE NERVOUS SYSTEM AND VOICE PATHOLOGY

The following section is a brief review of the major systems involved in phonation. More complete information about the nervous system can be found in Chapter 12. Ward et al. (1981) discuss the role of the afferent or sensory system in the control of phonation. Our discussion here will concentrate on the efferent or motor system involved in the control of phonation (Fig. 5.1).

In the cortex, area 4 of the precentral gyrus is very important in the control of vocalization. Neurons from this and other areas of the cortex converge to form the corticobulbar tracts. These tracts pass through the internal capsule and cerebral peduncle and eventually comprise what is known as the pyramidal tracts. At the upper part of the medulla, many fibers cross over (decussate) to the opposite side and continue down to the nucleus ambiguus in the brainstem. As discussed in Chapter 12, the nucleus ambiguus houses the motor nuclei for the 9th, 10th, and 11th cranial nerves. Thus, lesions anywhere along this pathway may involve the precentral cortex, the corticobulbar tracts, the internal capsule or the cerebral peduncles, the medulla, the brainstem, or the nucleus ambiguus itself, causing differential effects on phonation.

The extrapyramidal system consists of the reticular substance, corpus striatum (with the caudate and lenticular nuclei), and the basal ganglia (specifically the globus pallidus and the substantia nigra) (Ward, Hanson, & Berci, 1981). Lesions here will affect the coordination of laryngeal function. Athetoid movements are characteristic of patients with lesions in these areas. Degeneration of the basal ganglia and the reticular substance produce the symptoms typical of parkinsonism (see later section on Parkinsonism for a more complete discussion of this disease). The Shy-Drager syndrome, in which there is progressive abductor paralysis of the larynx, is thought to be a disease affecting the extrapyramidal system, as well as the motor nuclei of the vagus (see later section on Shy-Drager syndrome for a more complete discussion of this disease).

Lesions in the cerebellum affect the coordination of motor function and result in slurred speech and problems with coordination of the various speech systems, as well as nonspeech symptoms, such as ataxia, nystagmus, and gait problems. The voice may exhibit a breathy quality, or it may exhibit spastic behavior. In the Arnold-Chiari syndrome, for example, the vocal folds may typically demonstrate involuntary abduction (see later section on Arnold-Chiari Malformation for a more complete discussion).

Lower motor neuron problems occur in the brainstem and medulla. There are many syndromes that result from lesions in the medulla and in which voice will be affected, as will the functioning of the palate, pharynx, tongue, face, and other body

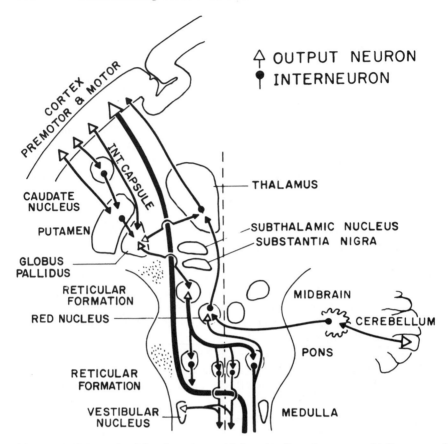

*Figure 5.1.* Schematic of the direct (pyramidal) and indirect (extrapyramidal) motor pathways. The direct reaches the neurons in the spinal cord without an intervening synapse (shown by heavy black line). The indirect has many synapses on its way to the lower motor neurons, with stops in the basal ganglia and reticular formation. Not shown are collaterals from the pyramidal system to the tegmentum of the pons and the midbrain, where they can interact with the extrapyramidal system.

parts. Lesions in the nucleus ambiguus may produce classic symptoms of a combined paralysis of the superior and recurrent laryngeal nerves, resulting in flaccid vocal folds. Such lesions, depending on their extent, may also affect the palate and pharynx.

Finally, there can be an interruption of control in the peripheral nerves supplying the larynx itself. Such disturbance can result from lesions or injury to the superior laryngeal nerve, the recurrent laryngeal nerve, or both. Furthermore, the lesions may be either unilateral or bilateral. Again, the specific symptoms presented by the patient will help to determine the proper diagnosis and locus of the problem.

There are voice problems in which neurological involvement is suspected but cannot be determined with certainty. Some of these problems may involve diffuse areas of the brain, and no specific single site of lesion can be determined. In other instances, the etiology is unknown or described as idiopathic in nature. However, "unknown" or "idiopathic" is not a diagnosis. It should signify a temporary condition during which further data are gathered in the search for the diagnosis. A more precise diagnosis may result from additional testing, but occasionally the simple passage of time reveals additional symptoms that help to refine the diagnosis; in some cases, a more specific diagnosis may remain undetermined or unknown.

In the following discussion about specific neurological problems that affect the voice, a primary vocal symptom will be stated. In most cases, this refers to the most frequently reported symptom for that disease, as reported by Aronson, Brown, Litin, and Pearson (1968b).In some cases, other studies were used to identify the primary vocal symptom. There will usually be additional voice symptoms associated with each neurological problem. These will be discussed for each disease in the section entitled "Perceptual Voice Signs and Symptoms."

## UPPER MOTOR NEURON DISORDERS (CORTICAL AND PYRAMIDAL)

### Supra- or Pseudobulbar Palsy

PRIMARY VOICE SYMPTOM: HOARSENESS OR HARSHNESS

DESCRIPTION AND ETIOLOGY

Two major pathway systems converge on the lower motor neurons for control of muscles that affect voice and speech. These are the pyramidal and extrapyramidal tracts. Selected damage to the extrapyramidal or indirect pathway[1] usually results in spasticity and increased muscle reflexes. Selected damage to the direct or pyramidal pathway results in a loss of function, especially for skilled movements. The pyramidal system is said to be the newer system phylogenetically. Both pathways are located very close to each other anatomically and lesions in these pathways would most likely affect both pathways and voluntary movement in four ways: spasticity, weakness, limitation of range, and a slowing of movement. The disease known as pseudobulbar palsy results when lesions affect these two systems.

Pseudobulbar palsy is actually a misnomer. The symptoms of the problem are in some instances very similar to those of bulbar disease (muscle weakness), and yet the evidence for bulbar lesions is equivocal. Langworthy and Hesser (1940) recommended the term "supranuclear bulbar paralysis." Aring (1965) agreed, believing that the term had an anatomical basis, locating the lesions rostral to the appropriate cranial motor nerve nuclei. However, the term "pseudobulbar palsy" has remained in use.

Pseudobulbar palsy results from progressive lesions that occur bilaterally in the corticobulbar tracts. These lesions occur most frequently in the internal capsules (Aring, 1965; Langworthy & Hesser, 1940), although there may be pontine or midbrain lesions. These lesions are usually the result of a stroke, although other reported causes have been cerebral palsy, brain injuries, multiple sclerosis, and arteriosclerosis (Darley, Aronson, & Brown, 1975; Langworthy & Hesser, 1940). The chief symptoms are difficulties with speech and swallowing, plus emotional lability. The latter presents a unique feature of this problem. Patients may show bursts of laughter or crying in the presence of very mild stimuli or no stimuli at all. It is as if the patient's higher centers have released their control of these responses, and they appear uncontrolled. Kreindler and Pruskauer-Apostol (1971) documented these unusual behaviors, and Aronson (1990) emphasized that reduced thresholds for crying and laughter are critical cues in the diagnosis of this disorder.

---

[1]Indirect refers to the fact that information traveling along this pathway encounters many synapses or connection points along its way to the final destination. The direct pathway or pyramidal system has a single, continuous pathway from the motor cortex to the lower motor neurons in the spinal cord or nuclei in the brainstem.

## PERCEPTUAL VOICE SIGNS AND SYMPTOMS

A major sign of pseudobulbar palsy is the dysarthria of speech, as documented by Darley and his colleagues (Darley, Aronson, & Brown, 1969a, 1969b, 1975). They grouped perceptual signs into clusters of the dysarthric symptoms that best characterize a particular type of neurological dysfunction. The important perceptual signs in pseudobulbar palsy are reported to be (using Darley, Aronson, and Brown's terminology) (*a*) prosodic excess (relates to rate and stress characteristics of speech), (*b*) prosodic insufficiency (monopitch, monoloudness, reduced stress, short phrases), (*c*) articulatory-resonatory incompetence (imprecise consonants, distorted vowels, hypernasality), and (*d*) phonatory stenosis (harsh voice, strain/struggle, pitch breaks).

Aronson et al. (1968a) rated the voice characteristics of 30 patients with pseudobulbar palsy (Darley, Aronson, & Brown, 1969a, 1969b) and found that 97% of the patients were considered to have monopitch and harsh voices, 87% had a too-low pitch level, 67% demonstrated considerable strain and struggle in phonation, and 30% exhibited pitch breaks and voice tremor. (These voice signs of pseudobulbar palsy are shown in Fig. 5.2.) Aring (1965) commented that the speech of a patient with pseudobulbar palsy is nasal, monotonic, with soft intensity and rapid rate, making it difficult to understand.

## ACOUSTIC SIGNS

There have been few data reported on the acoustic characteristics of patients with pseudobulbar palsy other than a study by Kammermeier (1969), who reported a mean fundamental frequency of 124.1 Hz in male subjects with a mean age of 61.7 years. When compared to the mean fundamental frequency ($F_0$) values reported for normal adult male speakers by Mysak (1959) (mean frequency = 124.3 Hz, mean age = 73.3 years) and Hollien and Shipp (1972) (mean frequency = 112 Hz, mean age = 64.6 years), the pseudobulbar subjects produced fundamental frequencies that were equal to or slightly higher than normal speakers. Kammermeier (1969) reported reduced

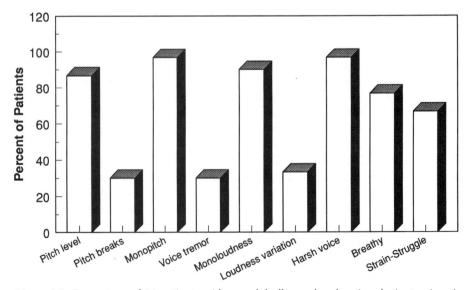

*Figure 5.2.* Percentage of 30 patients with pseudobulbar palsy showing deviant voice signs. Voice tremor was rated during contextual speech.

variability of fundamental frequency in pseudobulbar patients, as well as reduced intensity variation. These findings may be related to the perception of monopitch and monoloudness.

It appears that patients with pseudobulbar palsy exhibit normal or near-normal average fundamental frequency, reduced fundamental frequency variation, and reduced intensity variation.

## MEASURABLE PHYSIOLOGICAL SIGNS

We know of no data on the measurable physiological characteristics of the speech of patients with pseudobulbar palsy. Higher than normal subglottal pressures might be expected because of the hypertonicity and strain/struggle characteristics of the voice. If breathy, the patient would probably exhibit greater than normal airflows. If the range and force of movement of the vocal folds are affected, this might be reflected in slow opening and closing times of the vocal folds and perhaps a short closed phase due to the inability to maintain sufficient muscle forces.

## OBSERVABLE PHYSIOLOGICAL SIGNS

### Laryngoscopy

According to Darley et al. (1975), no laryngeal abnormalities have been reported. However, it is possible that vocal fold hyperadduction as well as hypofunction of other laryngeal structures might be observable, utilizing the improved instruments available today for laryngoscopic examination. Further study of these characteristics is needed.

### Stroboscopy

Again, there appear to be no reports on stroboscopic signs in patients with pseudobulbar palsy. When vocal fold hypertonicity is present, typical findings, according to Kitzing (1985), would include reduced vocal fold amplitudes, diminished mucosal waves, and excessive glottal closure. However, if the muscles have reduced force and movement, glottal closure may not be complete, and there may be asymmetry and aperiodicity of vocal fold movement.

## PATHOPHYSIOLOGY

Pseudobulbar palsy results in a loss of muscle coordination and a release of inhibition of the lower centers. The latter condition results in hyperactivity of the muscle reflexes and spasticity. In speech, pseudobulbar palsy patients will show a reduction in the force and range of the muscle movement (Darley, Aronson, & Brown, 1969b). In addition, the release of the lower motor centers results in hypertonicity of the vocal folds. Pseudobulbar palsy seems to be a condition in which both muscle weakness and muscle hyperactivity coexist, with differential effects on the motor act being performed. Hypertonicity would be consistent with the perception of harshness in the voice, as well as the strain and struggle to speak. It is not necessarily consistent with the perception of a low pitch level or the findings that the fundamental frequency of these patients is within the normal range. These findings might be understood by hypothesizing that the cricothyroid is minimally affected in pseudobulbar palsy but that the other adductors or abductors of the larynx are affected differentially. Breathiness (noted in 14 out of 30 patients with pseudobulbar palsy studied by Darley et al. [1969b]) would be produced by excessive opening of the vocal folds or perhaps by hypertonicity of the abductor muscle of the larynx (posterior cricothyroid). Hyperactivity in the adductors would have an effect similar to hypertonicity and would be consistent with strain/struggle quality, as well as excessive hoarseness or harshness. The specific voice signs (perceptual, acoustic, or physiological) noted in a patient with pseudobulbar palsy may reflect lesions at different locations along the long pathway from the brain to the ultimate motor neurons controlling the muscles of the larynx.

## EXTRAPYRAMIDAL DISORDERS

### *Parkinsonism*

#### PRIMARY VOICE SYMPTOM: MONOPITCH

#### DESCRIPTION AND ETIOLOGY

Parkinson's disease (PD) is a progressive, degenerative disease of the central nervous system affecting the basal ganglia, specifically the substantia nigra. There is also a decrease of dopamine in the caudate nucleus and the putamen. The disease results in rigidity, resting tremor, and reduced range of movement in the limbs, neck, and head. The general characteristic of PD is a slowness of movement and loss of automatic movements, referred to as bradykinesia (Brin, Fahn, Blitzer, Ramig, & Stewart, 1992). Bradykinesia also encompasses the masked facies or absence of facial expression, decreased dye blinking, decreased spontaneous swallowing, and difficulty in initiating movement or command that are features of PD. The amplitude of voluntary movement as well as impaired postural and righting reflexes are impaired (Hoehn & Yahr, 1967). All movements may be affected. It is important to realize that the muscles are not paralyzed but rather are hypokinetic and lack the dynamic aspects of movement. Respiratory movements are also affected producing a shallow and irregular respiratory cycle sometimes at twice the normal frequency (Ramig & Gould, 1986). Patients may have a limited vital capacity and inspiratory capacity. These respiratory deficits may affect the patient's ability to produce speech of normal loudness and utterance length. Laryngeal muscle involvement may affect the ability to initiate phonation, produce adequate loudness, and vary pitch.

Although the etiology of any particular case of PD is usually unknown, there are several causes that have been hypothesized or been directly linked to the disease. Some cases of PD have been traced to a disease called encephalitis lethargica which occurred in small epidemics in the 1920s. The last reported cases of this disease were in the 1940s (Duvoisin, 1976). With the recognition of post-encephalitic parkinsonism, the concept of multiple etiologies for the disease became understood. Other possible etiologies include an undetermined slow-growing virus, head trauma, toxic buildup, drugs, vascular trauma, or carbon monoxide poisoning (Darley, Aronson, & Brown, 1975). Iatrogenic PD is caused by antipsychotic phenothiazine drugs. It is usually reversible by withdrawal of the drug or sometimes by reduction in dosage.

Patients with Parkinson's disease may be classified into at least two distinct groups. The first, often referred to as idiopathic Parkinson's disease (IPD) displays the classic symptoms of this disease. The second group, often referred to as Parkinson Plus Syndrome (PPS) involves multiple symptom atrophy. One of these syndromes is called Shy-Drager and will be discussed separately. The speech and voice deficits in PPS are usually more severe and they deteriorate faster than in patients with IPD.

Parkinson's patients can be staged according to the severity of the symptoms as discussed by Hoehn and Yahr (1967). The scale used is arbitrary but is based on the level of clinical disability observed. The stages and their definition are displayed in Table 5.1. According to the data presented by Hoehn and Yahr there is a tendency for staging to be correlated with the duration of the illness ($r = 0.97$). Other rating systems have also been proposed to assess the physical status and limitations and daily living

*Table 5.1.* Stages of Degree of Severity for Patients with Parkinson's Disease (After Hoehn and Yahr, 1967)

| Stage | Description |
| --- | --- |
| I | Unilateral involvement only |
| II | Bilateral or midline involvement |
| III | Impaired righting reflexes (unsteadiness in turning or sudden change from a standing position) |
| IV | Severely disabling disease; patient can walk or stand but is otherwise incapacitated |
| V | Patient confined to bed or wheelchair |

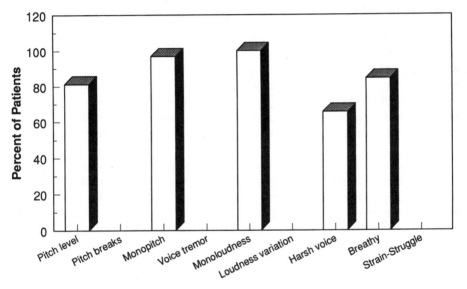

*Figure 5.3.* Percentage of 32 patients with Parkinson's disease showing deviant voice signs. Voice tremor was rated during contextual speech.

problems that might be encountered (Martínez-Martín & Bermejo-Pareja, 1988). Speech and voice disorders are present in 75% of persons with PD and virtually 100% will develop problems in these areas as the disease progresses into the more debilitating stages (Oxtoby, 1982; Streifler & Hofman, 1984)

## PERCEPTUAL VOICE SIGNS AND SYMPTOMS

The most frequently rated voice dimensions, as reported by Aronson et al. (1968b) (Fig. 5.3), were monopitch, excessively low pitch, and harshness. According to Aronson et al. (1968b), variability of loudness is reduced, but rate of speech is highly variable, sometimes with fast bursts and at other times a slow rate. The reduced variability of vocal loudness, pitch, and rate are thought to be the consequence of muscle rigidity and hypokinesia. Speech production is also affected by slurring and phoneme misarticulations, again associated directly with the physical symptoms described.

In a study of 200 patients with Parkinson's disease, Logemann, Fisher, Boches, and Blonsky (1978) found that 87% showed some laryngeal dysfunction and that 45% had laryngeal dysfunction as the only symptom. The specific voice signs these authors reported were breathiness (15%), roughness (29%), hoarseness (45%), and tremulousness (13.5%). Ramig (1995) reports that reduced vocal loudness is a classic speech symptom along with those noted previously. This vocal loudness reduction may be one of the first signs of PD (Aronson, 1985).

## ACOUSTIC SIGNS

Canter (1963) reported a rather extensive study on the acoustic characteristics of intensity, pitch, and duration of patients with Parkinson's disease. He found no differences between a group of 11 Parkinson's patients and 17 control subjects on average intensity in a reading passage. Furthermore, the range of SPLs in the passage for the two groups was very similar. Patients with PD were found to have a higher mean fundamental frequency (129 Hz) as compared to the control group (106 Hz), and frequency variability in the Parkinson's group was found to be much less than for the control group (0.5 octave versus 0.86 octave). There were no differences between the two groups on vowel duration, number of pauses, mean pause length, or mean syllable length. There was a tendency for the ranges of these measures to be higher in the PD patients.

There is a discrepancy between the Aronson et al. (1968a) study and the Canter (1963) study with respect to pitch and fundamental frequency. Aronson et al. reported a very low pitch level, but Canter reported a higher than normal fundamental frequency level. Pitch and fundamental frequency are not synonymous, although they are related. During speech, judgments of pitch can be influenced by other characteristics of the signal, including degrees of roughness and breathiness. It appears that in patients with Parkinson's disease, the pitch of the voice is perceived to be very low but the actual fundamental frequency is equal to or slightly higher than normal.

In a later study, Canter (1965) measured minimum and maximum intensity levels, pitch range, and maximum phonation time in 17 patients with PD. The patients showed a higher SPL at their minimum intensity level ("quiet") and a lower maximum intensity level ("shouted") than the control group. The PD patients had a higher low fundamental frequency (100 Hz versus 80 Hz for controls) and a lowered maximum fundamental frequency level (200 Hz versus 260 Hz for controls). Finally, the PD patients had a much shorter maximum phonation time (9.5 seconds) compared to the control subjects (20.6 seconds). Thus, all ranges of function were reduced.

Logemann et al. (1978) reported that of all symptoms affecting the speech of patients with PD, voice symptoms were reported most frequently, with articulation errors being the next most often cited symptom. Consonants (stops, fricatives, and affricatives) are most often affected by errors in place and manner. The severity of the disease appeared to be related to the speech errors exhibited. Although a severity-to-voice-symptom relationship might be expected to be present, data are not available to document it.

More recently, there have been several studies reporting on the acoustic characteristics of the voices of patients with Parkinson's disease (Kent et al., 1994; King, Ramig, Lemke, & Horii, 1994; Ramig, Scherer, Klasner, Titze, & Horii, 1990; Zwirner, Murry, & Woodson, 1991). All report fundamental frequencies within the normal range (Table 5.2). However, they show greater than normal variation of fundamental frequency in sustained vowels (Zwirner, Murry, & Woodson, 1991).

Ludlow, Coulter, and Gentges (1983) found no significant differences of vocal jitter between their group of seven patients with PD and seven age and sex matched normal controls (jitter ratios of 7.21 and 5.92 respectively). However, Ramig and colleagues (Ramig, Scherer, Titze, & Ringel, 1988) reported a jitter value of their patients that was more than twice as large as their control group (1.26% versus 0.53%). On the other hand, Kent et al. (1994) failed to find a statistically significant difference on the same measure.

Table 5.2. Reported Fundamental Frequency Levels for Patients with Parkinson's Disease

| | Ludlow et al 1983 | Ramig et al 1989 | Zwirner et al 1991 | Kent et al 1994 |
|---|---|---|---|---|
| *Measure* | | | | |
| Mean | 163.9 | 128 | 120 | 140.7 |
| SD | 34.5 | 16 | 21 | 45.29 |
| N | 7[a] | 8 | 12 | 22 |
| *Jitter (%)* | | | | |
| Mean | | 1.26 | | |
| SD | | 1.05 | | |
| *Jitter (ms)* | | | | |
| Mean | | | 0.1 | 0.17 |
| SD | | | 0.1 | 0.17 |
| *Jitter Ratio* | | | | |
| Mean | 7.21 | | | |
| SD | 2.97 | | | |
| *Reported Shimmer for Parkinson's Patients* | | | | |
| Mean | | 5.18 | 6 | 5.42 |
| SD | | 3.43 | 6.6 | 3.2 |
| *Reported Signal-to-Noise Ratios for Parkinson's Patients* | | | | |
| Mean | | 14.75 | 17.5 | 18.85 |
| SD | | 2.97 | 4.5 | 4.64 |

[a]includes 4 males and 3 females

Shimmer has been reported to range between 5% and 6% in patients with Parkinson's disease; however, the significance of this range is difficult to evaluate since in one study (Zwirner, Murry, & Woodson, 1991) the normal control group had a mean shimmer of 4.1% whereas in another study (Kent et al., 1994) the normal control group shimmer was 7%. In the Ramig study (1988), the youngest control group had a mean shimmer of about 2%, the oldest group about 2.5%.

Signal-to-noise ratio (SNR) ranged between 14 and 19 dB for the Parkinson's patients (Table 5.2). Normal SNRs were reported to be between 17 and 25 dB. Thus it appears that patients with Parkinson's disease have slightly lower SNR than normal. One might interpret this finding to mean that Parkinson's patients have slightly nosier voice production.

Available acoustic data suggest that in patients with Parkinson's disease, the mean fundamental frequency is similar to normal speakers but the variability of fundamental frequency within a speech segment is increased, probably reflecting loss of control of the motor act. Jitter and shimmer are also increased whereas SNR is slightly decreased.

## MEASURABLE PHYSIOLOGICAL SIGNS

Patients with PD appear to produce higher resting and background activity in the interarytenoid and posterior cricoarytenoid muscles (Guidi, Bannister, & Gibson, 1981). Lip muscles also show greater resting and background activity levels, and the degree of activity seems to be related to the side of the body most affected by the disease (Leanderson, Meyerson, & Persson, 1972).

## OBSERVABLE PHYSIOLOGICAL SIGNS

### Laryngoscopy

Cisler (1927) reported diminished vocal fold movement, and Schilling (1925) described a rigor of the vocal folds. Darley et al. (1969b) reported no abnormal laryngoscopic signs.

The most extensive description of laryngoscopic signs in PD patients was reported by Hanson, Gerratt, and Ward (1984). They studied 32 patients, of whom 30 had abnormal laryngoscopic signs. The most prominent sign was bowed vocal folds, and the vocal folds appeared to vibrate with greater amplitude. In 26 patients, varying degrees of laryngeal asymmetry were observed. Many patients showed a characteristic pattern consisting of a more posterior position of the vocal process, a more posterior and lateral position of the apex of the arytenoid, and a more contracted ventricular fold than seen in normal speakers. These signs were associated with the side of the body affected by the disease. Many patients also showed overclosure of the vocal folds, and 5 of the 32 exhibited an extreme degree of supraglottal constriction.

### Stroboscopy

There have been two reports on the stroboscopic signs of Parkinson's disease (Perez, Ramig, Smith, & Dromey, 1994; Smith, Ramig, Dromey, Perez, & Samandari, 1994). Smith et al. (1994) studied 22 patients with the idiopathic form of Parkinson's disease (IPD). Both flexible and rigid endoscopes were used to view and record the laryngeal images as the patients produced a sustained /ee/. The images were visually rated by four experienced raters on glottal closure configuration, degree of glottal incompetence, and laryngeal hyperfunction. The results of the glottal closure configuration ratings are shown in Figure 5.4. The severity of glottal incompetence was in the mild range. As a group, the patients showed mild false fold and anterior-posterior approximation. Interestingly, although Hanson et al. (1984) found that the overwhelming ma-

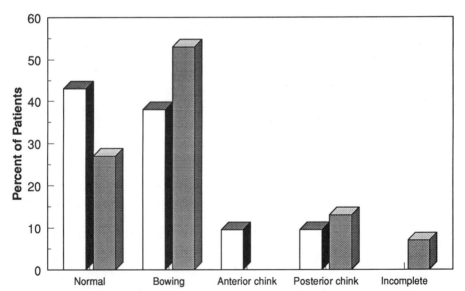

*Figure 5.4.* Glottal closure patterns of patients with Parkinson's disease as rated from stroboscopic video images. Open bars show data collected from flexible scope recordings whereas filled bars show data collected from rigid scope recordings.

jority of their patients had a bowed vocal fold configuration, Smith et al. reported that about 50% of their patients exhibited such a pattern. The exact percentage depended on the type of scope used to make the recording, i.e., flexible or rigid.

Perez et al. (1994) rated tremor, phase closure, symmetry, amplitude of vocal fold lateral excursion, and excursion of the mucosal wave in 22 patients with IPD. A majority of the patients (53%) exhibited tremor on at least one of the three experimental conditions. The incidence of tremor in each experimental condition is shown in Figure 5.5.

The incidence of abnormal strobe findings is shown in Figure 5.6. Many patients showed abnormal phase closure and phase symmetry, probably due to the hypotonic characteristics of Parkinson's patients.

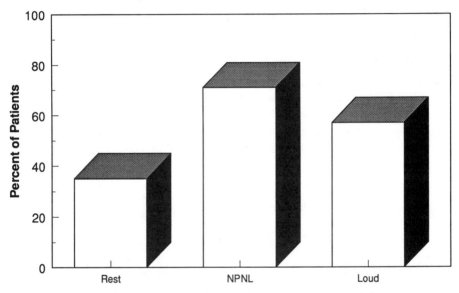

*Figure 5.5.* Incidence of tremor in structures of the larynx at rest and during phonation at conditions of normal loudness and normal pitch (NPNL) and loud voice among 22 patients with Parkinson's disease.

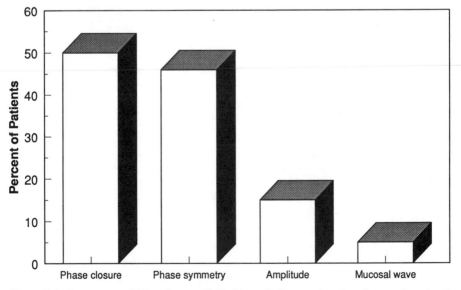

*Figure 5.6.* Percentage of 22 patients with Parkinson's disease showing abnormal strobe signs during phonation at normal loudness and normal pitch.

In spite of tremor, the stroboscopic signs of patients with Parkinson's disease can be rated successfully. These patients may show a variety of closure configurations including bowing, anterior chinks, posterior chinks, and incomplete. Some may show a normal closure pattern. The severity of closure probably depends on the degree of severity of the disease but in the early stages, one might expect mild symptoms, symptoms that might be correlated with the weak intensity voice often heard in these patients.

## PATHOPHYSIOLOGY

Muscle rigidity and squeezing of structures within the larynx may produce a symptom of strain/struggle in the voice. Unequal tensions in the vocal folds, as noted by Hanson et al. (1984), would be expected to produce aperiodicity, resulting in hoarseness or roughness in the voice. In more advanced stages of the disease process, patients often have much difficulty with chewing and swallowing. Management of saliva and drooling also are problematic. The typical characteristics of PD are mirrored in speech and voice production. Difficulty in initiating movement is seen in initiating speech attempts as it is in initiating walking. Muscle rigidity and hypokinesia are seen in the reduced range of motion of the speech mechanism, which results in reduced loudness (rigidity of respiratory and laryngeal muscles), monotone (rigidity of laryngeal muscles), and imprecise articulation (rigidity of all oral articulators). Tremor may be heard in the voice as well as seen in the extremities.

## *Shy-Drager Syndrome*

### PRIMARY VOICE SYMPTOM: HOARSENESS

### DESCRIPTION AND ETIOLOGY

Shy-Drager syndrome is a variant of Parkinson's disease, sometimes referred to as Parkinson's Plus. It is a disease of later middle age and affects males more often than females. The major characteristic of Shy-Drager is generalized autonomic nervous system failure. It is considered one of the degenerative neurological disorders that is characterized by multiple system atrophy, not all of which include autonomic nervous system dysfunction. The initial symptoms are postural hypotension (decrease of blood pressure when the patient stands), impotence, and sphincter problems. In their study of 12 patients with Shy-Drager syndrome, Hanson, Ludlow, and Bassich (1983) reported symptoms of weakness of the accessory muscles of respiration, respiratory obstruction, limited movement of the soft palate, and dysphagia. They suggest that these symptoms are indicative of extrapyramidal, pyramidal, and bulbar involvement.

Shy-Drager syndrome was first described in two cases by Shy and Drager (1960). In one case, they were able to examine the brain after the patient's death and reported changes in the spinal cord, autonomic ganglia, and medulla (i.e., marked changes in the inferior olives) and a reduced number of Purkinje cells in the cerebellum, as well as extensive changes in the substantia nigra and the caudate nucleus of the basal ganglia.

Williams, Hanson, and Calne (1979) reported on 12 cases of Shy-Drager syndrome in which 8 had moderate to severe bilateral abductor paresis or paralysis of the vocal folds. Two patients, upon initial examination, showed a unilateral paresis, but these patients eventually developed bilateral paralysis as the disease progressed. They concluded that the combination of vocal fold paralysis and respiratory difficulties in some of their patients may be consistent with a lesion in the nucleus ambiguus and the retrofacial nucleus. Denervation of the posterior cricoarytenoid muscle, the muscle

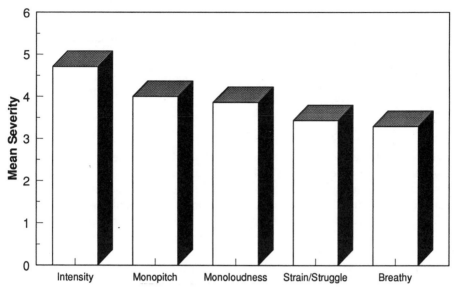

*Figure 5.7.* Rated severity of voice signs in 7 patients with Shy-Drager syndrome.

primarily responsible for vocal fold abduction, has been reported in Shy-Drager patients who had bilateral abductor vocal fold paralysis (Guidi, Bannister, & Gibson, 1981).

Linebaugh (1979) reviewed 35 patients with Shy-Drager syndrome who presented with a dysarthria. He identified three major types of dysarthria: ataxic, hypokinetic, and mixed. Fifteen of the 35 presented with ataxic dysarthria, which involves the cerebellum and affects the accuracy, force, range, and timing of speech movements; 11 exhibited a hypokinetic dysarthria in which the extrapyramidal system was affected, resulting in muscular rigidity; and nine showed a mixed dysarthria involving combinations of the extrapyramidal, cerebellar, and pyramidal systems. Linebaugh presented examples of patients with these various types and commented on how careful listening can help to distinguish among them.

## PERCEPTUAL VOICE SIGNS AND SYMPTOMS

The most complete description and study of the speech signs and symptoms of Shy-Drager syndrome was presented by Hanson, Ludlow, and Bassich (1983). They rated the speech of 12 Shy-Drager syndrome patients, using scales reported previously by Darley et al. (1969a). Shy-Drager syndrome patients were rated most severe on scales of rate of speaking (variable rate and rate[2]). The mean ratings on five voice scales are shown in Figure 5.7. The format of this figure is different from that of Figures 5.2 and 5.3. Hanson, Ludlow, and Bassich (1983) did not report the proportion of patients with aberrant ratings on the scales used, probably because of the small number of patients. Rather, the mean ratings were reported using a seven-point scale on which 1 means normal and 7 means very severe. Other speech scales on which these patients were rated as severe included intensity (this scale may relate to the overall level of voice), imprecise consonants, reduced stress, monopitch, and monoloudness. These authors performed a discriminant analysis of these ratings to determine if they could separate groups of Shy-Drager syndrome patients from Parkinsonism patients who

---

[2]Variable rate was defined as a rate of speaking that alternates between slow and fast. Rate was defined as a rate of speaking that is abnormally slow or abnormally rapid.

exhibit some of the same symptoms and from a group of normal subjects. Three scales did a very good job of distinguishing among these groups and included strain/struggle, glottal fry (a low pitch, popping sound), and monopitch. Shy-Drager patients were rated higher on impaired function on the scales of strain/struggle and glottal fry than the PD patients but lower (less impaired) on monopitch. Perceptual speech scales may be useful in distinguishing the Shy-Drager syndrome from IPD and normal speakers.

## ACOUSTIC SIGNS

Various indices of perturbation were reported by Ludlow and her colleagues (1983) for a group of seven patients with Shy-Drager, four male and three female. Measurements included perturbation (in msec), DLT (perturbation after removal of fundamental frequency due to linear trend), a diplophonia ratio, fundamental frequency, and duration of phonation. As a group, the Shy-Drager patients had a mean $f_0$ of 160.3 Hz compared to a $f_0$ of 127.6 Hz for age and sex matched controls; the difference was statistically significant suggesting perhaps greater vocal fold tension and/or muscle rigidity.[3] There were no statistically significant differences between the Shy-Drager and normal controls on any measure of frequency perturbation. The data provided some evidence of diplophonia, at least for two of the subjects. Although not statistically significant, the patients' diplophonia ratio was somewhat higher (1.418) than the normal controls' (1.046).

## MEASURABLE PHYSIOLOGICAL SIGNS

In a study of activity in the laryngeal muscles, Guidi et al. (1981) reported that all five of their Shy-Drager patients showed denervation of the posterior cricoarytenoid muscle, and two of the five showed fibrillation potentials in the interarytenoid muscle. Histological studies have shown marked atrophy of the posterior cricoarytenoid muscle (Bannister, Gibson, Michaels, & Oppenheimer, 1981). Interestingly, there was little evidence of cell losses in the nucleus ambiguus, suggesting a possible biochemical abnormality (Ludlow, Coulter, & Gentges, 1983). These electromyographic characteristics were very different from the muscle activity recorded in patients with IPD.

## OBSERVABLE PHYSIOLOGICAL SIGNS

The primary laryngoscopic sign seen in Shy-Drager syndrome is bilateral abductor vocal fold paresis. Hanson, Ludlow, and Bassich (1983) reported that 11 of their 12 patients presented moderate to severe abductor paresis (also reported by Williams, Hanson, & Calne, 1979). Longridge (1987) reported a case of Shy-Drager with bilateral vocal fold paralysis but did not specify whether it was of the adductor or abductor type.

We know of no studies in which the stroboscopic signs of patients with Shy-Drager syndrome have been reported.

## PATHOPHYSIOLOGY

Shy-Drager syndrome is a disease involving the pyramidal, extrapyramidal, and cerebellar systems. It may also involve atrophy of neurons in the brainstem and part

---

[3]This finding is somewhat strange because the group included males and females: it is well known that male fundamental frequencies are much lower than female fundamental frequencies. The statistical results may be accurate if the authors tested only the differences of fundamental frequency between the patient groups and their age and sex matched controls.

of the spinal cord (Bannister & Oppenheimer, 1972). It affects the control and coordination of speech and voice. Lesions that affect the upper motor neurons will result in the loss of muscle coordination. Lesions in the cerebellum will also affect muscle coordination, whereas lesions in the medulla and brainstem will affect the motor nuclei of the muscles serving the larynx, producing problems of muscle tone and function. Interestingly, the disease affects the neurons that control abductory function and not adductory function. The hyperadduction that results in strain/struggle in speech is produced by lesions higher in the brain. In many respects the disease is similar to IPD, but with its own unique features. The outlook for patients with Shy-Drager syndrome is bleak, with few surviving more than 5 or 10 years (Thomas & Schirger, 1970). The course of the disease is a steady increase in neuromuscular impairment that will eventually affect the respiratory muscles and compromise respiratory function.

## Amyotrophic Lateral Sclerosis (ALS)

### PRIMARY VOICE SYMPTOM: HOARSENESS OR STRAIN/STRUGGLE

### DESCRIPTION AND ETIOLOGY

Amyotrophic lateral sclerosis (ALS or Lou Gehrig's disease) is a progressive, degenerative disease of the central nervous system that involves both upper and lower motor neurons. As a result, the patient with amyotrophic lateral sclerosis may have symptoms such as spasticity (upper motor neuron symptom) along with muscle weakness (a symptom of lower motor neuron lesions). The lower motor neuron lesions usually affect the ventral horn cells. The incidence of amyotrophic lateral sclerosis is about 0.4 to 1.8 per 100,000 people (Janzen, Rae, & Hudson, 1988). The initial manifestation is muscle weakness, cramps, and fasciculation. The disease usually affects people later in life, although reports of early onset are known.

In the study by Carpenter, McDonald, and Howard (1988), 28% of 123 patients with amyotrophic lateral sclerosis presented symptoms in the head, neck, larynx, or voice. The mean age of these patients was 61, and the ratio between males and females was about equal. Of the patients presenting head/neck symptoms, 68% exhibited slurred speech, 14% had hoarseness, and 13% presented with dysphagia. On physical exam, the patients presented muscle weakness and fasciculation in various areas, as shown in Table 5.3. In many patients, excessive drooling may exist and presents unique problems for management.

Table 5.3. Percent of Patients with ALS Presenting Physical Abnormalities in the Head and Neck Region

| Area | Weakness | Fasciculations |
|---|---|---|
| Tongue | 66 | 54 |
| Extremities | 66 | 30 |
| Neck | 41 | 10 |
| Face | 2 | 38 |
| Palate and pharynx | 2 | 32 |
| Masseter muscle | 8 | 2 |

Speech signs in ALS include flaccid dysarthria or spastic dysarthria or both. A more detailed list of speech signs is presented in Table 5.4. There are many possible etiologies for this condition. Aronson (1990) listed infection, malignancy, and genetic defects. Janzen et al. (1988) added toxins, autoimmunity problems, and metabolic deficiencies. There is no effective treatment, although certain drugs have been used to ease the symptoms.

## PERCEPTUAL VOICE SIGNS AND SYMPTOMS

The primary symptom is hoarseness or harshness, with slurred speech as an additional symptom. In their classic study of the perceptual characteristics of dysarthria, Darley et al. (1969a) listed imprecise consonants, hypernasality, harsh voice, slow rate, and monopitch as the prominent speech characteristics in their group of 30 subjects with amyotrophic lateral sclerosis. Figure 5.8 presents a summary of the voice signs and symptoms found in a group of patients with amyotrophic lateral sclerosis patients, as reported by Aronson et al. (1968b). Similar speech and voice symptoms were reported by Carrow, Mauldin, and Shamblin (1974).

## ACOUSTIC SIGNS

Caruso and Burton (1987) reported that the stop gaps in stop consonant syllables and vowel duration were much longer in the speech of patients with amyotrophic lateral sclerosis than in normal speakers. Voice onset time in the two groups was very similar. These authors suggest that laryngeal structures may move more slowly in amyotrophic lateral sclerosis than in normal speakers. They point out that because the nucleus ambiguus is often affected, the neural control of adduction and abduction by the vocal folds may be impaired.

In a study primarily concerned with patients with other neurologic problems, Ramig et al. (1988) reported on the changes of $f_0$, jitter, shimmer, and harmonics-to-noise ratio (HNR) of a 69-year-old male recorded four times over a period of 6

*Table 5.4.* Frequency of Speech Deviations in Patients with ALS

|  | Percent |
| --- | --- |
| Harsh voice | 79.75 |
| Hypernasality | 74.68 |
| Breathy voice | 64.56 |
| Voice tremor | 63.29 |
| Strain/struggle voice | 59.49 |
| Imprecise consonants | 56.96 |
| Reduced intelligibility | 46.84 |
| Slow rate | 46.84 |
| Phonemes prolonged | 45.57 |
| Audible inspiration | 40.51 |
| Continuous phonation | 37.97 |
| High pitch | 37.97 |
| Phrases short | 36.71 |
| Inappropriate silences | 32.91 |
| Nasal emission | 30.28 |
| Vowels distorted | 24.05 |
| Low pitch | 7.59 |
| Fast rate | 2.53 |

months. Shimmer and HNR were most sensitive to the changes that occurred over the 6-month period. At the end of the recording sessions, the subject displayed greater acoustic instability. Additional data on this subject were reported by Ramig et al. (1990). The coefficient of amplitude and the coefficient of frequency, measures that reflect the long-term stability of phonation, were also greater for the patient than for his control. These data are consistent with the notion that ALS patients exhibit decreased phonatory control that is exacerbated by the progression of the disease.

Kent et al. (1991) reported abnormalities of fundamental frequency and perturbation in their group of 10 female patients with ALS. Kent et al. (1991) found that the fundamental frequency of their male patients with ALS (N = 32) was somewhat higher than the normal controls (127.4 Hz versus 112.8 Hz) (Table 5.5).

Strand, Buder, Yorkston, and Ramig (1993) also reported on fundamental frequency, intensity, jitter, shimmer, and SNR of four adult females with ALS. Although the patient data were different from the normal controls, the patients did show considerable variation of fundamental frequency both in sustained phonation and in phrase samples. All four patients exhibited greater jitter and shimmer than the control subject. One interesting facet of this study is the report of the perceptual voice characteristics of the four patients that should be considered when interpreting the acoustic data. One patient was characterized as having a strained-struggled voice quality whereas another exhibited breathy phonation with low volume. The other two subjects exhibited harsh voice quality with fluctuations of intensity and frequency.

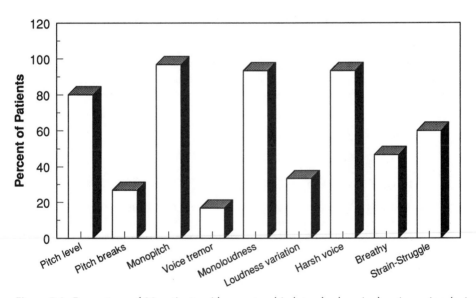

*Figure 5.8.* Percentage of 30 patients with amyotrophic lateral sclerosis showing voice deviations. Voice tremor was rated during contextual speech.

*Table 5.5.* Acoustic Measures in ALS

|  | Males | | Females | |
| --- | --- | --- | --- | --- |
|  | *ALS* | *Control* | *ALS* | *Control* |
| Fundamental frequency | 127.4 | 112.8 | 179 | 194.5 |
| Jitter (msec) | 0.11 | 0.12 | 0.24 | 0.07 |
| Shimmer (%) | 5.3 | 7 | 18.53 | 2.61 |
| SNR (dB) | 19.32 | 16.87 | 13.08 | 21.38 |

The group was heterogeneous and one should expect variation in the acoustic data. Such was the case in this report. ALS is a mixed dysarthria; some patients can exhibit symptoms characteristic of spasticity whereas others can exhibit a flaccid dysarthria. The acoustic features of each type of dysarthria are very different.

## MEASURABLE PHYSIOLOGICAL SIGNS

There have been no data reported on the physiological characteristics of the speech of ALS patients. However, electromyographic studies have been reported on nonlaryngeal muscles and reveal sporadic action potentials, a reduction in the number of potentials, and fibrillation. Similar findings might be expected in the laryngeal muscles.

## OBSERVABLE PHYSIOLOGICAL SIGNS

The larynx in amyotrophic lateral sclerosis usually presents a normal appearance (Aronson, 1990). However, it is possible to observe hyperadduction if the major component in the disease is spasticity. If the major component is flaccidity, one might expect incomplete closure, bowing and/or slower speed of vocal fold movement.

There have been no data reported on stroboscopic signs specifically in amyotrophic lateral sclerosis patients. However, signs typical of flaccid paralysis (reduced mucosal wave, incomplete closure) or those associated with problems affecting the upper motor neurons (spastic characteristics such as hyperadduction) would be consistent with the nature of the effects of the disease.

## PATHOPHYSIOLOGY

Amyotrophic lateral sclerosis impairs central nervous system control of the muscles of the larynx. Furthermore, if the lower motor neurons are affected, muscle tone and strength are affected. Patients may exhibit spastic phases or flaccid phases depending on the precise areas affected. Spastic effects might result in a strain/struggle type of voice whereas flaccid effects might reduce the efficiency of glottal valving.

## Huntington's Chorea (HC)

### PRIMARY VOICE SYMPTOM: HOARSENESS

### DESCRIPTION AND ETIOLOGY

Chorea refers to a hyperkinetic disorder in which there are abrupt, jerky, purposeless, movements of the head, neck, or limbs. There are several variants, including Sydenham's chorea (which is often associated with children) and Huntington's chorea (more often associated with adulthood). There are many causes of chorea, including trauma, neoplasms, cerebrovascular disorders, infection, compromised immune system, metabolic disturbances, intoxications, and drugs (Padberg & Bruyn, 1986). Some forms are linked to hereditary causes.

Huntington's chorea is a disease of the basal ganglia with an incidence of 4–7 per 100,000 (Merritt, 1979). It has a genetic basis; the child of an affected person has a 50% chance of developing the disease. It usually appears in the 3rd through 5th decades of life (average age = 38) (Brin, Fahn, Blitzer, Ramig, & Stewart, 1992), although it has been reported to appear as early as age 5 and as late as age 70 (Merritt, 1979). The basic signs are choreiform movements and progressive mental deterioration. The abnormal movements appear to increase with heightened emotional levels, are dramatically reduced during sleep, and affect any voluntary movements. Mentally, a patient with Huntington's chorea experiences a progressive loss of memory and intellectual capacity.

Ramig (1986) reasoned that generalized instability of muscle contraction (involuntary contractions, variable tone or tremor) would be expected to affect the muscles of the larynx. Therefore, disorders of phonation associated with Huntington's chorea would be likely.

## PERCEPTUAL VOICE SIGNS AND SYMPTOMS

The most prominent perceptual voice sign is harshness, followed by monopitch and strain/struggle voice quality (Aronson, 1990; Aronson, Brown, Litin, & Pearson, 1968a). Figure 5.9 presents the percentage of patients exhibiting the various voice signs rated by Darley et al. (1969a).

## ACOUSTIC SIGNS

Jarema, Kennedy, and Shoulson (1985) studied some acoustic characteristics in 12 adults with Huntington's chorea. There were 7 females with a mean age of 44 years and 5 males with a mean age of 42 years. The authors also collected these data for a normal-speaking group. They measured habitual (mean) fundamental frequency and intensity during sustained vowel production and obtained estimates of phonational range and maximum phonation time. Their data on fundamental frequency and vocal intensity are summarized in Table 5.6. There is no statistically significant difference

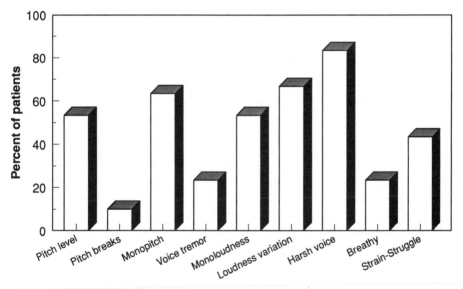

Figure 5.9. Percentage of 30 patients with Huntington's chorea showing voice deviations. Voice tremor was rated during contextual speech.

Table 5.6. Fundamental Frequency and Intensity Characteristics of the Speech of Patients with Huntington's Chorea

| | Female | | Male | |
|---|---|---|---|---|
| | Patient | Normal | Patient | Normal |
| Fundamental frequency (Hz) | | | | |
| Habitual | 166 | 182 | 106 | 103 |
| Low | 155 | 143 | 92 | 83 |
| High | 592 | 716 | 390 | 422 |
| Intensity (dB SPL) | | | | |
| Habitual | 71 | 71 | 74 | 72 |
| Soft | 68 | 66 | 71 | 66 |
| Loud | 100 | 108 | 104 | 106 |

between the patient and normal-speaking groups on habitual fundamental frequency. Although there were some restrictions at both ends of the patients' phonational and dynamic ranges, the differences compared to the normal control group were not statistically significant. The male patients in the study were found to produce shorter maximum phonation times (15 seconds) than the normal male speakers (23 seconds), but this difference was not statistically significant. However, the female patient phonation times (14 seconds versus 23 seconds) were significantly shorter than those for the normal group.

Ramig (1986) also measured some acoustic features in the speech of eight patients, four males and four females. She noted frequent abrupt low-frequency segments during a sustained vowel (sudden drop of fundamental frequency, then a return to almost the same fundamental frequency), voice arrests, and reduced duration of the sustained vowels /ah/, /ee/, and /oo/. Voice arrests (370–510 msec in mean duration) occurred in six of the eight patients. Mean vowel durations for the patients ranged from 0.50 to 9.75 seconds, whereas mean normal vowel durations on the same task were 14.61 seconds.

A later report by Ramig et al. (1988) reported further acoustic data on these eight patients. The patient group did not show large cycle-to-cycle variation but rather abrupt drops of fundamental frequency. Low-frequency segments occurred 102 times in the 27 vowel segments produced by these patients. Furthermore, another group of patients at risk for Huntington's chorea showed 34 instances of low-frequency drops in 90 vowel segments. These abrupt low-frequency segments support the hypothesis of increased phonatory instability in these patients.

Another study (Zwirner, Murry, & Woodson, 1991) compared measurements of fundamental frequency, standard deviation of fundamental frequency, jitter, shimmer, and SNR of 13 patients with Huntington's chorea. There was no statistically significant difference between the patients and normal controls on fundamental frequency. Frequency variability was much greater for the patient group as was jitter. Shimmer and SNR were different from the normal group but the difference was not statistically significant. Another interesting finding was the lack of a significant correlation between perceptual ratings of voice severity and any measure of perturbation or variability (standard deviation of fundamental frequency, jitter, shimmer, SNR).

## MEASURABLE PHYSIOLOGICAL SIGNS

Few measurable physiological data have been reported on voice in chorea. Jarema, Kennedy, and Shoulson (1985) measured airflow rates during sustained vowel production for their 12 adults with Huntington's chorea and found much higher flow rates (220 ml/sec for females, 320 ml/sec for males) than for their normal control subjects (178 ml/sec for females, 254 ml/sec for males). These data would suggest increased breathiness in patients with Huntington's chorea.

Ramig (1986) suggested that the previously noted voice arrests had to be associated with sudden adductory or abductory movements of the vocal folds, as they occurred much too fast to be produced by articulatory movements. This could be seen as indirect evidence of either hyper- or hypotense vocal folds.

## OBSERVABLE PHYSIOLOGICAL SIGNS

Usually, the larynges of patients with Huntington's chorea appear normal (Aronson, 1990). However, close observation may reveal short periods of adductory or abductory movement, especially in patients exhibiting voice arrests. Sudden shifts of fundamental frequency (usually downward) may be accompanied by jerky movements of the vocal folds. Further research is needed on the laryngoscopic signs of Huntington's chorea.

No data have been reported on the stroboscopic signs in Huntington's chorea. Because the movements in Huntington's chorea are very jerky and irregular, visualization of the larynx with stroboscopy might be difficult in some patients.

### PATHOPHYSIOLOGY

The jerky, sudden, and abrupt movements of Huntington's chorea would seriously interfere with the production of smooth, controlled sound. Patients have decreased phonatory stability. Sudden adduction of the vocal folds may result in intensity bursts or voice arrests. Sudden abductory bursts would be accompanied by excessive airflow and breathiness or aphonic episodes. It is possible for a patient to exhibit both conditions, although one or the other characteristic will probably be the most prominent.

## CEREBELLAR DISORDERS

### *Cerebellar Ataxia*

#### PRIMARY VOICE SYMPTOM: HOARSENESS

#### DESCRIPTION AND ETIOLOGY

Cerebellar ataxia is a disorder of the cerebellum. Its accompanying speech disorder is called ataxic dysphonia or, more generally, ataxic dysarthria. A lesion in the cerebellum results in a loss of muscle coordination and movement. Fulton and Dow (1937) considered two kinds of speech defects in cerebellar lesions: (*a*) errors in the rate, range, direction, and force of movements and (*b*) hypotonia. Kent, Netsell, and Abbs (1979) presented some acoustic evidence for scanning speech and suggested that it may be the result of the cerebellum's failing to properly integrate movements, or it may be due to an alteration in the motor programming plan of the cerebellum. In their study of ataxic dysarthria, Brown, Darley, and Aronson (1970) concluded that excess and equal stress plus irregular articulatory breakdown were the speech scales most suggestive of this condition.

The etiology of dysphonia in ataxic dysarthria is varied. In their study, Brown et al. (1970) reported that 3 patients had a neoplasm, 1 had experienced trauma, 1 had an infarct, 1 was thought to have multiple sclerosis, and 24 were diagnosed with cerebellar degeneration. They suggested that the important areas of the cerebellum serving speech were the vermis and the adjacent paravermis. Lechtenberg and Gilman (1978) implicate the left cerebellar hemisphere as important for the control of speech. Based on that implication, Kent, Netsell, and Abbs (1979) hypothesized that the right cerebral hemisphere must send its information to the left cerebellar hemisphere, making both hemispheres responsible for the control of speech prosody. If true, one might expect patients with ataxic dysarthria to have greater difficulty in the control of the suprasegmental features of speech (i.e., stress and intonation), both of which involve the vocal folds.

#### PERCEPTUAL VOICE SIGNS AND SYMPTOMS

In their rating study of the speech of patients with various kinds of neuromuscular diseases, Aronson et al. (1968a) noted the voice features of harshness, monopitch, too-low pitch, strain/struggle, and pitch breaks as prevalent in ataxic dysarthria. The percentage of patients showing these perceptual signs of the voice is shown in Figure 5.10.

Aronson (1990) noted that some ataxics may exhibit normal voice quality but that many will show harshness, monopitch, and monoloudness as characteristic perceptual features.

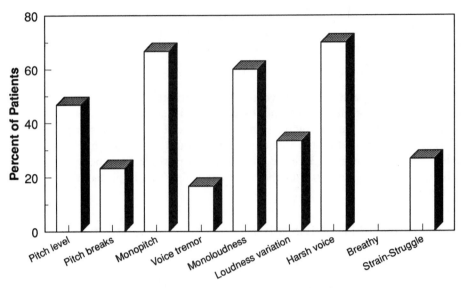

*Figure 5.10.* Percentage of 30 patients with ataxic dysarthria showing voice deviations. Voice tremor was rated during contextual speech.

## ACOUSTIC SIGNS

Kent, Netsell, and Abbs (1979) reported a study on the acoustic characteristics of the speech of five ataxic patients. They found abnormally long vowel and segment durations and strongly suggested that there were aberrations in the control of fundamental frequency. In an earlier study, Kent and Netsell (1975) reported on the speech characteristics of a female ataxic patient. Among other variables, they examined fundamental frequency contours during the production of words and sentences. They noted that many fundamental frequency contours had a monotone appearance, while others had marked variability of fundamental frequency. They suggested that ataxics may have more difficulty controlling fundamental frequency during speech than they have in articulating the phonemes. They also noted spectrographic evidence of harshness and/or vocal fry.

The fundamental frequency of ataxic dysphonics is very similar to normal speakers (Zwirner, Murry, & Woodson, 1991); however, the standard deviation of fundamental frequency of these patients was over three times as large (1.3 versus 6.1 Hz). Jitter was also much larger than normal. Patients also showed a difference of shimmer and SNR compared to the normal controls but the differences were not statistically significant.

These data support the notion of Kent and Netsell (1975) that persons with cerebellar ataxia have difficulty controlling fundamental frequency. Both the standard deviation of fundamental frequency and jitter reflect frequency variability and both are much larger than normal. Patients with cerebellar ataxia can produce the desired fundamental frequency but they have difficulty controlling it.

## MEASURABLE PHYSIOLOGICAL SIGNS

There appear to be no data available in the literature concerning the measurable physiological characteristics of the voice of ataxic patients. In their single-subject analysis, Kent and Netsell (1975) reported that cineradiographic analysis of the oral cavity during speech revealed abnormal but small anteroposterior lingual adjustments. Furthermore, they found that the patient's articulatory movements were longer in duration than normal movements. Thus, valving movements of the vocal folds might show abnormally long durations.

Brown et al. (1970) reported that electromyographic recordings were made on 6 of their 30 patients with ataxic dysarthria but failed to specify which muscles were studied. They reported normal electromyographic patterns in two patients, evidence of a motor lesion in one patient, and evidence of a peripheral neuropathy in three patients. Similar abnormalities might be found in the laryngeal muscles, although not in all patients.

### OBSERVABLE PHYSIOLOGICAL SIGNS

Aronson (1990) expects to find a normal-appearing larynx in patients with ataxic dysphonia. Evidence of reduced speed of adduction or abduction during valving and movements of the vocal folds might be observed on careful study. There are no reported data on the stroboscopic signs in patients with ataxic dysphonia.

### PATHOPHYSIOLOGY

Ataxic dysphonia or dysarthria seems to be characterized by hypotonia and an incoordination of muscles. Hypotonia manifests itself as a delay in the generation of a force, a reduced rate of muscular contraction, and a reduced range of movement (Brown, Darley, & Aronson, 1970; Kent & Netsell, 1975; Kent, Netsell, & Abbs, 1979). Reduced muscle activity may account for the reduced fundamental frequency range during conversational speech, since in order to increase vocal pitch, cricothyroid muscle activity must be increased. Reduced muscle tone may also account for hoarseness in ataxic voices because of tension differences between the two vocal folds. Hypotonicity will have a similar effect on the control of intensity, although few data have been reported on this acoustic variable. Incoordination of phonation may be manifested by difficulty in controlling the magnitude and extent of laryngeal movements as well as the control of the magnitude and extent of articulatory movements.

## *Arnold-Chiari Malformation (Chiari II Malformation)*

The Arnold-Chiari malformation is a congenital anomaly of the hindbrain where the brainstem and cerebellum are squeezed into the cervical portion of the spinal column, causing injury to the cerebellum, medulla, and lower cranial nerves (Bralley, Bull, Gore, & Edgerton, 1978; Merritt, 1979). It was first described by Arnold (1894) and more extensively by Chiari (1896). There are actually four types of malformations originally discussed by Chiari. Types I and II are often referred to as the Arnold-Chiari type (Bamberger-Bozo, 1987; Salam & Adams, 1978). Type I is one in which only the cerebellar tonsils are displaced. Types III and IV are much more severe and in some cases incompatible with life. In type II, malformation of the medulla, cerebellum, and mesencephalon are encountered usually with a lumbar meningomyelocele. Interestingly, many of the clinical manifestations of type II occur after birth (Bamberger-Bozo, 1987). Infants will usually have difficulty swallowing, apneic episodes, laryngeal paralysis, stridor, and occasionally arm weakness. Most laryngeal paralysis is the abductor type.

In some cases, this malformation can result in vocal fold paralysis (Rullan, 1991) in which voice symptoms will appear that are similar to cerebellar ataxia (discussed earlier) or to lesions affecting the medulla or the peripheral nerves as they leave the cranium and causing flaccid paralysis. In the latter case, perceptual, acoustic, and physiological signs as seen in recurrent nerve paralysis would be expected (see "Peripheral Nerve Lesions" for a more complete discussion.)

## LOWER MOTOR NEURON DISORDERS (BRAINSTEM AND MEDULLA)

### *Spasmodic Dysphonia*

#### PRIMARY VOICE SYMPTOM: STRAIN/STRUGGLE

#### DESCRIPTION AND ETIOLOGY

Spasmodic dysphonia, according to Ludlow (1995), is a "focal dystonia affecting laryngeal muscle control during speech" (p. 436). It has received much attention over the past 15–20 years, perhaps out of proportion to its incidence. It is a relatively rare voice disorder, although judging from the many reports in the literature it appears that its numbers have increased. Perhaps this is due to the availability of methods of providing some form of symptom relief or to increased awareness of and knowledge about the disorder. Spasmodic dysphonia seems to occur equally in men and women (Aronson, Brown, Litin, & Pearson, 1968b), with onset most frequently in middle age, although we have seen patients as young as 20 years with a history of onset in the teens.

The nature of the onset of spasmodic dysphonia is variable. In some patients, onset is associated with a major upper respiratory infection (Aronson, Brown, Litin, & Pearson, 1968b), in others a traumatic emotional event is identified (Aronson, 1990; Brodnitz, 1976), and in still other patients the onset is insidious, beginning as a mild hoarseness and progressing to interrupted, strained phonation. The progression of symptoms may be rapid or may take place over a number of years.

In the past, thinking about the etiology of spasmodic dysphonia has taken two major forms (Aronson, 1990; Salamy & Sessions, 1980). Some authors have advocated a psychological origin (Arnold, 1959; Block, 1965; Brodnitz, 1976; Heaver, 1959; Henschen & Burton, 1978) , whereas others have implicated a neurological origin (Aminoff, Dedo, & Izdebski, 1978; Aronson, Brown, Litin, & Pearson, 1968a, 1968b; Blitzer & Brin, 1992; Rabuzzi & McCall, 1972; Robe, Brumlik, & Moore, 1960; Shaefer, 1983).

One rationale for the psychological etiology is that patients often report a traumatic emotional event closely associated with the awareness of the onset of symptoms. Brodnitz (1976) described the case of a woman whose symptoms appeared after her husband tried to kill her. Other patients have reported severe marital crises, an accident, the death of a loved one, or the threat of loss of a job preceding the onset of the symptoms. Another reason may be the difficulty in differentiating the symptoms and signs of spasmodic dysphonia from those found in certain manifestations of psychogenic or muscle tension dysphonias. Advocates of the psychological etiology theory point to some success in therapy (voice or psychiatric) or to relief of symptoms with the use of tranquilizing or neuroleptic drugs (Brodnitz, 1976) as positive evidence of the correctness of the theory. Advocates of a neurological etiology would suggest that these patients had perhaps been incorrectly diagnosed.

Advocates of the neurological etiology of spasmodic dysphonia point to the sizable body of evidence of associated neurological signs in these patients (Aronson, Brown, Litin, & Pearson, 1968b) and to the documented existence of abnormal findings in various tests of brain function (Aminoff, Dedo, & Izdebski, 1978; Dordain & Dordain, 1972; Finitzo-Hieber, Freeman, Gerling, Dobson, & Schaeffer, 1982; Robe, Brumlik, & Moore, 1960; Shaefer, 1983). Many of these authors also point out that there has been little actual documentation of symptom relief as a result of voice therapy or in response to psychiatric treatment. Reports of successful treatment have been anecdotal (Cooper & Cooper, 1977), and, moreover, the lack of success of these treatment protocols for patients with spasmodic dysphonia has been extensively noted (Aronson, 1990). On the other hand, there have been reports of symptom relief in patients with spasmodic dysphonia who have undergone a recurrent nerve section (Dedo, 1976; Dedo & Izdebski, 1981, 1983; Izdebski, Dedo, & Shipp, 1981) or BOTOX injection (Blitzer, Brin, Stewart, Aviv, & Fahn, 1992; Ford, Bless, & Patel, 1992; Ludlow, 1990; Shaefer et al., 1992; Woo, Colton, Casper, & Brewer, 1992; Zwirner, Murry, Swenson, & Woodson, 1991).

Recently, there appears to be a general consensus in the literature that spasmodic dysphonia is a problem with a neurological substrate. The exact locus of the dysfunction is not clear although many point to the basal ganglia or associated structures as the most likely location (Blitzer & Brin, 1992; Izdebski, 1992; Swenson, Zwirner, Murry, & Woodson, 1992). The problem probably has many causes (Izdebski, 1992) and may be linked to other neurological disorders (Swenson, Zwirner, Murry, & Woodson, 1992). Aronson (1990) believes that spasmodic dysphonia should be considered a disorder that may have either a neurological or a psychological etiology. In some cases, the etiology may be in doubt or idiopathic.

Izdebski (1992) presented a model of spasmodic dysphonia in which sudden or sustained increases of muscle activity occur, probably in response to faulty processing of afferent information about various events within the larynx such as the variation of air pressures during phonation. The symptoms are absent in vegetative tasks and in speech tasks that do not involve phonation. Thus, in a whisper, symptoms are absent or minimal because there is no variation of air pressures or vocal fold movement. Effective treatment should focus on reducing the afferent information to the central processing unit (e.g., basal ganglia) or by reducing the motor response because of faulty input processing. Section or crush of the recurrent laryngeal nerve would potentially remove sensory input as well as motor control. Injection of botulinum toxin (BOTOX) reduces the motor response to any faulty input. The focal nature of spasmodic dysphonia (that is, involvement of only a few muscles) suggests that specific therapeutic techniques should be most effective in obtaining symptom relief. Perhaps, this explains why the use of drugs systemically has been reported to have little lasting effect on the amelioration of the symptoms in spasmodic dysphonia.

Another distinction that should be made concerning this problem is whether the symptoms are indicative of an adductor (closing) type of disorder or an abductor (opening) type of disorder. The specific symptoms of each form are quite different (discussed later in "Perceptual Voice Symptoms and Signs"). Presumably, the underlying pathophysiology will also differ, and the form of treatment should differ. Some authors (Hartman & Aronson, 1981; Shipp, Mueller, & Zwitman, 1980) have even suggested that abductor spasmodic dysphonia is so dissimilar to the adductor type that it should be given a name more indicative of its pathophysiology. Hartman and Aronson (1981) have suggested the term "intermittent breathy dysphonia," whereas Shipp et al. (1980) advocate the term "intermittent abductory dysphonia."

Another common name for spasmodic dysphonia is spastic dysphonia. Many believe that the use of the term "spastic" is inappropriate. "Spastic" implies lesions in the corticobulbar or corticospinal (pyramidal) systems. That does not seem to be the case in this disorder. Current evidence suggests that the underlying disease state in spasmodic dysphonia affects structures in the extrapyramidal system. Aronson et al. (1968b) suggested that the term "spasmodic" would be more appropriate.

## PERCEPTUAL VOICE SIGNS AND SYMPTOMS

### *Adductor Spasmodic Dysphonia*

The most characteristic symptom (and sign) is the struggle and strain to talk, in association with intermittent stoppages of voice (Aronson, 1990; Aronson, Brown, Litin, & Pearson, 1968b; Brodnitz, 1976). Associated symptoms may include hoarseness, harshness, and tremor (Fig. 5.11). Other patients present with a creaking, choked, tense, or squeezed voice with extreme tension noted in the entire speech production system. Perceptual signs include strain/struggle, sudden interruption of voicing, tension, loudness and pitch variations, pitch breaks, and stoppages of phonation. According to Ludlow (1995), voice stoppages occur primarily in vowel productions.

### *Abductor Spasmodic Dysphonia*

Descriptions of the abductor type of spasmodic dysphonia vary. Some authors describe intermittent episodes of breathy dysphonia, drops in pitch, and vowel prolongations (Hartman & Aronson, 1981; Merson & Ginsberg, 1979; Zwitman, 1979). Aronson (1973, 1990) states that in many respects it is the mirror image of adductor spasmodic dysphonia. Ludlow (1995) describes the perceptual attribute characteristic of the abductor type of spasmodic dysphonia as a delay in voice onset following production of voiceless consonants. Close attention to the episodes of voice interruption in these patients confirms the preponderance of difficulty associated with the transition from voiceless to voiced phonemes.

## ACOUSTIC SIGNS

There have been considerable data reported in the literature about the various acoustic signs accompanying spasmodic dysphonia.

### *Fundamental Frequency*

Davis, Boone, Carroll, Davenzia, and Harrison (1988) reported the average fundamental frequencies during a reading passage for 16 female and 7 male patients with

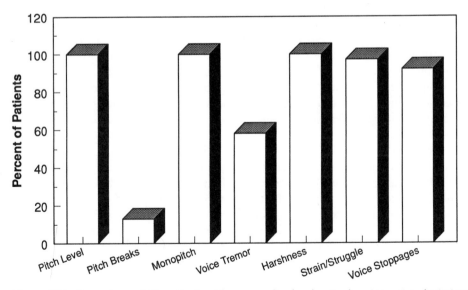

*Figure 5.11.* Percentage of 31 patients with spasmodic dysphonia showing voice deviations. Voice tremor was rated during contextual speech.

adductor spasmodic dysphonia and compared these data to those of a set of control subjects. The female patients had a mean fundamental frequency of 162 Hz compared to a mean fundamental frequency of 175 Hz for the 17 female control subjects. The male patients had a mean fundamental frequency of 134 Hz compared to a mean fundamental frequency of 106 Hz for 7 male controls. These authors also reported that the spasmodic dysphonia patients had a much greater variation of fundamental frequency during the passage than the controls (21.89 semitones [ST] for females and 14.79 ST for males compared to 12.29 ST for normal females and 11.89 ST for normal males).

Fritzell, Feuer, Haglund, Knutsson, and Schiratski (1982) analyzed the distribution of fundamental frequency in the voices of four patients (three males and one female) reading a short passage. Mean fundamental frequency ranged from 111 to 238 Hz. The distribution of fundamental frequency was bimodal, with a major peak centered above 200 Hz and a minor peak centered around 150 Hz. These patients underwent section of the recurrent laryngeal nerve for relief of symptoms (see Chapter 8). Postsurgically, the fundamental frequency distribution was much lower (mean fundamental frequencies ranged from 125 to 171 Hz) and the distribution was unimodal.

Merson and Ginsberg (1979) reported mean fundamental frequencies of 161.3 Hz and 203.8 Hz for two female patients with abductor spasmodic dysphonia reading a sentence.

### Vocal Intensity

Hartman and Aronson (1981) reported the amplitude variations observed in the speech of 17 abductor-type spasmodic dysphonia patients. They found a steady but random variation of amplitude in some patients, rhythmic variation in other patients, and evidence of moments of breathiness in still other patients. We know of no data on vocal intensity in the adductor type of spasmodic dysphonia. It has been our experience, however, that some of these patients use much-reduced intensity levels in conversation, even to the point of aphonic whisper. This is perhaps a compensatory behavior adopted in order to avoid voice stoppages.

### Long-Term Average Spectrum

Izdebski (1984) measured the long-term average spectrum (LTAS, a spectrum computed over a sentence or paragraph) in 23 patients with adductor spasmodic dysphonia. Figure 5.12 illustrates his results. The solid line shows the spectrum of a female speaker before surgery (recurrent nerve section), and the dotted line shows the same patient after surgery. Note the high levels of high frequency energy in the speech before surgery, but the dramatic decrease of high frequency energy after surgery.

Fritzell et al. (1982) analyzed the LTAS in the voices of four patients reading a short passage. They reported only a slight difference of spectral shape and levels after surgery. Because there was no control group, it is not known whether the levels of energy at the higher frequencies were greater than normal. Informal comparisons of the data presented by Fritzell et al. (1982) to those presented by Hammarberg, Fritzell, Gauffin, and Sundberg (1986) for normal speakers suggests that the patient group exhibited greater than normal energy levels in the high frequencies.

Hartman, Abbs, and Vishwanat (1988) observed pronounced peaks between 4 and 7 Hz in the spectrum of sustained /ah/s produced by four patients with adductor spasmodic dysphonia. These peaks may be indicative of vocal tremor. The finding of low-frequency tremor in the frequency spectrum of these patients is of interest. Wolfe and Bacon (1976), using spectrographic analysis of a patient with adductor spasmodic dysphonia, showed a breakdown in the harmonic structure of vowels, dark areas on the

*Figure 5.12.* Long-time average spectra of a female patient with spasmodic dysphonia before and after recurrent nerve section.

spectrogram (indicating greater loudness), and sudden changes of gray levels on the spectrogram, indicating the irregular variation of voicing present in adductor spasmodic dysphonia (Fig. 5.13). They also reported spectrographic findings for a patient with what appears to be abductor spasmodic dysphonia, in which there is evidence of interruptions of voicing, as well as irregularly spaced vertical striations indicating a variation of voicing associated with the strain and struggle to speak. Zwitman (1979) reported similar findings for two patients with abductor spasmodic dysphonia. He also reported that voiceless stops seem to be distinguished from voiced stops by a sustained frication during the voiceless stops. Some of the spectrographic features of abductor spasmodic dysphonia can be seen in Figure 5.13.

### MEASURABLE PHYSIOLOGICAL SIGNS

Several studies have reported airflows and air pressures for spasmodic dysphonia patients. Hirano, Koike, and von Leden (1968) reported flows within the normal range for their eight spasmodic dysphonia patients, whereas other studies have reported low (Casper, Colton, & Brewer, 1985; Davis, Boone, Carroll, Darvenzia, & Harrison, 1988; Farmakides & Boone, 1960; Hirano, 1974, 1981b; Hollien, Dew, & Phillips, 1971; Javkin, Antonanzas-Barros, & Maddieson, 1987) to very low flows (Briant, Blair, Cole, & Singer, 1983; Garrett & Healey, 1987; Hill, 1938; Hollien, 1975). In adductor spasmodic dysphonia, patients may exhibit strain during voicing, which may produce small glottal apertures through which air can flow. Low flows would be expected in this situation. On the other hand, in abductor spasmodic dysphonia, high flows would be expected as a result of the impaired glottal closure, which allows large quantities of airflow. Merson and Ginsberg (1979) reported such large flows in two patients with abductor spasmodic dysphonia (e.g., 321 ml/sec on a sustained /ah/ vowel, 400 ml/sec and 435 ml/sec during sentence production for two patients). We have shown very low average flow rates in patients with adductor spasmodic dysphonia (72 ml/sec) (Woo, Colton, Casper, & Brewer, 1992). Airflow rates increased after nerve section (232 ml/sec) or BOTOX (138 ml/sec).

*Figure 5.13.* Broad band spectrogram of a patient with abductor-type spasmodic dysphonia (left panel) and adductor-type spasmodic dysphonia (right panel). The utterance was the word "colors."

Shipp, Izdebski, Schutte, and Morrissey (1988) studied subglottal air pressure magnitudes in two patients with adductor spasmodic dysphonia. They reported much higher pressures (13–14 cm/H$_2$O) than normal (about 6 cm/H$_2$O). These very high pressures are consistent with patients' reports of the increased effort required to speak. The elevated pressures in combination with the low flows suggest increased glottal resistance during voicing for patients with adductor spasmodic dysphonia.

## OBSERVABLE PHYSIOLOGICAL SIGNS

### Laryngoscopy

Anatomically, the larynx appears essentially normal. However, during phonation it is possible to observe the hyperadduction of the adductor type of spasmodic dysphonia or the inefficient closure of the vocal folds in the abductor variety. Hartman and Aronson (1981) reported the appearance of bowed vocal folds in 2 of 17 patients with otherwise normal-looking vocal folds. Hartman et al. (1988) reported the observations of quick adductory movements of the true vocal folds, the ventricular folds, and much of the supraglottal structures in one patient; small, irregular movements of the true vocal folds in another patient; and, in a third patient, periodic laryngospasms. In the study reported by Davis et al. (1988), most patients had normal laryngoscopic exams, but interruption of voicing was reported to occur in seven patients due to action of the true vocal folds, in two patients tremor seemed to cause the interruption, and in four other patients the ventricular folds appeared to cause the voice stoppage. Blitzer and Brin (1992) advocate the use of flexible fiberoptic laryngoscopy to study the hyperadduction characteristics of spasmodic dysphonia.

### Stroboscopy

Few data have been reported on the vibratory characteristics of patients with spasmodic dysphonia as seen via stroboscopy. Fritzell et al. (1982) report that stroboscopy was carried out prior to recurrent nerve section, but no data were presented. Postsurgically, two patients showed symmetrical vocal fold vibrations, indicating a return of function to the muscle. Because patients with spasmodic dysphonia have difficulty in sustaining phonation, stroboscopic visualization of the vocal folds might be unproductive.

## PATHOPHYSIOLOGY

The pathophysiology of both adductor and abductor spasmodic dysphonia is not well understood. High levels of muscle activity are seen in the thyroarytenoid muscles of some, but not all, patients with adductor spasmodic dysphonia. Muscle hypertonia or hypotonia for various groups of speakers (i.e., adductor spasmodic dysphonia, abductor spasmodic dysphonia, and normal speakers) has not been well studied or compared. The mechanism for spasmodic bursts of increased activity in specific muscles is not clear.

The spasm activity of the vocal folds, be it adductory or abductory, will have a pronounced effect on the production of sound. Excessive adductory forces will require greater than normal pressures to force the vocal folds apart during phonation. Greater air pressures will be associated with greater sound pressure levels and a more rapid opening and closing phase of the vocal folds. Rapid closing phases are associated with the production of greater energy in the higher frequencies and high energy, high frequency spectra. The intermittent nature of the problem will produce wide variations of spectrum and fundamental frequency unless some compensatory mechanism is employed in the attempt to maintain a steady, smooth flow of speech. In abductory spasmodic dysphonia, the sudden spasm results in a sudden increase of airflow and relatively short closed times. The combination of rapid airflows and short closed time would be expected to produce much less energy in the higher frequencies of the spectrum. The voice will be perceived as intermittently breathy and weak. Again, there are periods of normal vocal fold vibration, but it is the sudden, unexpected stoppages that create havoc in the production of voice and speech.

## OTHER CONSIDERATIONS

In many patients with spasmodic dysphonia, other neurological signs will appear, including voice tremor, jaw or facial jerks, hand or limb tremor, hyperreflexia, sucking reflex, torticollis, or asymmetries in the face or palate (Aronson, Brown, Litin, & Pearson, 1968b; Davis, Boone, Carroll, Darvenzia, & Harrison, 1988). The high incidence of tremor in spasmodic dysphonia patients suggests that perhaps a proportion of patients diagnosed with spasmodic dysphonia are in fact patients with essential tremor (Aronson, Brown, Litin, & Pearson, 1968a). On the other hand, it is possible that in some cases spasmodic dysphonia is another manifestation of essential tremor (Aronson & Hartman, 1981; Davis, Boone, Carroll, Darvenzia, & Harrison, 1988). At the very least, the frequency of occurrence of additional neurological signs suggests that spasmodic dysphonia may have as one etiology a neurological substrate somewhere in the brain, probably in the extrapyramidal system (Charcot, 1881).

Sharbrough, Stockard, and Aronson (1975) reported brainstem abnormalities in 7 of their 18 spasmodic dysphonia patients. They concluded that spasmodic dysphonia is "a symptom due to organic CNS disease which, in some cases, incidentally produces asymptomatic slowing of conduction within the brainstem auditory pathway" (p. 200).

Patients with spasmodic dysphonia may show abnormal auditory brainstem responses (Finitzo-Hieber, Freeman, Gerling, Dobson, & Schaeffer, 1982); that is, the capacity of the brainstem to conduct impulses is impaired. Further, spasmodic dysphonia may be a disease involving multiple cranial nerves that when stressed break down and disrupt the speech system (Shaefer, 1983). Such a notion may explain why patients with spasmodic dysphonia present such variable symptoms.

Blitzer and his colleagues (Blitzer & Brin, 1991, 1992; Blitzer, Brin, Fahn, & Lovelace, 1988; Blitzer, Lovelace, Brin, Fahn, & Fink, 1985; Brin, Fahn, Blitzer, Ramig, & Stewart, 1992) placed spasmodic dysphonia as a member of the family of dystonias. Dystonias are characterized by uncontrolled spasmodic muscle contractions. Dystonias may begin at any age but many patients show either an early onset (before age 26) or late onset. They may be focal (restricted to a few muscles), segmental (involving a group of muscles), or general (involving larger areas of the body). Examples of focal dystonias are blepharospasm (involuntary eye closures), torticollis (neck twisting), and writer's cramp. Focal dystonias are apparent during the execution of a task and are not usually seen when the affected structure is at rest. Blitzer and his colleagues believe that spasmodic dysphonia is an action induced dystonia involving the larynx. They found tremor in only 25% of their patients and question the hypothesis proposed by Aronson (Aronson & Hartman, 1981) that some spasmodic dysphonias are a manifestation of essential tremor. The tremor is irregular and can sometimes be reduced through compensatory maneuvers (Brin, Fahn, Blitzer, Ramig, & Stewart, 1992; Folkins, 1978; Kinney, Kado, & Royner, 1972). Brin states:

> Adductor spasmodic dysphonia is characterized by abnormal involuntary co-contraction of the vocalis muscle complex muscles (sic) resulting in inappropriate adduction of the vocal folds. As an action-induced, "task specific," or "functional" movement disorder, the muscles and anatomical structures are normal at rest but move inappropriately with action. Conversely, abductor SD is characterized by action-induced inappropriate co-contraction of the posterior cricoarytenoid muscles during the action of speaking, resulting in inappropriate abduction of the vocal cords. (Brin, Fahn, Blitzer, Ramig, & Stewart, 1992)

Dystonias can be induced by trauma, may have a genetic link and show a variety of midbrain, brainstem abnormalities. Often, there is a psychological component which may have developed in response to the dystonia and the patient's efforts to deal with the problem.

Spasmodic dysphonia has been very resistant to treatment. Drugs do not alleviate the symptoms in most patients; surgery of the recurrent laryngeal nerve has been shown to have limited success; speech therapy and/or psychotherapy do little to relieve the symptoms. BOTOX injection offers some relief but is not a true long-term solution to the problem.

## DIFFERENTIATING SPASMODIC DYSPHONIA FROM OTHER DYSPHONIAS

Although a number of features of spasmodic dysphonia, psychogenic dysphonia, and musculoskeletal tension (hyperfunctional) dysphonia may be similar in some respects, careful history taking, examination, and analysis of characteristics of speech production will reveal unique features of each. Patients with psychogenic problems will frequently reveal a long history marked by the presence of stress; those with hyperfunctional dysphonia may report a clearly defined period of increased stresses and tensions; and the patient with spasmodic dysphonia will more frequently report increased stress since the onset of the symptoms.

The voice symptoms in the patient with psychogenic problems may be variable with return of normal voice for hours, days, or even weeks at a time; may be slightly bizarre in their presentations; show no pattern of phonemic variability; are not present in reflexive acts with associated phonation; show a consistent "phonatory set" during flexible endoscopic laryngeal examination; and often respond well to voice therapy. In contrast, patients with spasmodic dysphonia present with minimal variability and no instances of normal voice for an appreciable length of time. The symptoms are usually in keeping with the underlying nature of the problem (not bizarre); are spasmodic, not constant, in presentation and can be visualized to be so on laryngoscopic examination; show a pattern of phonemic variability (hyperadduction on voiced segments or difficulty in voiceless to voiced transition); have voice arrests as a very characteristic feature; and do not respond well to voice therapy.

Persons with hyperfunctional dysphonia usually present with symptoms that tend to be fairly consistent; do not vary phonemically; are characterized by consistent rather than episodic vocal tension, which is visible on examination but is responsive to alteration through guided probes and suggestions; and respond well to voice therapy.

## Essential Tremor

### PRIMARY VOICE SYMPTOM: TREMOR

### CLASSIFICATION OF TREMOR

There are various types of tremor that may have differing etiologies (central, peripheral, or both), characteristic timing features, and unique characteristics of presentation. Tremor may be present as an isolated symptom or it may be one characteristic of a more generalized neurological disorder.

Tremor is characterized by relatively regular, involuntary movements of the distal or proximal muscles. Everyone has some degree of normal tremor, which ranges in frequency from 6 to 12 Hz. Abnormal tremor has a lower frequency range, larger amplitudes, and may interfere with purposeful movements. Tremor may occur while a structure is at rest (resting tremor) or in action (action tremor). Action tremor may consist of postural tremor (when holding a structure in position), contraction tremor, and/or intention tremor (Brin, Fahn, Blitzer, Ramig, & Stewart, 1992). It may be focal or more generalized.

Essential tremor is a disorder of the central nervous system that may result in tremor in the head, limbs, tongue, palate, and larynx. It tends to start in the hands and then progresses to the arms, head, neck, face, and so on (Brown & Simonson, 1963). "Essential tremor is typically absent at rest, maximal during maintenance of a posture, attenuated during movement and often accentuated at the termination of movement" (Brin, Fahn, Blitzer, Ramig, & Stewart, 1992; Emanuel & Sansone, 1969). Typically, the frequency of tremor in patients with essential tremor is between 3 and 7 Hz (Brin, Fahn, Blitzer, Ramig, & Stewart, 1992).

### DESCRIPTION AND ETIOLOGY

In some patients voice tremor may be the primary or sole characteristic. In the Brown and Simonson study (1963), only 6 of 31 essential tremor patients exhibited isolated voice tremor, while the remaining 25 had, in addition to voice tremor, tremor in the head or extremities or both. Some have reported voice tremor in 10–20% of their patients (Brin, Fahn, Blitzer, Ramig, & Stewart, 1992). Lou and Jankovic (1991), reporting on 350 patients with essential tremor, found only one case of voice tremor as the sole symptom, gradual onset of tremor, and frequent occurrence of family members with some kind of tremor. Seventeen patients had associated neurological signs, including a positive sucking reflex, spasmodic torticollis, bilateral facial spasms, incoordination, and diadochokinesis.

Larsson and Sjogren (1960) reported that essential tremor occurred more frequently in males, with a mean age of onset of 48 years. Aronson and Hartman (1981) reported the mean age of onset at 57 years. They also found extralaryngeal tremor in 93% of their patients. In their study of 678 patients with essential tremor, Koller, Busenbark, and Miner (1994) found that about 49% were female and 51% male. The average age of onset was 45.3 years. About 90% of the patients had tremor affecting either hand; about 20% had head tremor with smaller numbers of patients with tremors of the leg, chin, trunk, and tongue.

Thus, essential tremor seems to be associated with aging, although the reasons for this are unclear. The highest prevalence is in the 7th decade of life. Heredity may affect the development of the tremor. About one half of patients with essential tremor have a history of an affected family member (Young, 1986). In sudden onset cases, Brown and Simonson (1963) suggested that some kind of arterial disease may have been responsible.

It is difficult to determine the locus of the central nervous system lesion that causes essential tremor. Critchley (1949) suggested that the extrapyramidal system is involved, but it is possible that other structures might be affected. Brin et al. (1992) suggest that tremor may be the result of oscillation in the olivocerebellar tracts. Young (1986) noted that a ventrolateral thalamotomy reduced or eliminated the tremor. There may be a possibility of dysfunction in the cerebellum as a cause of the tremor (Young, 1986).

## PERCEPTUAL VOICE SIGNS AND SYMPTOMS

The most prominent voice symptom and sign is tremor, a regular modulation of frequency or intensity, that is most noticeable during prolonged production of a vowel but is also apparent during contextual speech. In 100% of their patients with essential tremor, Aronson et al. (1968b) reported tremor on a sustained /ah/ vowel, (only tremor in contextual speech is shown in Figure 5.14) as well as harshness and strain/struggle. Figure 5.14 presents a summary of the voice symptoms in essential tremor as reported in the Aronson et al. (1968b) study.

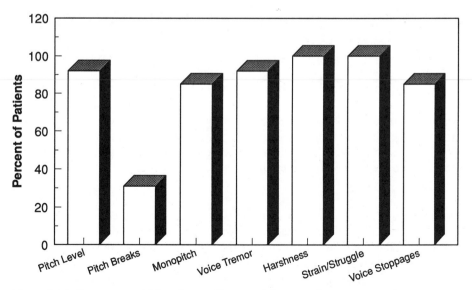

*Figure 5.14.* Percentage of 26 patients with essential tremor showing voice deviations. Voice tremor was rated during contextual speech.

In general, the voice of essential tremor patients may be described as sounding quavery and tremulous. Some patients will have a relatively constant and noticeable tremor during speech. Some may have such severe tremor that stoppage of voice occurs, as reported by Ardran, Kinsbourne, and Rushworth (1966).

## ACOUSTIC SIGNS

There are few data on many of the acoustic signs in essential tremor. Most studies have concentrated on the variation of amplitude during sustained vowel production. Brown and Simonson (1963) measured the rate of tremor from oscillograms of 23 patients. Tremor frequencies of 5–6 Hz were measured in most patients. Ardran et al. (1966) reported spectrographic evidence of low-amplitude noise during the production of monosyllabic words by a single patient. This noise, they suggested, gave evidence of breathiness in the patients' speech. Aronson and Hartman (1981) analyzed the tremor in oscillograms of 14 patients with essential tremor and reported a mean tremor frequency of 5.7 Hz. Lebrun, Devreux, Rousseau, and Darimont (1982) reported a tremor frequency of 4 Hz in the voice of their 84-year-old patient. They also observed erratic voice breaks and arrests.

## MEASURABLE PHYSIOLOGICAL SIGNS

There have been few data reported on the measurable physiological characteristics of patients with essential tremor. Ardran et al. (1966) performed electromyograms on the cricothyroid and hyoglossus muscles of a 72-year-old female patient. They showed that at rest, both muscles had regular variation in activity at about a rate of 5–6 Hz. They comment that this was low-level activity that did not result in movement of the structures. This variation in muscle activity was not entirely regular and disappeared occasionally. Furthermore, the variation of activity between the hyoglossus and the cricothyroid muscle was not synchronized. There was also resting tremor in the electromyogram of the pectoralis major and external intercostal muscles in this patient. However, these disappeared when the patient contracted these muscles.

## OBSERVABLE PHYSIOLOGICAL SIGNS

By and large, the larynges of patients with essential tremor will show normal structure and movement. Rhythmic movement of one or more structures may sometimes be observed during phonation and/or at rest. Brown and Simonson (1963) reported normal-appearing larynges in 13 of their essential tremor patients and vocal fold bowing in 1 patient. However, 17 of their patients were not examined laryngoscopically.

We know of no data on the stroboscopic signs in essential tremor. Obtaining good stroboscopic recordings may be very difficult since the tremor makes tracking of the fundamental frequency difficult. However, newer stroboscopic equipment appears to be able to track vibration in the presence of tremor. In some patients we have observed with tremor, it has not been possible to obtain good stroboscopic pictures that would permit reliable observation of the significant stroboscopic signs.

## PATHOPHYSIOLOGY

The rhythmically changing activity in the muscles of the larynx create varying degrees of tension in the vocal folds and lead to a rhythmic change in fundamental frequency. Furthermore, the degree of adduction varies systematically in synchrony with the variation of muscle activity, creating a rhythmic change in the force of adduction. This results in variations of subglottal air pressure and thus of vocal intensity. If the tremor is severe, the adductory force could become large enough to completely stop voice production. Voice stoppages are also characteristic of spasmodic dysphonia. As discussed earlier (see "Spasmodic Dysphonia, Other Considerations"), Aronson and Hartman (1981) and others have suggested that some forms of spasmodic dysphonia may have essential tremor as their etiology. Medication has been used to treat essential tremor with mixed results. Propranolol (sometimes in conjunction with diazepam), primidone, and clonazepam have been used. Brin, Fahn, Blitzer, Ramig, and Stewart (1992), however, report limited success in using these drugs with essential tremor. The voice tremor characteristics of patients with spasmodic dysphonia and those with essential tremor are different (Brin, Fahn, Blitzer, Ramig, & Stewart, 1992).

## Miscellaneous Syndromes

Lesions in the upper neck or the medulla result in various syndromes that have paralysis of the vocal folds as one characteristic. There is involvement of the recurrent and superior laryngeal nerves, with a characteristic combined paralysis of the vocal folds. Other cranial nerves are usually also affected in these syndromes. Table 5.7 presents a summary of syndromes as discussed by Ballenger (1985). Note how often these syndromes include some effect on the pharynx, palate, and tongue, as well as the larynx.

*Table 5.7.* Miscellaneous Medulla Syndromes Affecting the Vocal Folds

| Name | Effect | Etiology |
|------|--------|----------|
| Wallenberg's | Paralysis of half of larynx, pharynx, palate, loss of sensation to the face, vestibular dysfunction, ataxia, Horner's syndrome | Infarction of posterior inferior cerebellar artery |
| Babinski-Nageotte | Similar to Wallenberg's, including paralysis of tongue, loss of position and vibratory sense | Similar to Wallenberg's, plus involvement of medial bulbar area |
| Cestan-Chenais | Similar to Babinski-Nageotte, except little or no involvement proximal to nucleus ambiguus | Infarction of vertebral artery below the posterior inferior cerebellar artery |
| Avellis' | Causes laryngeal, pharyngeal, and palatal paralysis with dysphonia and dysphagia | Vascular or inflammatory lesion in medulla; lesion in nucleus ambiguus of vagus, plus cranial part of spinal accessory |
| Hughlings-Jackson | Results in ipsilateral paralysis of the soft palate, pharynx, larynx, tongue, and sternocleidomastoid muscles | Intramedullary lesion or a lesion high in the lateral pharyngeal space; affects vagus, spinal accessory, and hypoglossal nerves |
| Schmidt's | Ipsilateral paralysis of soft palate, pharynx, larynx, sternomastoid, and trapezius muscles | Vascular lesion in caudal part of medulla |
| Mackenzie | Unilateral paralysis of soft palate, pharynx, larynx, and tongue | Vascular lesion in medulla |
| Bonnier's | General weakness | Lesion in Deiters' nucleus or associated vestibular tracts |

# GENERALIZED CENTRAL NERVOUS SYSTEM DAMAGE OF UNKNOWN LOCATIONS

## Gilles de la Tourette Syndrome

Gilles de la Tourette syndrome develops in early childhood, usually between age 2 and 13. It is characterized by twitching and grimacing, with tics of the face and eyes being the most common symptom (Golden, 1977; Merritt, 1975). The tics may later spread to the limbs. The speech of these individuals is characterized by unusual noises, explosive outbursts, and the unexpected utterance of profanities. Contrary to most belief, coprolalia (foul explicatives), and echolalia are not frequently heard in childhood. The disease increases in severity during childhood, but the symptoms may diminish in adulthood. The disease can usually be controlled by the use of the drug haloperidol, although there have been reports of unwanted side effects in some patients. Lang and Marsden (1983) reported a case in which spasmodic dysphonia developed during the use of haloperidol and persisted after removal of the drug.

Gilles de la Tourette syndrome, although interesting and unusual, does not present any unique challenges for the speech pathologist insofar as the voice is concerned. The symptoms are not under voluntary control and cannot be altered or controlled through a behavioral approach. It would appear that pharmacological treatment can be effective in reducing or eliminating the symptoms.

## Multiple Sclerosis

### PRIMARY VOICE SYMPTOMS: IMPAIRED LOUDNESS CONTROL AND HOARSENESS

### DESCRIPTION AND ETIOLOGY

Multiple sclerosis was first described by Charcot (1881), who referred to it as disseminated sclerosis. It is a disease characterized by multiple scarring (sclerosis) of the white matter in the brain, brainstem, and spinal cord. The initial symptoms of the disease may be very mild. As it progresses, the severity of the symptoms may increase, yet intermittently there may be long periods of remission or latency during which the person may seem well, but then the symptoms return. In the United States, the incidence of multiple sclerosis is about 50 per 100,000. It is much more common in the temperate regions of the northern and southern hemispheres, with the incidence dropping markedly close to the equator. The male-female ratio is unclear. The disease frequently develops in young adulthood, although it has been suggested that the onset of the very slowly progressing symptoms occurs in childhood but only becomes apparent in the adult (Millar, 1971).

Approximately 50% of patients with multiple sclerosis initially seek medical attention because of ENT symptoms, including vertigo (25%), nystagmus (40–70%), dysarthria (20%), or dysphagia (10-15%) (Garfinkle & Kimmelman, 1982; Ward, Cannon, & Lindsay, 1965). Bilateral abductor paralysis of the vocal folds may also occur. Noffsinger, Olsen, Carhart, Hart, and Sahgal (1972) documented many of the auditory and vestibular system dysfunctions in patients with multiple sclerosis. Of course, a patient may present more than one of these symptoms.

The reported loci of central nervous system involvement are not consistent. In a study of 234 multiple sclerosis patients, 85% were reported to have pyramidal involvement, followed by cerebellar (77%) and brainstem (73%) involvement (Kurtzke, Beebe, Nagler, Auth, & Kurland, 1972). Multiple system involvement was also noted by Garfinkle and Kimmelman (1982). Patients with multiple sclerosis present a variety of neurological signs. Some of these are summarized in Table 5.8, based on the data presented by Darley, Brown, and Goldstein (1972).

It has been stated that the cardinal signs of multiple sclerosis are scanning speech, nystagmus, and intention tremor (Ivers & Goldstein, 1963). However, available data suggest that speech/voice problems, although sometimes present, are not pervasive. Darley et al. (1972) found that 59% of their 168 patients presented normal speech patterns, and another 29% had minimal speech impairment. Table 5.9 presents a summary of the speech and voice symptoms in their patients. These authors also noted that the severity of speech difficulty increased with an increase in the severity of the neurological deficit. They concluded that dysarthria was not characteristic of multiple sclerosis speech, nor was scanning speech. Kurtzke et al. (1972) reported that scanning speech was present in only 18.9% of their 525 male patients with multiple sclerosis.

## PERCEPTUAL VOICE SIGNS AND SYMPTOMS

The primary voice symptoms associated with multiple sclerosis are impaired loudness control and harshness (Darley, Brown, & Goldstein, 1972; Farmakides & Boone, 1960). Hypernasality is also prominent (Farmakides & Boone, 1960), while impaired pitch control, inappropriate pitch level, and breathiness can occur less frequently. Speech characteristics include a slowing of speech rate, defective articulation (Darley, Brown, & Goldstein, 1972; Jensen, 1960), impaired emphasis (scanning speech), and occasionally poor respiratory control.

## ACOUSTIC SIGNS

The range of fundamental frequencies produced by patients with multiple sclerosis appears to be very similar to that of normal speakers, with the possible exception of a slightly greater fundamental frequency range and larger variability of fundamental frequency (Zemlin, 1962).

*Table 5.8.* Neurological Signs in Multiple Sclerosis

| Neurological Sign | Percent |
|---|---|
| Finger to finger/toe to finger tests | 82 |
| Dysdiadochokinesis | 71 |
| Impairment of posterior column sense | 60 |
| Pyramidal signs (sucking reflex, Hoffman's sign, Babinski's sign, increased muscle-stretch reflexes | 92 |
| Muscular weakness | 9 |

*Table 5.9.* Speech Deviations in Multiple Sclerosis

| | Percent |
|---|---|
| Normal speech performance | 59 |
| Defective speech performance | 41 |
| Impaired loudness control | 77 |
| Harshness | 72 |
| Defective articulation | 46 |
| Impaired emphasis | 39 |
| Impaired pitch control | 37 |
| Hypernasality | 24 |
| Inappropriate pitch level | 24 |
| Breathiness | 22 |

## MEASURABLE PHYSIOLOGICAL SIGNS

We know of no data on the measurable phonatory physiological characteristics of patients with multiple sclerosis. If harshness is present, suggestive of vocal fold hypertonicity, low flows and high subglottal pressures might be expected. The vibratory cycle of the vocal folds is probably highly variable because of the harshness and impaired muscle control.

## OBSERVABLE PHYSIOLOGICAL SIGNS

In most patients, the larynx would be expected to appear normal. In patients with abductor paralysis, vocal fold opening should be impaired, and the patient may present problems related to air intake. There may be reduced range of motion of the vocal folds and momentary stoppages of vocal fold motion.

We know of no data on the stroboscopic signs in multiple sclerosis. We might expect to find good closure of the vocal folds (unless the patient is very breathy), but there may be a reduction of the amplitude of vibration and perhaps poor phase symmetry.

## PATHOPHYSIOLOGY

Multiple sclerosis is characterized by increasing incoordination, spasticity, and weakness of the muscles in the body. When the laryngeal musculature is affected, these same characteristics might be evidenced by impaired phonatory coordination and control and by reduced range and force of movement. Spasticity and muscle weakness will affect the ability of the vocal folds to adduct smoothly and to maintain the proper adductory forces needed for phonation. Weakness of vocal fold adduction may mean an inability to produce the proper subglottal pressures needed for speech. This will manifest itself in reduced vocal loudness. The spastic characteristic of multiple sclerosis may impair the ability to maintain control over vocal fold adduction and therefore may result in uneven vocal loudness. Poor coordination of the vocal folds may produce aperiodicity of vibration and lead to greater perceived hoarseness/harshness. The rate of movement of the vocal folds may also be impaired similarly to the impaired rate of speaking (Jensen, 1960).

Treatment may involve various drugs to produce relief of symptoms such as spasticity, fatigue, neurobehavioral disorders, paroxysmal disorders, pain, bladder dysfunction, and cerebellar dysfunction (Mitchell, 1993).

# DISORDERS OF MUSCLE AND MYONEURAL JUNCTION

## *Myasthenia Gravis*

### PRIMARY VOICE SYMPTOM: BREATHINESS

### DESCRIPTION AND ETIOLOGY

Patients with myasthenia gravis show a characteristic weakening of the striated muscles and a prolonged return of function after activation. Muscles innervated by cranial nerves seem most susceptible to this disease. The disease is relatively rare, with an incidence between 2 to 10 per 100,000 (Garfinkle & Kimmelman, 1982). It tends to affect the sexes differentially in terms of incidence and age of onset. It occurs twice as often in females and much earlier than in males. Onset for females is reported in the 3rd decade of life, while in males it is during the 6th decade (Garfinkle & Kimmelman, 1982).

Patients with myasthenia gravis tend to show bulbar symptoms, with the earliest and most common being ptosis or drooping of the eyelids (Grob, 1961). Other symptoms include diplopia, weakness of the legs, fatigue, dysphagia, dysphonia, and blurred vision. All patients will not exhibit all symptoms. Furthermore, these symptoms are not unique to myasthenia gravis but are encountered in other disease states. The symptom of diplopia, for example, can be associated with infection, glioma of the brainstem, multiple sclerosis, toxicity, aneurysms, tumors, and trauma (Baker, 1958). Paralysis or muscle weakness can also be a sign of poliomyelitis or brainstem glioma in children. In adults, paralysis can be a sign of poliomyelitis, Guillain-Barré syndrome, brainstem glioma, cerebellopontine angle tumor, cerebral artery occlusion, amyotrophic lateral sclerosis, and pseudobulbar palsy or tumor (Tucker & Lavertu, 1992; Stuart, 1965). Carpenter, McDonald, and Howard (1979) emphasized the differential diagnosis of myasthenia gravis, amyotrophic lateral sclerosis, and multiple sclerosis. The unique features of myasthenia gravis are fatigability, fluctuation of function, and restoration of function after rest. These features do not occur, for example, in amyotrophic lateral sclerosis or multiple sclerosis. The voice symptoms of myasthenia gravis, because of their variability, have been mistaken for hysterical aphonia (Ball & Lloyd, 1971).

Some myasthenia gravis patients may present with voice or speech dysfunction as their initial symptom. Wolski (1967) reported a case of myasthenia gravis in which nasality was the initial presenting symptom. Colton and Brewer (1985) and Levine, Hatlali, and Zaggy (1985) each reported a case diagnosed as myasthenia gravis that presented unusual fiberoptic laryngoscopic findings.

Myasthenia gravis seems to be a disease of the myoneural junction. It may result from inadequate release of acetylcholine or other aberrant chemical activity at the myoneural junction (Osserman, 1958).

## PERCEPTUAL VOICE SIGNS AND SYMPTOMS

The primary symptom of myasthenia gravis is the general fatigability of muscle functions in the head, neck, tongue, pharynx, and larynx. Voice signs include hoarseness, breathy voice, and vocal weakness (Carpenter, McDonald, & Howard, 1979). In one study, 60% of myasthenia gravis patients presented voice symptoms (Rontal, Rontal, Leuchter, & Rolnick, 1978). The following voice characteristics were reported in ratings of 11 patients with myasthenia gravis: hypernasality, nasal emission, inspiratory voice, dysphonia, intermittent aphonia, and aspirate voice (Maxwell & Locke, 1969). Interestingly, these symptoms were completely eliminated with pharmacological treatment.

## ACOUSTIC SIGNS

Few studies have been reported about the acoustic characteristics of voice in patients with myasthenia gravis. In a study of 11 females and 1 male with myasthenia gravis, average fundamental frequency of speech was found to be very similar to normal expectations in both medicated and unmedicated states (Maxwell & Locke, 1969).

Rontal et al. (1978) presented spectrographic evidence of aperiodicity and high frequency noise in the speech of patients with myasthenia gravis.

## MEASURABLE PHYSIOLOGICAL SIGNS

Electromyographic studies have shown a characteristic decrement of activity with repetitive stimulation (Warren, Gutmann, & Cody, 1977). We have studied the airflow and electroglottogram characteristics of a patient with myasthenia gravis. The data are shown in Figure 5.15. Note the extremely long opening phase of the airflow waveform cycles, with a rather slow (but faster than the opening phase) closing phase. The electroglottogram waveform seems to mirror these slow opening and closing phases of the vocal folds. The airflow/slope ratio (ratio of the closing slope to the opening slope) and the electroglottogram closing time were significantly greater than for normal subjects.

## OBSERVABLE PHYSIOLOGICAL SIGNS

The characteristic sign seen in laryngoscopic evaluations is sluggishness of vocal fold abduction. Continued phonation by a patient with myasthenia gravis over a period of time may show increasing weakness of arytenoid and vocal fold motion. Normal movement will return, however, with sufficient rest.

There have been no data reported on the stroboscopic signs associated with myasthenia gravis. Normal mucosal waves but reduced amplitude of motion might be expected.

## PATHOPHYSIOLOGY

Muscle weakness will be expected to affect the patient's ability to raise the vocal pitch and produce loud voice. However, these changes may occur only when the mechanism has fatigued following phonation over a period of time. The inability to maintain the proper tension in the vocal folds will result in increased aperiodicity and the inability to maintain good glottal closure. These conditions will produce roughness or hoarseness and breathiness in the voice. Drugs can help relieve some of the symptoms of myasthenia gravis. Neostigmine and pyridostigmine (Mestinon) are often prescribed. Immunosuppressive drugs are often used. In some cases a thymectomy is performed. Plasma pheresis may also bring improvement (Sanders and Scopetta, 1994).

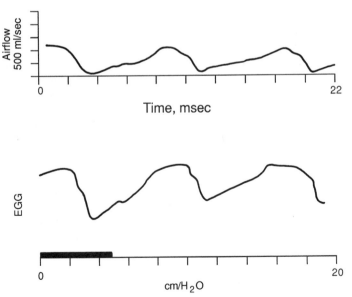

*Figure 5.15.* Inverse filtered airflow and electroglottogram (EGG) waveforms for a 65-year-old female with myasthenia gravis. Note the extremely long opening phase of the vocal folds and the slow closing phase. The electroglottogram waveform mirrors these slow variations of vibration. Lung pressure was within normal limits.

## Lesions of the Peripheral Nerves

### PRIMARY VOICE SYMPTOM: BREATHINESS

### DESCRIPTION AND ETIOLOGY

Lesions that affect the vagus nerve somewhere along its course from the base of the skull to the larynx will result in a paresis (weakness) or paralysis of muscles in the larynx. These peripheral lesions of the vagus are the most common cause of vocal fold paralysis. The intrinsic laryngeal muscles affected will depend on the exact location of the lesion. Recall that the superior laryngeal nerve (SLN) of the vagus controls the cricothyroid muscles, whereas the recurrent laryngeal nerve (RLN) controls the remaining muscles of the larynx. The SLN branches off from the vagus high in the neck. The RLN branches off somewhat below the SLN. A paralysis of all the muscles suggests that the lesion is high in the neck or in the brainstem itself. Lesions affecting only the RLN will be much lower in the neck or as far down as the thorax.

Lesions of the SLN or RLN may affect the position of the vocal folds. In RLN paralysis, the lesion may be unilateral or bilateral and may be of the adductor or abductor type, depending on the muscles affected. In the instance of a unilateral adductor paralysis, the affected vocal fold will not be actively moved toward the midline when phonation commences. When the glottis cannot be completely closed, the quality of the voice produced will be weak and breathy. In bilateral adductor paralysis, neither vocal fold will be capable of moving to the midline, thus making phonation impossible. The position of the paralyzed vocal folds, that is, how far apart they are, will depend partly on whether or not the SLN is affected. The SLN innervates the cricothyroid muscle, which when contracted tends to contribute to adduction of the vocal folds, in addition to tensing them to create a rise of vocal pitch. Paralysis of this muscle in addition to muscles controlled by the RLN will further reduce the adductory forces of the vocal folds, thereby increasing their distance from each other over what it might be with an RLN lesion alone. Other factors, such as degree of fibrosis of the affected fold, tension of the conus elasticus, and freedom of joint movement may also affect the final position of the vocal folds after paralysis of the RLN or SLN (Ballenger, 1985).

Lesions may also affect the abductory function of the vocal folds, which opens the airway for inspiration. Such lesions affect the recurrent laryngeal nerve and specifically the posterior cricoarytenoid muscle, which may produce unilateral or bilateral abductory paralysis. Bilateral abductor paralysis in which the vocal folds remain in an adducted posture causes serious respiratory problems (dyspnea), for which most patients will require a tracheotomy.

The etiology of vocal fold paralysis is varied and, as mentioned previously, can include lesions in the brainstem itself. These high vagal lesions (from the nodose ganglion up) will affect all laryngeal muscles, as well as muscles supplied by other cranial nerves. The lesions include tumors at the base of the skull, carcinoma of the nasopharynx, or trauma. A listing of some of the lesions in this area that could affect the larynx is shown in Table 5.10.

The possible etiologies of low vagal lesions are even more numerous. Neuritis is a frequent cause and occurs with upper respiratory infection, infectious mononucleosis, sarcoidosis, and infections of the parapharyngeal spaces (Ballenger, 1985). Neoplasms in the neck, bronchi, and chest may invade and affect the nerve. Mechanical stretching or compression of the nerve may also result in paralysis of the laryngeal musculature. Among the most common etiologies are acute external trauma to the neck, surgery, and idiopathic etiologies (Ballenger, 1985; Tucker, 1980). In their report on unilateral

*Table 5.10.* Miscellaneous Peripheral Syndromes Resulting in Laryngeal Paralysis

| Name | Effect | Etiology |
|---|---|---|
| Collet-Sicard | Last four cranial nerves | Tumor, meningitis, or trauma to posterior cranial fossa |
| Vernet's | Nerves 9, 10, 11; dysphagia and dysphonia | Lesion in jugular fossa |
| Villarets | Like Vernet's, including sympathetic paralysis and Horner's syndrome | Lesion in retroparotid or lateral pharyngeal space |
| Tapia's | Ipsilateral paralysis of tongue and larynx | Neoplasm where hypoglossal crosses vagus and internal carotid |
| Gard-Gignoux | Paralysis of vocal folds, weakness of trapezius and sternomastoid muscles | 11th and vagus below nodose ganglion |
| Klinkert | Paralysis of recurrent and phrenic nerves | Lesion in root of neck or mediastinum |

*Figure 5.16.* Etiology of vocal fold paralysis in adults. **A,** Unilateral paralysis. **B,** Bilateral paralysis.

vocal fold paralysis, Terris, Arnstein, and Nguyen (1992) reviewed 84 of their own cases as well as summaries reported in the literature for a total of 1019 cases. Their results are presented in Figure 5.16. Etiologies of bilateral adductor paralysis were presented by Tucker (1980) and are also shown in Figure 5.16. Thyroidectomy is a relatively rare cause of a unilateral paralysis (13.64% of all cases but 55.4% of surgical cases), but the major cause of bilateral paralysis.

Cohen, Geller, Birns, and Thompson (1982) reported on the causes of laryngeal nerve paralysis in children, the symptoms of which will usually be observed shortly after birth. In some cases, however, the symptoms may be so minor that a vocal fold paralysis may not be recognized until many years later. Such was the case of K. B. reported in Chapter 2. The major cause of vocal fold paralysis in children is birth trauma (19%), with central nervous system disease the next most common etiology. The other causes of paralysis in children are shown in Figure 5.17. Also shown in this

*Figure 5.17.* Etiology and symptoms of peripheral nerve paralysis in a study of children (N = 50 male and 41 female subjects).

figure are the presenting ENT signs. Interestingly, 65% of infants with laryngeal paralysis had a normal delivery; 38% of these had unilateral paralysis, whereas 62% had bilateral abductor paralysis.

## PERCEPTUAL VOICE SIGNS AND SYMPTOMS

The most common perceptual symptoms of unilateral paralysis are breathiness and hoarseness. Occasionally diplophonia may be present. Bilateral paralysis of the adductor type will cause severe breathiness or aphonia, but near-normal voice may be present in the abductor type. An additional perceptual sign of bilateral abductor paralysis is inspiratory stridor that results from the passage of ingressive air over approximated vocal folds that are incapable of opening.

## ACOUSTIC SIGNS

Acoustically, increased aperiodicity (jitter and shimmer), a reduced pitch range, reduced variability of pitch, higher noise levels, and a reduced vocal intensity range are found.

Murry (1978) reported the fundamental frequency characteristics of 20 patients with unilateral paralysis of the vocal folds as they read a standard reading passage. The patient group had a mean fundamental frequency of 127 Hz, whereas a group of 20 normal speakers had a mean fundamental frequency of 121.9 Hz. This difference was not statistically significant. The variability of fundamental frequency (pitch sigma) between the two groups of subjects was also not significant.

Davis (1981) reported pitch perturbation quotient (PPQ), or jitter, and amplitude perturbation quotient (APQ), or shimmer, values for two patients with unilateral paralysis of the vocal folds. The average PPQ was 9.165% for the patients versus 0.42% for a group of 10 normal speakers. The APQ was 12.96% for the patient group and 6.14% for the 10 normal speakers. It is difficult to generalize about these findings based on only two subjects, but they appear to be in the direction hypothesized. That is, patients with unilateral paralysis will show greater frequency and amplitude perturbation than speakers with normal-functioning vocal folds.

Kim, Kakita, and Hirano (1982) carried out spectrographic analysis of some acoustic characteristics of the voices of 10 persons with unilateral RLN paralysis. They were unable to obtain accurate measures of fundamental frequency probably due to the large amount of aperiodicity in the voice. The only difference between the patient and the normal group on amplitude variation and extent (a rough analog of shimmer) occurred between males. Other differences measured in these spectrograms included higher harmonic energy in the patient group, as well as greater noise energy. These latter features may correlate with the greater breathiness and noise levels that are present in many patients with unilateral recurrent nerve paralysis.

## MEASURABLE PHYSIOLOGICAL SIGNS

There have been several investigations concerned with the measurement of average airflow during the speech of patients with vocal fold paralysis. Hirano (1981a) summarized several of these studies, noting that the mean flow rates in paralysis are much higher than normal, although they range from a low of 35 ml/sec to a high of 1150 ml/sec (see Table 3.3, p. 30, in Hirano, 1981a). Normal-speaking males produce rates of about 110 ml/sec, females about 94 ml/sec (Koike & Hirano, 1968). Yanagihara and von Leden (1967) reported a mean flow rate of 442.2 ml/sec for their 10 patients with unilateral paralysis, whereas Iwata et al. reported a mean flow of 353 ml/sec for their group of 19 unilateral paralysis patients. Hirano, Koike, and von Leden (1968) reported a mean flow rate of 312.8 ml/sec for their 10 patients with bilateral paralysis. Thus, it would appear that higher mean flow rates occur in unilateral paralysis than in bilateral paralysis.

Based on their analysis of EGG waveforms of paralysis patients, Hanson, Gerrat, Karin and Berke (1988) were able to differentiate among four etiologies of unilateral vocal fold paralysis. Vagal lesions produced an open quotient that was much smaller than the other etiologies studied (Figure 5.18). Measures of speed quotient showed greater variation among the four etiologies studied (Figure 5.19). Perhaps, measure-

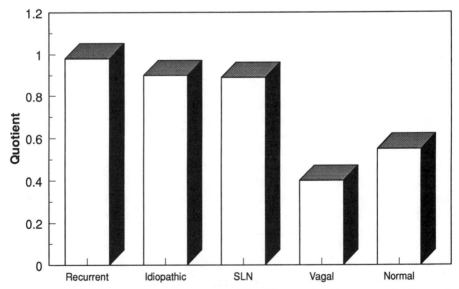

*Figure 5.18.* Open quotient measurements of four forms of unilateral vocal fold paralysis compared to a group of normal control subjects.

ments such as these and others yet to be tried could be used to differentiate the type of etiology responsible for a paralysis of a vocal fold.

We have recorded the inverse filtered flow characteristics and electroglottograms of several patients with unilateral paralysis. One patient is shown in Figure 5.20. This is the same female (K. B.) whose case was presented in Chapter 2. Note the high levels of offset flow (from baseline to lowest point on the airflow waveform), which were much greater than for the normal subjects. The airflow waveform is variable, perhaps indicative of the greater aperiodicity of the vocal folds. This increased aperiodicity is also evident in the electroglottographic trace shown below the airflow trace.

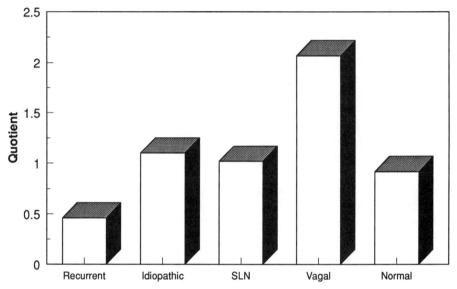

*Figure 5.19.* Speed quotient measurements of different forms of unilateral vocal fold paralysis compared to a group of normal control subjects.

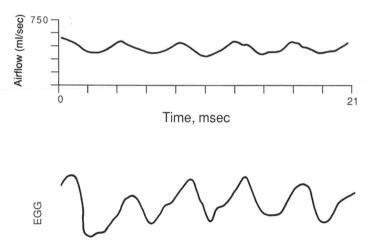

*Figure 5.20.* Inverse filtered airflow and electroglottogram (EGG) waveforms for patient K. B., a female with a congenital unilateral vocal fold paralysis. Note the large airflow offset, indicative of a large leak through the vocal folds. The electroglottogram also exhibits unusual waveforms with marked change from one cycle to the next. Due to technical problems, we were unable to record the lung pressure used with this phonation.

Kuroki (1969) studied the subglottal pressures produced by patients with unilateral and bilateral recurrent nerve paralysis. Most patients with unilateral paralysis produced higher than normal subglottal pressures (normal, about 6–8 cm/H$_2$O), and two bilateral paralysis patients showed much higher than normal subglottal pressures. This might be expected in view of the air loss during phonation and the natural tendency for the speaker to attempt to compensate for this loss with greater driving pressures below the vocal folds. On the other hand, patients with vocal fold paralysis may produce greater pressures (and therefore greater flows) because of their inability to achieve glottal closure during the vibratory cycle.

## OBSERVABLE PHYSIOLOGICAL SIGNS

### Laryngoscopy

The typical laryngoscopic view in unilateral paralysis is that of one relatively immobile vocal fold that does not adduct during phonation, while the unaffected fold moves to the midline. There may be some apparent movement of the affected vocal fold caused by movements of other structures, or by contraction of the cricothyroid (assuming an intact SLN), which will tend to exert some adductory force on the vocal folds (as described earlier), or perhaps the affected fold is driven by air pressure. Movement in the pyriform sinus on the affected side may be reduced or absent (Brewer & Gould, 1974) in patients with unilateral vocal fold paralysis. Differences in the horizontal level of the two vocal folds has been reported by Isshiki and Ishikawa (1976). About one-half of their 56 patients showed a higher level of the paralyzed vocal fold. Reasons for this level difference may include (*a*) the position of the arytenoid on the paralyzed side, (*b*) effects of the extrinsic muscles, and (*c*) the possibility of a paralyzed cricothyroid muscle which would affect the tension that can be placed on the affected fold. It should be noted, however, that others have failed to find a consistent level difference (Adran, Demp, & Marland, 1954; Ballantyne & Groves, 1978; Casper, Colton, & Brewer, 1985; Lee, 1973).

### Stroboscopy

Hirano, Feder, and Bless (1983) discussed some of the stroboscopic signs seen in patients with peripheral nerve paralysis. These signs will vary depending on the severity of involvement and the type of problem, that is, superior or recurrent nerve involvement, or both. A summary of the important signs they report for unilateral adductor paralysis is presented in Table 5.11.

Kitzing (1985) reported that stroboscopic signs in vocal fold paresis include vocal fold asymmetry and aperiodicity, greater than normal vibratory amplitudes, absence of a mucosal wave, and incomplete glottal closure. These signs are consistent with the nature of the disease and the perceptual, acoustic, physiological, and laryngoscopic signs discussed earlier.

*Table 5.11.* Stroboscopic Signs in Laryngeal Paralysis

1. Abnormal vibration with predominant vertical movements
2. Large irregular amplitudes
3. Poor vocal fold closure
4. Asymmetrical vibration
5. Affected fold seems to flutter
6. Absence of edge deflections (upward, on affected fold)

We have observed many of these same signs. The paralyzed fold vibrates occasionally but not at the same rate nor in the same way as the unaffected fold. There is an anterioposterior (or the reverse) ripple-like motion on the affected side. We have observed a mucosal wave on the affected fold although it is usually not as regular as the unaffected side. Amplitude of vibration of the affected fold sometimes appears to be increased. Most often, the paralyzed fold and the nonparalyzed fold produce an aperiodic motion. There are a variety of glottal closure patterns observed but most often we have observed incomplete closure (22/39 patients).

The location of the pathology in vocal fold paralysis is in the muscle, i.e., the thyroarytenoid muscle has little or no neural control (Hirano & Bless, 1993). There may be glottal incompetence with a bowed fold sometimes seen. The stiffness of the cover and the transition layers are normal. The stiffness of the body is decreased.

Sercarz and his colleagues (Sercarz, Berke, Ming, Gerratt, & Natividad, 1992) reported on stroboscopic findings in three normal speakers whose recurrent and/or superior laryngeal nerves were paralyzed with drugs as well as 20 patients with unilateral paralysis. Their most significant finding was the asymmetry of traveling wave motion in the paralyzed larynx. The normal fold has the fastest traveling wave; the difference of wave velocity produced a phase asymmetry of vibration.

### PATHOPHYSIOLOGY

A paralyzed vocal fold may affect adduction or abduction of the vocal folds. Voice problems are most commonly associated with unilateral adductor paralysis. In bilateral adductor paralysis, the patient may be aphonic, but the patient's primary and potentially life-threatening problem in need of urgent attention will be loss of protection of the airway and the attendant risk of aspiration. The incidence of unilateral vocal fold paralysis is much greater than that of bilateral paralysis.

One problem encountered in the diagnosis of vocal fold paralysis is whether or not there is a true paralysis of the fold or if the immobility of the vocal fold is due to fixation of the arytenoid joint or a dislocated arytenoid (Rontal & Rontal, 1986). The diagnostician must carefully explore these other possibilities either indirectly by observing other structures in the larynx (e.g., the pyriform sinus) or by directly manipulating the arytenoid to test its mobility. EMG evaluation of muscle electrical activity may also assist in making the correct diagnosis. Most important of all is a complete and careful case history (Woo, Colton, Brewer, & Casper, 1991).

In unilateral paralysis, the affected fold cannot move to the midline and assist in closure of the glottis. Because of this incomplete closure, greater than normal airflows and a weak voice will be produced. The affected fold may also exhibit muscle tensions vastly different from the unaffected cord, resulting in asymmetrical tension and increased aperiodicity in the voice. This will be perceived as roughness or hoarseness. A difference in level between the two folds may also contribute to the increased aperiodicity and excessive airflow, although its precise effect remains unknown.

## AN UNUSUAL CASE OF UNILATERAL VOCAL FOLD PARALYSIS

R. C. is a 52-year-old male who awoke one morning with pain and pronounced weakness in both arms, slightly more pronounced on the right with impaired manual dexterity in the right hand that prevented simple acts such as eating, writing, etc. After visiting his general practitioner, he was referred to a neurologist who performed routine neurological tests and conduction velocity tests on nerves in the right arm. The diagnosis was Guillain-Barré syndrome (acute inflammatory demyelinating polyneuropathy), and R. C. was hospitalized immediately. On the day after hospitalization, R. C. developed a breathy and hoarse voice quality consistent with a unilateral vocal fold paralysis. Also, he developed mild dysphagia. A flexible fiberoptic laryngeal examination was conducted two days later and revealed a left vocal fold paralysis.

Guillain-Barré is a neuropathy (Dowling, Blumberg, & Cook, 1987) that affects somewhere between 0.6 to 2 individuals per 100,000 population. It is the body's reaction to a virus that the person may have had up to 8 weeks prior to the onset of symptoms. (R. C. reported a mild upper respiratory infection about 2 months previous to onset and a very mild, one day illness about 5 days previous to onset.) The affected individual's immune system develops antibodies in reaction to the virus that begin to attack the myelin sheaths of nerves, primarily peripheral nerves. It is probably an autoimmune T cell-mediated disease (Taft, 1988). No nerve is safe, including those that control respiration, the heart, and other vital functions. The classic symptoms of Guillain-Barré begin with weakness in the legs and ascend to the trunk, arms, head, and neck. However, other variants of the disease exist as evinced by R. C. How far the demyelinating extends and what systems are affected is unpredictable. Until quite recently persons with this diagnosis were hospitalized so that the progression of the disease could be monitored and appropriate life-saving intervention, such as respiratory assistance, could be introduced as necessary.

R. C. was hospitalized not only to monitor the progress of the disease, but also to start him on a treatment program of plasmapheresis (Guillain-Barré Syndrome Study Group, 1985). This treatment has been found to be an effective method of interrupting the course of the disease in some patients. During the plasmapheresis treatments, each of which can take several hours, blood is continuously extracted from the body; the white and red blood cells are separated from the plasma; the plasma is discarded; and the red and white cells are mixed with human albumen and pumped back into the patient. The theory is that the antibody causing the problem attaches itself to a protein in the plasma. Removing the plasma removes the offending antibody. R. C. remained in the hospital for 8 days and completed four plasmapheresis treatments. He did not develop any additional symptoms; indeed, the dysphagia and the acute arm pain had resolved. He still had arm weakness, vocal fold paralysis, and fatigue. He was then discharged to recuperate at home for another 2 weeks. During this time, he received two additional pheresis treatments as an outpatient. He returned to work about 22 days after the onset of the first symptom. The vocal fold paralysis persisted for about 6 weeks after its onset. R. C. recovered full use of his voice and at 3 months post onset had only mild soreness in his arms, especially his right, secondary to remyelination.

Vocal fold paralysis is a rare complication of Guillain-Barré syndrome. It appears to respond to the treatment for the disease itself, i.e., plasmapheresis. Early diagnosis and immediate treatment appear to be critical, and patients can often experience full recovery of function with time. The presentation of vocal fold paralysis must be viewed as potentially one sign of an underlying problem that may have life threatening implications. A thorough history is critical to alert the examiner to areas that need further exploration. It is essential to rule out the presence of more diffuse disease, the presence of a neck, thoracic, or lung lesion, that might be impinging on the nerve (RLN), the possibility of joint ankylosis or dislocation, and possible psychogenicity.

## SUMMARY

Vocal fold vibration depends on an intact neurological system in order to maintain the proper tension in the vocal folds, produce the proper airflow and air pressures needed for voicing, and adduct or abduct the vocal folds in accord with the requirements of the speaking act. Disruption of this control will affect the normal vibration of the vocal folds. This disruption may occur either in the central or the peripheral nervous system. When lesions occur in the peripheral nervous system, the phonatory system will show signs of denervation and flaccidity. The muscles controlled by the nerves will fail to receive the proper innervation and will not contract.

When lesions occur within the central nervous system, the phonatory system may show signs of flaccidity or hyperfunction depending on the site of the lesion(s). Lesions high in the central nervous system but not in the cortex affecting the pyramidal or extrapyramidal systems will produce hypertonia and exaggerated reflexes. Lesions in the cerebellum will produce deficits in the control of muscles, especially groups of muscles needed for the complex motor act of speech. The signs and symptoms of phonatory difficulty that develop will depend on the site of lesion. A good working knowledge of the appropriate physical signs and symptoms as well as the voice signs and symptoms is needed before the clinician can properly diagnose and/or understand the nature of the difficulty presented by a patient. In this chapter we have presented an overview of many different neurological problems in which voice may be affected, including Parkinson's disease, myasthenia gravis, amyotrophic lateral sclerosis, Shy-Drager syndrome, multiple sclerosis, cerebellar ataxia, spasmodic dysphonia, essential tremor, and many of the problems that may affect the recurrent and superior laryngeal nerves when they exit the central nervous system or as they travel in the neck and thorax to their ultimate destinations.

*Chapter 6*

# Voice Problems Associated with Organic Disease, Trauma, and the Geriatric Voice

The conditions discussed in this chapter represent organic disease states that have an effect on phonation. The etiology of these conditions is unrelated to ways in which the voice has been used, and their treatment is primarily medical and/or surgical. It is important for clinicians to be familiar with these conditions and their effect on phonatory physiology, and to be prepared to offer the appropriate level of service as the need for it becomes timely. It is often the case that the speech-language pathologist provides presurgical treatment counseling, and secondarily is called upon to provide voice therapy along with or subsequent to medical or surgical intervention. The conditions include keratosis, granulomas, pachydermia laryngis, ankylosis of the cricoarytenoid joint, papillomas, carcinoma and other malignancies, blunt or penetrating trauma, and chemical or heat trauma. A section on the voice of the geriatric individual is included in this chapter.

## BENIGN LESIONS

### Keratosis

PRIMARY VOICE SYMPTOM: HOARSENESS

DESCRIPTION AND ETIOLOGY

Keratosis refers to epithelial lesions in which there is abnormal tissue growth on the vocal folds (Fig. 6.1). This usually originates in epithelium but may enter the superficial layer of the lamina propria. Other terms may be used to describe this condition, including leukoplakia, hyperkeratosis, keratosis with cellular atypia, and dyskeratosis. Two kinds of lesions may be seen: flat, white, plaque-like lesions (leukoplakia) or irregular growth of epithelium that results in a warty lesion (papillary keratosis). There is a full spectrum of premalignant laryngeal tissue changes observed in smokers that are not seen in nonsmokers (U.S. Dept. of Health and Human Services, 1985). These lesions must be carefully monitored.

Smoking, environmental pollutants, and other factors have been implicated in the development of keratotic epithelium on the vocal folds. These lesions tend to occur more often in males than females. Recently, gastroesophageal reflux disease (GERD) has also been implicated as an etiology of these tissue changes (Koufman, 1991). The lesions may be unilateral or bilateral but are usually asymmetric in appearance. The glottal edge is often rough.

### PERCEPTUAL SIGNS AND SYMPTOMS

The primary symptom is hoarseness or roughness in the voice.

### ACOUSTIC SIGNS

There are few data available on the acoustic characteristics of patients with keratosis of the vocal folds. Due to the growths on the vocal folds, greater than normal frequency and amplitude perturbation as well as greater than normal spectral noise would be expected.

### MEASURABLE PHYSIOLOGICAL SIGNS

Minimal measurable physiological data exist on patients with keratosis of the vocal folds. Iwata, von Leden, and Williams (1972) reported a mean airflow rate of 227 ml/sec for patients with leukoplakia of the vocal folds. Lesions that might have a similar effect (papilloma, epithelial hyperplasia) also show greater than normal airflows (see Table 3.6 in Hirano, 1981b).

### OBSERVABLE PHYSIOLOGICAL SIGNS

In patients with leukoplakia, there will be whitish plaque-like lesions on the mucosal surface of the vocal folds. These may be limited in extent or may cover almost the entire vocal fold. Ballenger (1985) reports that another form of this lesion, papillary keratosis, may show a piling up of small, reddish epithelium or an irregular mucosa covered by keratin.

Because these lesions can be so variable in extent and in location on the folds, their stroboscopic appearance will vary. Vocal fold edges may be rough and result in an irregularly shaped glottic chink on vocal fold closure. There will be asymmetric behavior and aperiodicity. In extensive lesions, diminished amplitude of lateral vocal fold excursion and limited mucosal wave, especially over the sites occupied by the lesion, are seen. In instances of early and superficial hyperkeratosis, it is possible to observe a fairly normal mucosal wave. This stroboscopic feature may help to distinguish keratosis from cancer. Deeper invasion of the underlying structures occurs in carcinoma limiting vibratory behavior to a greater extent.

*Figure 6.1.* Hyperkeratosis of the vocal folds. See color plate.

PATHOPHYSIOLOGY

Keratotic-type lesions, for the most part, affect the cover, increasing its mass and stiffness.

## Granulomas

PRIMARY VOICE SYMPTOM: HOARSENESS

DESCRIPTION AND ETIOLOGY

Granulomas most commonly are a complication of intubation (Fig. 6.2). Their development may be an early complication occurring at some point between intubation and extubation, or a late complication, the morbid sequelae of extubation (Balestrieri & Watson, 1982). The passing of an intubation tube between the vocal processes may be necessary in order to provide access to the airway for purposes of delivering anesthesia and maintaining appropriate oxygenation during a surgical procedure. Intubation may also be necessary in nonsurgical situations to maintain adequate oxygen supply for persons in need of respiratory assistance. Contact between the tube and the vocal processes may occur at the time of intubation or with the tube in situ. During such

*Figure 6.2.* Granuloma involving the posterior part of the glottis. **A,** The granuloma during respiration. **B,** During phonation. See color plate.

contact the mucosal perichondrium of the vocal processes may be traumatized, causing a small ulcer to appear on the vocal process. The bare process will eventually be covered by granulation tissue, which will become epithelialized and present as a granuloma. The condition is surprisingly uncommon in light of the frequency with which intubation is required, and spontaneous resolution occurs within a few weeks in most cases. The incidence of granuloma is dependent on factors such as duration of intubation, the method of intubation, the patient's age and general condition, nursing techniques, and other factors. All reported cases have occurred in patients 15 years or older, and women are more prone to develop an intubation granuloma because of small laryngeal size and a thinner mucosal layer covering the vocal processes (Snow, Marano, & Balogh, 1966).

Endotracheal intubation is being accepted for longer and longer periods of time. Although it is not a benign procedure, mortality and morbidity rates, when compared to the option of tracheotomy, are much lower. Weymuller (1988) presents a thorough review of the pertinent factors relating to endotracheal injury, its nature, the biomechanical factors of the tube itself, and the efforts made to prevent injury from the procedure.

### PERCEPTUAL SIGNS AND SYMPTOMS

The symptoms of granuloma are breathiness and hoarseness. Some may not affect phonation due to their location.

### ACOUSTIC SIGNS

There are no data on the acoustic characteristics of patients with granulomas. Greater than normal frequency and amplitude perturbation would be expected, and depending on the severity of the hoarseness, greater than normal spectral noise could be present.

### MEASURABLE PHYSIOLOGICAL SIGNS

Normal airflow rates have been reported in patients with contact granulomas (see Table 3.7 in Hirano, 1981b). Few other physiological data are available on the physiological characteristics associated with granulomas of the vocal folds.

### OBSERVABLE PHYSIOLOGICAL SIGNS

Granulomas manifest themselves laryngoscopically as irregularly shaped masses of tissue either at the site of the vocal processes of the arytenoids (if an intubation granuloma) or elsewhere on the vocal folds or larynx (Friedman, 1973).

The vocal folds will show normal stroboscopic signs unless the granuloma appears on the vocal fold margins. In that case, glottic closure may be incomplete and we would expect to see reduced amplitude of lateral excursion of the affected vocal fold(s) and some degree of disturbance of the mucosal wave.

### PATHOPHYSIOLOGY

Intubation granulomas primarily affect the mucosa of the vocal processes of the arytenoids.

## *Pachydermia Laryngis*

### PRIMARY VOCAL SYMPTOM: HOARSENESS

### DESCRIPTION AND ETIOLOGY

This is a relatively rare problem whose etiology is unknown. Some suspect smoking to be the major cause and others suspect irritation caused by GERD. Pachydermia laryngis is characterized by a thickening of the epithelium with acanthosis and keratosis (Ballenger, 1985). Clinically it appears as a whitish mass of tissue in the interarytenoid space. The membranous vocal folds may also be injected and thickened. Conservative treatment usually consists of cessation of smoking and alcohol use and treatment (behavioral and pharmacological) of the GERD. Surgical removal may be necessary.

### PERCEPTUAL SIGNS AND SYMPTOMS

Hoarseness will be a primary perceptual sign of this disease.

### ACOUSTIC SIGNS

There are few data on the acoustic signs for this vocal problem. A lower fundamental frequency may be expected if the vocal folds are thickened sufficiently.

### MEASURABLE PHYSIOLOGICAL SIGNS

We have no knowledge of physiological data on this vocal problem. One might expect that if the lesion interfered with glottal closure, excessive airflows would result.

### OBSERVABLE PHYSIOLOGICAL SIGNS

On direct or indirect laryngoscopy, the vocal folds may look thickened and rough, and there is an excess of rough, uneven tissue present in the interarytenoid space.

We know of no data concerning the stroboscopic signs associated with pachydermia laryngis. However, we would expect that glottal closure might be compromised, and mucosal wave and amplitude may be reduced due to the thickened mucosa.

## *Papilloma*

### PRIMARY VOICE SYMPTOM: HOARSENESS

### DESCRIPTION AND ETIOLOGY

Papilloma is a rather common benign tumor that starts in the epithelium and is thought to be caused by a virus, probably of the papovavirus group. It occurs in both children and adults. In children it is referred to as juvenile papilloma, and it is very resistant to eradication. Surgical excision is required, as papillomas tend to proliferate and can obstruct the airway. It is not uncommon for children with this problem to require multiple surgical excisions before the condition runs its course. If juvenile papilloma persists or begins in adulthood, it continues to be a condition that is highly resistant to treatment. The papilloma may occur in various parts of the larynx: subglottally, at the level of the vocal folds, and supraglottally. It is sometimes necessary for children with aggressive papilloma growth to undergo tracheotomy. When the papillomas have ceased recurring, or perhaps between episodes of recurrence, voice therapy may be appropriate in order to maintain or restore the best possible voice production. The prognosis will depend largely on the state of the vocal fold mucosa.

### PERCEPTUAL SIGNS AND SYMPTOMS

Hoarseness is the primary symptom and sign of the voice disorder caused by this condition. Because of the sometimes extensive involvement of the true vocal folds, a low pitch level might also be evident, although there are no data to support this hypothesis.

## MEASURABLE PHYSIOLOGICAL SIGNS

We know of no measurable physiological data reported for individuals with papillomas of the vocal folds. However, because of the increased stiffness of the cords we might expect greater expiratory air pressures.

## OBSERVABLE PHYSIOLOGICAL SIGNS

### *Laryngoscopy*

A papilloma will typically present as a whitish cluster of tissue, somewhat comparable in texture to a raspberry. An example of the laryngoscopic appearance of a papilloma is shown in Figure 6.3. In Figure 6.4 multiple papillomas are evident, illustrating the potentially extensive nature of the disease.

### *Stroboscopy*

Papillomas will often interfere with glottal closure. To what extent this is true will depend on the extent of the lesion. The increased stiffness created by the lesion will

*Figure 6.3.* Papilloma of the vocal folds. See color plate.

*Figure 6.4.* Multiple papillomas of the vocal folds. See color plate.

impede horizontal excursion of the folds and mucosal wave will be absent in the area of the lesions. When multiple surgical excisions have been required for vocal fold papilloma, the membranous cover of the vocal folds may have been sufficiently damaged to interfere with amplitude and vibratory behavior.

## PATHOPHYSIOLOGY

Papillomas affect vocal fold vibration by increasing the mass and the stiffness of the vocal folds and altering the biomechanical characteristics of the mucosa. Although they can be removed surgically the lesions tend to recur, especially in children (Bastian, 1986). Treatment with interferon has been tried but with inconclusive results (Benjamin, Gatenby, Kitchen, Harrison, Cameron, & Basten, 1988).

## *Ankylosis of the Cricoarytenoid Joint*

### PRIMARY VOICE SYMPTOM: HOARSENESS

### DESCRIPTION AND ETIOLOGY

Fixation of the cricoarytenoid joint may be due to several causes, including arthritis, trauma, or joint disease. Ankylosis of the cricoarytenoid joint is sometimes difficult to distinguish from paralysis of the vocal folds. Clinically they appear very similar (Cummings, 1986). However, pain may be a symptom of ankylosis due to arthritis and would usually not be a symptom of paralysis. An attempt to manipulate the joint under direct laryngoscopy may be necessary in order to distinguish between the two conditions. Treatment of ankylosis requires surgical arytenoidectomy or arytenoidopexy (Ballenger, 1985). Voice therapy is usually not helpful.

### PERCEPTUAL SIGNS AND SYMPTOMS

The primary perceptual symptoms of unilateral arytenoid fixation are hoarseness and breathiness secondary to the anticipated inadequacy of posterior vocal fold closure. In the event that the condition is bilateral, stridor may be present, and the patient may display symptoms of dyspnea.

### ACOUSTIC SIGNS

We know of no experimental data concerning the acoustic characteristics of voice in the presence of cricoarytenoid ankylosis. In unilateral ankylosis, these might include increased frequency and amplitude perturbation (jitter and shimmer), reduced phonational and dynamic ranges, increased spectral noise, and reduced phonation time. Acoustic signs in bilateral ankylosis may be minimal.

### MEASURABLE PHYSIOLOGICAL SIGNS

Physiological signs of ankylosis are not documented. As with unilateral vocal fold paralysis, if the glottis is not fully adducted during phonation, we would expect increased airflows and an electroglottogram that would reveal the incomplete closure and reduced closed time. On the other hand, in the bilateral condition, airflows might be expected to be reduced, and the electrogram should reveal minimal vocal fold opening phase.

### OBSERVABLE PHYSIOLOGICAL SIGNS

As noted previously, the laryngeal appearance of ankylosis might be difficult to distinguish from vocal fold paralysis. If unilateral, we would expect to observe lack of movement of the arytenoid and incomplete glottal closure. In bilateral ankylosis, the position of both arytenoids would be fixed and unmoving, resulting also in lack of either adduction or abduction of the folds. We have observed that in paralysis, movement in the opening of the pyriform sinuses may be absent, while in ankylosis such movement continues to be present. If the cause of ankylosis is an arthritic condition (usually rheumatoid arthritis), mucosal edema, inflammation, or both may be seen in the area of the cricoarytenoid joint.

We know of no data on the stroboscopic signs of a fixed arytenoid. One might expect to see incomplete glottal closure, but minimal aberrations in the vibratory motion of the vocal folds.

### PATHOPHYSIOLOGY

The movement of the ankylosed arytenoid cartilage(s) is reduced or absent. The glottis may be incompletely adducted, or, in the case of bilateral ankylosis, it may be neither fully adducted nor abducted.

## VASCULAR DISORDERS

### *Hemorrhage*

#### PRIMARY VOICE SYMPTOM

Hoarseness, occasional or intermittent aphonia, and loss of pitch range

#### DESCRIPTION AND ETIOLOGY

Hemorrhage into the vocal fold is usually unilateral, although it may be bilateral. It can involve the full length of the vocal fold or portions of the fold. The hemorrhagic area appears reddish in color with significant swelling. Hemorrhage is most frequently the result of a single episode of traumatic voice use or laryngeal trauma, or it can result from the combination of heavy voice use and use of anticoagulants and salicylates (such as aspirin), or extended use of inhaled steroids.

#### PERCEPTUAL SIGNS AND SYMPTOMS

Patients may complain of pain particularly at the time of the precipitating event. Dryness, vocal fatigue and loss of upper range are among the perceptual symptoms that accompany the primary symptom and sign of hoarseness. Depending on the severity of the bleed, the voice may be intermittently aphonic and it may require added effort for voicing to be produced. Vocal fold hemorrhage occurs more frequently in females than in males and usually in adults.

#### ACOUSTIC SIGNS

Although there are no data for this population, we would anticipate increased shimmer and jitter related to the hoarseness that is perceptible. We would also expect decreased signal-to-noise ratio, restricted pitch, and dynamic ranges.

#### MEASURABLE PHYSIOLOGICAL SIGNS

We would expect subglottic air pressures to be increased as the patient must exert greater effort to produce phonation. Increased air flows may also be noted as a result of the limitations in laryngeal valving due to stiffness of the hemorrhagic cord.

#### OBSERVABLE PHYSIOLOGICAL SIGNS

As noted in the description, hemorrhage is visible when the vocal folds are visualized by the apparent redness of the area of the fold involved, the significant swelling present and the stiffness of the cord. A prominent blood vessel may be seen.

Under stroboscopic observation, stiffness of the hemorrhagic vocal fold or part thereof is apparent with reduced amplitude of the involved fold and absence of mucosal wave in the area of the hemorrhage. Glottal closure may vary in degree depending on the amount of stiffness and swelling. The vocal fold edge usually remains straight as long as the hemorrhage has not organized into a specific lesion such as a hemorrhagic polyp. Because the lesion is usually unilateral, asymmetry of movement between the vocal folds would be apparent as would aperiodicity.

### PATHOPHYSIOLOGY

Rupture of blood vessels results in bleeding into the submucosal layer. This produces extreme swelling of that area decreasing the efficiency of the vibratory behavior of the vocal folds. The mass and stiffness of the cover are increased.

## Varix and Ectasia

### PRIMARY VOICE SYMPTOM: HOARSENESS

### DESCRIPTION AND ETIOLOGY

A varix is seen as a prominent, distended, lengthened, and tortuous blood vessel on the surface of the vocal fold. The location of a varix may be either on the superior surface of the fold or on the free edge of the fold. A varix is often visualized following resorption of a hemorrhage or in conjunction with a hemorrhagic polyp. We have also observed varices in the absence of a known previous hemorrhage. The etiology seems to be related to vocal abuse or trauma and usually results from a single or focused short term episode of abuse.

Ectasia is defined as a dilation of a small vessel. Occasionally, vascular microectasias are seen on the surface of the vocal folds, which may affect vibration in that location.

### ACOUSTIC SIGNS

These signs will vary depending on the size and location of the varix or ectasia. When hoarseness is present we would anticipate increased shimmer and jitter magnitudes.

### MEASURABLE PHYSIOLOGICAL SIGNS

Airflow should not necessarily show any change from normal unless the varix is large or ectasias are extensive enough to create vocal fold stiffness and interfere with glottal closure.

### OBSERVABLE PHYSIOLOGICAL SIGNS

#### Laryngoscopy

Varices and ectasias may be seen on the surface of the vocal folds as increased vascularity not normally present. When a hemorrhagic polyp is present, it is often possible to visualize a prominent blood vessel leading directly to the polyp suggesting that the vessel is "feeding" the polyp and is a factor in its presence.

#### Stroboscopy

The area of the varix or the ectasia may appear stiffened with reduced mucosal wave. The effect on vibratory behavior of the fold will be in direct relation to the location and the extent of the varix or the ectasia. A small varix on the superior surface of the fold may have minimal effect on the vibratory characteristics of that fold, whereas, a large vessel along the edge or even on the superior surface of the fold will limit mucosal wave and perhaps amplitude of lateral excursion of the fold. Glottal closure pattern will also vary depending upon the size and location of the lesion.

### PATHOPHYSIOLOGY

The varix is usually in the submucosal layer and the amount of distortion of that layer will depend on its size. A large varix or large cluster of small vessels will increase stiffness and mass of the cover. If a varix is the residual effect of a hemorrhage, full resorption of the hemorrhage may not have occurred and the behavior of the fold will be affected by that as well.

## Contact Ulcer

### PRIMARY VOICE SYMPTOM: HOARSENESS

### DESCRIPTION AND ETIOLOGY

A contact ulcer is a small ulceration that develops on the medial surface of the vocal processes of the arytenoid cartilages. The ulceration may be unilateral or bilateral and may present a "cup and saucer" appearance, with a protuberance on one side and a crater or concavity on the other. Continued irritation results in an ulceration on one side and the production of granulation tissue on the other.

The thinking about the etiology of contact ulcers has undergone major change within the recent past. The traditional view had been that contact ulcers occurred predominantly in adult males with an average age of 50 years (Peacher, 1947) who engaged in a great deal of forceful, aggressive speaking, the so-called type A personality.

In support of that view, von Leden and Moore (1960) described some of the anatomical and physiological variations of phonation that could contribute to the formation of a contact ulcer. They pointed out that at low pitches the arytenoids oscillate vigorously, in a rocking-type motion. Thus, at low pitches it is more likely that the arytenoids would be subjected to greater trauma. They also observed that at low pitches there is greater vocal fold approximation, the approximation is prolonged, and it tends to persist beyond the vibratory phase of the vocal folds. Greater loudness will also increase the degree of approximation as well as its duration. Harsh, guttural sounds will increase the force of approximation of the vocal folds, as will other nonphonatory acts (throat clearing, etc.). Voice therapy was a treatment course often followed but with little documentation of its efficacy. Contact ulcers were often surgically excised, but they showed a propensity to recur.

In a study relating gastric reflux to contact ulcer, Cherry and Margulies (1968) studied three patients who showed evidence of peptic ulcer. All were treated with antacids, reduced food intake at night, and elevation of the head during sleep, and all experienced resolution of the ulcer. Delahunty and Cherry (1968) demonstrated that continued exposure of the arytenoid vocal processes to stomach acids would create ulcers and granulation tissue in dogs in about a month's time. Histologically, these lesions exhibited epithelial necrosis with an organized fibrous exudate beneath. Submucosal edema and nonspecific inflammation were also described. In a control condition, saliva was applied to the arytenoids over the same time period, with no development of granulation tissue. Ward, Zwitman, Hanson, and Berci (1980) reported that contact ulcers result from constant throat clearing that is secondary to irritation of the mucosa due to gastroesophageal reflux (regurgitation of peptic acids, especially at night), and with less frequency to irritation from nasal secretions (postnasal drip). They further reported that of 28 cases, only 2 failed to respond to medical treatment. Feder and

Michell (1984) divided ulcers into two groups, hyperfunctional and hyperacidic. Watterson, Hensen-Magorian, and McFarlane (1988) reported that 51% of their patients with a contact ulcer also exhibited a hiatal hernia. It had been thought that hiatal hernia and GERD were two parts of the same problem. According to Bozymski (1993), most hiatal hernias are now thought to be normal variants of the anatomy. Thus, it would appear that the etiology of contact ulcers may be primarily related to reflux with hyperfunctional vocal abuse being a contributory factor.

Benjamin and Croxson (1985) reported clinical and histological similarities between contact ulcers and granulomas. They studied 16 patients, of whom 7 had postintubation granulomas and the remainder contact ulcers. The most common symptom of all patients was hoarseness. They concluded that contact ulcer was not a precursor to granulomas since the history of the problems was different and the patient with a granuloma did not present the profile of a patient with a contact ulcer. Recent literature has even more strongly implicated GERD as the primary etiology of contact ulcer, and, further, postnasal drip is also thought to be related to the same process of mucosal irritation resulting from the reflux of gastric juices (Bozymski, 1993; Deveney, Benner, & Cohen, 1993; Gaynor, 1991; Koufman, 1991; Wilson, Pryde, Cecilia, & MacIntyre, 1989).

## PERCEPTUAL SIGNS AND SYMPTOMS

The primary perceptual symptoms of a contact ulcer are constant throat clearing and vocal fatigue. There may be a breathy voice with some hoarseness, accompanied by discomfort or even severe, stabbing pain. The pain is usually unilateral and located in the area of the greater horn of the thyroid. The pain may radiate to the ear. There is usually the constant feeling of something in the throat, which accounts for the continual throat clearing.

## ACOUSTIC SIGNS

Depending on the severity of the voice symptoms, some increased frequency perturbation and spectral noise may be present in the voice.

## MEASURABLE PHYSIOLOGICAL SIGNS

Isshiki and von Leden (1964) reported a mean flow of 144 ml/sec for their group of patients with contact ulcers. This value is not much higher than would be expected in normal speakers. Increased air pressures might be expected due to the tendency to use higher than normal forces when speaking. Muscle activity levels should be within normal limits.

## OBSERVABLE PHYSIOLOGICAL SIGNS

Laryngoscopically, a contact ulcer will be visible as a buildup of pink or pinkish-white tissue on one of the vocal processes of the arytenoids. This usually occurs at the tip of the process, but it is possible to find such an outgrowth elsewhere on the vocal process or on the lower base of the arytenoid. On the contralateral process, there may be injection of the mucosa or a depression. This has been described as the "cup and saucer" appearance because the two processes fit together in that way. Inflammation of the arytenoids and the posterior pharyngeal wall may be seen. In the early stages of contact ulcer development, even prior to tissue outgrowth, a strand of mucus may be seen between the two processes. This is referred to as a contact ulcer diathesis.

Unless there are abnormal voice symptoms, normal stroboscopic features would be anticipated.

PATHOPHYSIOLOGY

Since the contact ulcer does not involve the membranous vocal fold, there will be little change in the mass or stiffness of the cover, transition layers, or body.

## Blunt or Penetrating Trauma

A variety of traumatic injuries may affect the larynx. These may include attempted strangulation, a penetrating neck wound, blunt trauma resulting from a blow to the neck or from the body's being hurled with force, and the neck's striking an object. In severe trauma, the structures of the larynx may be fractured or severely damaged, compromising the airway and resulting in vocal difficulty. An example of the effects of trauma to the vocal folds is shown in Figure 6.5.

Most cases of blunt or penetrating trauma require medical/surgical treatment. The most urgent concern is management of the airway. Subsequently there will be an attempt to repair or reconstruct the damaged structures. Voice restoration, following the completion of the repair, may be very difficult. A speech-language pathologist may be asked to help the patient achieve the best possible voice. In these cases, the speech-language pathologist should ask for and expect to receive detailed information about the altered laryngeal anatomy, in order to understand the constraints upon the system and to be able to plan the treatment approach accordingly.

## Inhalation and Thermal Trauma

There is a paucity of information in the literature about the long-term laryngeal and phonatory sequelae of the inhalation of gases, smoke, or steam. Inhalation injuries are usually referred to as chemical tracheobronchitis, a term that seems to exclude laryngeal and supraglottal effects of such injury even though they occur as frequently and almost always with greater severity (Hunt, Agee, & Pruitt, 1975; Miller, Gray, Cotton, & Myer, 1988). Hot fumes cause reflex closure of the glottis, which, in combination with the cooling capacity of the upper respiratory tract, protects the trachea and lower tract (Miller et al., 1988). Acute airway obstruction can result from either supraglottal

*Figure 6.5.* Trauma of the vocal folds. Note the obliteration of clear definition of either vocal fold due to the formation of a web that has grown after trauma. There is also excessive vascularization of the folds. See color plate.

or laryngeal edema, or both. Hunt et al. (1975) point out that laryngeal and supraglottal structures tend to show massive amounts of edema in a short period of time due to the loose attachment of the surface mucosa to the underlying basal layers.

During the acute stage, those who suffer inhalation injury are frequently at risk for survival, making their medical condition and treatment of the utmost urgency. The severe edema of the respiratory tract may appear immediately or may develop within a matter of hours and can quickly lead to airway obstruction and to death (Crapo, 1981; Cudmore & Vivori, 1981). Intubation or tracheotomy may be required. A risk of intubation is the possibility of damage to the already compromised mucosal tissue. Symptoms of inhalation trauma include swelling, inflammation, burns, or soot around the nose and mouth and in the oropharynx (even with minimal body surface injury), respiratory distress, stridor, wheezing, and hoarseness (Crapo, 1981). The symptoms will depend on the severity of the trauma, the type of fumes or gases inhaled, and the stage of the body's response to the trauma. The trauma may result not only from heat but also from the particles and toxic chemicals released as the burning material breaks down, and from the reduction in oxygen. The heat capacity of steam is 4000 times greater than that of air; thus, steam inhalation can quickly produce thermal burns of the respiratory tract. Steam inhalation burns may occur with a scald injury in young children. According to Cudmore and Vivori (1981), inhalation of hot, dry gases causes damage primarily to the upper airway (including the larynx) because there is a rapid decrease in temperature of the gases as soon as they enter the airway. Chemical damage to the entire airway results from inhalation of smoke. Smoke from the combustion of polyurethane foams is reported to be especially damaging (Dyer & Esch, 1976). This fact is all the more disturbing in view of the increased numbers of house fires resulting in more inhalation burns in children (Chisnall, 1977) and the increased use of plastics and polyurethane foam in homes.

Voice can only become a concern after the patient has survived the acute stage of trauma and has completed the major portion of treatment for the injuries sustained. If there has been extensive body surface burn in addition to the inhalation injuries, treatment may be quite lengthy. Only when the patient is sufficiently recovered is it appropriate to focus on aspects of vocal recovery. However, during the recovery period, consultation by the speech-language pathologist may be helpful in establishing the most efficacious means of communication for patients whose ability to communicate has been significantly compromised.

As noted previously, there is little documentation of the long-term effects of laryngeal trauma. Close, Catlin, and Cohn (1980), reporting on the chronic effects of ammonia inhalation burns, cite one case in which breathy phonation was present and showed some improvement with voice therapy. In another instance, severe and progressive hoarseness noted in the early post-trauma stage apparently resolved spontaneously. Recently 22 patients who had been treated in the regional burn unit at the SUNY Health Science Center over a 10-year period were examined for voice problems (Casper, Clark, & Kellman, unpublished data). Of these, 11 or 50% were judged by an experienced voice clinician to show some degree of voice abnormality that, according to patient reports, was not present prior to the trauma. Although most of the patients so identified had been either intubated or tracheotomized or both, some patients had not experienced either of these procedures. Thus, injury resulting from intubation or tracheotomy cannot fully account for the resulting voice abnormality.

In view of these findings, we would suspect that there are more residual voice problems in inhalation burn survivors than have previously been recognized. The pathophysiology is not well understood and may differ from patient to patient. There are many unanswered questions relative to phonatory function in this population, such as whether problems result from changes in laryngeal mucosa, peripheral nerve damage from the burn or from subsequent surgery, or central nervous system damage due to hypoxia.

Our experience in voice therapy with this population is very limited. Nevertheless, the case study of C. H. is instructive.

## Case Study

C. H. was a 17-year-old young man who had suffered extensive burns of the head, neck, face, hands, and upper body following the crash of an ultralight plane that he had been flying alone. He also suffered inhalation injury. His treatment course included two periods of intubation, the first for a week and the second for 4 days, with a 2-day intervening period. He survived a long and painful course of treatment and surgeries. Although now he was being followed as an outpatient, he faced further surgery in the future. He was in constant physical pain and discomfort, and his emotional pain due to his grotesquely deformed appearance was perhaps even greater. He was essentially aphonic, as he had been throughout the entire post-trauma course. Ear, nose, and throat examination was reported to be negative, with no observable reason for the aphonia. The vocal folds were reported to show good movement, although they did not adduct completely during speaking.

C. H. responded minimally to questions, offered no information spontaneously, and did not make eye contact with the clinician. He generally kept his eyes downcast or looked out of the window. Several sessions were required to work through this resistance and to establish a relationship. As he began to open up, C. H. talked more about the crash, and also about his parents, who were divorced. He was living with his mother; he would have preferred to have been with his father, but the accident had occurred during a time spent with the father, who was apparently finding the guilt related to the event overwhelming. C. H. was supposed to be returning to school but had thus far been resisting that because he saw himself as a "monster" whom others saw as disgusting. As therapy progressed, C. H. was increasingly willing to attempt voicing. Indeed, he was able to produce voice, but with a hoarse and somewhat breathy quality. The sound of this voice was just one more abnormality that he could not deal with, and his response had been to be aphonic. Work with C. H. continued for a period of time, during which he began to use voice routinely and with some improvement in quality. He was clearly in need of psychological counseling but had previously refused to consider such referral. Leading him to an acceptance of such counseling had been one of the goals of therapy, and, indeed, after his experience with us he was able to accept the support that had been offered and to recognize his need for continuation of such support. Although his voice quality was not "normal," C. H. was using voice routinely and finding that communication was easier.

The reason for C. H.'s hoarse voice quality was never fully understood. However, more testing, given his initial level of resistance and the subsequent determination of his very vulnerable psychological state, was not entirely necessary and might result in his withdrawal from further therapy. He made sufficient progress so that his voice was entirely usable, and although still hoarse, was not severely so. The reason for his aphonic presentation appeared to be primarily psychological. This case highlights the need to be alert to more than a single problem being present at one time, especially when there may be an obvious cause that might explain the problem.

## CARCINOMA AND OTHER TUMORS

### *Carcinoma*

#### PRIMARY VOICE SYMPTOM

The primary voice symptom of laryngeal cancer is hoarseness. Indeed, this is recognized as one of the seven warning signs of cancer.

#### DESCRIPTION AND ETIOLOGY

Cancer is one of the diseases that may affect the structures of the oral cavity, pharynx, and larynx. If allowed to proceed unchecked, it is life threatening. The incidence of laryngeal cancer is reported to be between 2% and 5% of all malignancies. Persistent hoarseness is well known as one of the primary symptoms of cancer. If a malignant lesion affects one or both vocal folds directly, hoarseness will result. Figure 6.6 shows a cancer involving both vocal folds. Laryngeal lesions that do not affect the vibratory characteristics of the vocal folds will not necessarily result in a change in the voice.

There are many possible etiologies for cancer, including smoking, environmental irritants, chemicals and other contaminants, metabolic disturbances, and unknown causes. According to the Surgeon General's report (U.S. Department of Health and Human Services, 1985), "Cigarette smoking is a major cause of cancers of the lung, larynx, oral cavity and esophagus" (p. vi). Furthermore, 50–70% of oral and laryngeal cancer deaths are associated with smoking. The report also states that a synergistic effect is created by the use of alcohol in conjunction with smoking that greatly increases the risk of oral and laryngeal cancers. The ratio of men to women who develop these cancers was reported to be 5 to 1 in 1985 (Ballenger, 1985), but that ratio has been narrowing steadily for the past 20 years. The carcinogenic effects of cigar and pipe smoke are similar to those of cigarette smoke.

The severity of the malignancy is evaluated using the "TNM" system or its variants (American Joint Committee for Cancer Staging and End Results Reporting, 1983). The T refers to the site of the primary tumor, the N indicates the involvement of lymph nodes, and the M signifies spread of the lesion to other parts of the body

*Figure 6.6.* Carcinoma of the vocal folds. See color plate.

(metastasis). Low numbers associated with each code indicate a lesser involvement; the numbers increase as severity or extent increase (Table 6.1). Thus, a patient described to have a T1N0M0 lesion has a locally confined tumor with neither node involvement nor any distant metastasis. Where the values of N and M are zero, the description is often truncated (e.g., T1 or T2 carcinoma) (Fig. 6.7).

### PERCEPTUAL SIGNS AND SYMPTOMS

Hoarseness is the primary sign and symptom (Stoicheff, Ciampi, Passi, & Frederickson, 1983). Other signs of cancer of the larynx may include (*a*) a lump in the neck, (*b*) a broadening of the larynx, detected on palpation; and (*c*) tenderness in the neck. Other symptoms may include dysphagia, odynophagia (pain on swallowing), and dyspnea.

*Table 6.1.* Classification of Glottal Cancers

| | | |
|---|---|---|
| *T: Location of Primary Tumor* | | |
| | Tx | Cannot be staged |
| | T0 | No evidence of tumor |
| | Tis | Carcinoma in situ |
| | T1 | Confined to vocal folds |
| | T2 | Supraglottal or subglottal extension, normal or impaired mobility |
| | T3 | Confined to larynx but with fixed cord |
| | T4 | Massive tumor |
| *N: Involvement of regional lymph nodes* | | |
| | Nx | Cannot be assessed |
| | N0 | No involvement |
| | N1 | A single small node on one side |
| | N2 | A single large or multiple small nodes on one side |
| | N3 | Massive nodes on one or both sides |
| *M: Distant metastasis* | | |
| | Mx | Cannot be assessed |
| | M0 | No known metastasis |
| | M1 | Metastasis present |

*Figure 6.7.* T1 carcinoma involving a single vocal fold. See color plate.

ACOUSTIC SIGNS

Cancer will affect the vibration of the vocal folds and therefore will affect the acoustic characteristics of the voice. The magnitude of the effect will depend on the extent of the carcinoma. Frequency and amplitude perturbation will be increased. For their sample of 5 cancer patients, Hecker and Kruel (1971) reported pitch perturbation quotients similar to normal (patients = 13.6 versus normal = 13.0) but much greater directional perturbation quotients (patient = 48.9; normal = 33.3). Lieberman (1963) had reported large perturbation values in an earlier study. Murry, Bone, and von Essen (1974) reported lower than normal phonational ranges for their one male subject with T1 carcinoma of the vocal folds. Colton, Reed, Sagerman, and Chung (1982) reported slightly higher fundamental frequencies for the vowels /ah/ and /ee/ for males with T1 or T2 carcinoma and much larger fundamental frequencies for both vowels produced by female patients with T1 cancer of the vocal folds (Figure 6.8). Pitch perturbation quotients were increased in both vowels for both male T1 and T2 cancer classification groups. However, female patients tended to show lower PPQs for the vowel /ah/ and similar PPQs for the vowel /ee/ when compared to the normal control group (Figure 6.9). Spectral noise levels are also increased. Colton, Sagerman, Chung, Young, and Reed (1978) reported elevated spectrum levels, especially in the higher frequencies, for their sample of five cancer patients. Similar findings were reported for a much larger group of patients with cancer (Colton et al., 1982). In the same study, both phonational and dynamic ranges were found to be lower in patients with laryngeal cancer than normal control subjects (Figure 6.10).

Measurement of the noise energy in the voices of patients with laryngeal cancer may be predictive of the severity of the cancer (Kasuya, Ogawa, Mashima, & Ebihara, 1986). Noise levels were measured in sustained vowels and a measure called normalized noise energy (NNE) was calculated for 64 samples of normal voice and 57 samples of patients with carcinoma of the vocal folds. NNE was effective in detecting 91% of the normal voices. In voices with carcinoma, NNE was effective in detecting T1 cancer about 77% of the time and always detected T2, T3, or T4 cancer. Thus, measurement of noise levels may be a very useful clinical technique for documenting the magnitude of the voice change of cancer patients and for following effects of treatment.

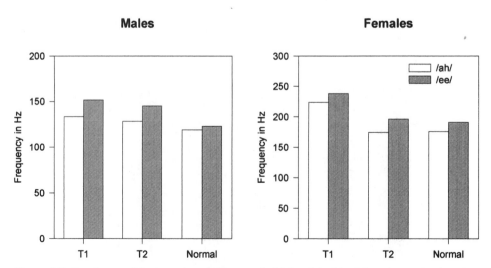

*Figure 6.8.* Fundamental frequencies of the vowels /ah/ and /ee/ for 38 males and 5 females with T1 cancer classification and 13 males and 7 females with T2 cancer classification compared to a normal control group of 35 males and 27 females.

### MEASURABLE PHYSIOLOGICAL SIGNS

There are very little data on the measurable physiological characteristics of patients with cancer. Airflows are generally increased with large leakage flows associated with large tumors that prevent complete vocal fold closure. Mean airflow rates are increased (Murry, Bone, & von Essen, 1974). EGG recordings will reflect reduced time of closure. Subglottal air pressures may be increased because of the increased stiffness of the vocal folds.

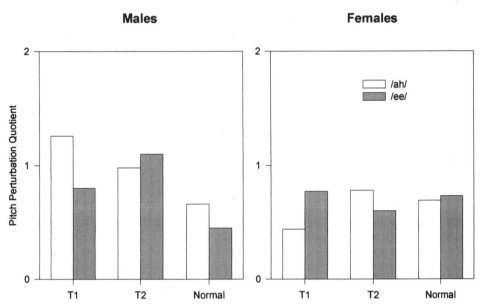

*Figure 6.9.* Pitch perturbation quotients for the vowels /ah/ and /ee/ for 38 males and 5 females with T1 cancer classification and 13 males and 7 females with T2 cancer classification compared to a normal control group of 35 males and 27 females.

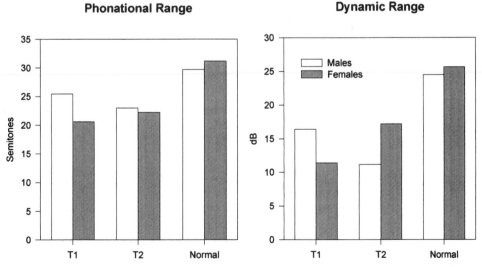

*Figure 6.10.* Phonational and dynamic ranges of 38 males and 5 females with T1 cancer classification and 13 males and 7 females with T2 cancer classification compared to a normal control group of 35 males and 27 females.

## OBSERVABLE PHYSIOLOGICAL SIGNS

### *Laryngoscopy*

Laryngoscopic examination may reveal anything from a small, well-defined tumor to a large and diffuse one involving any part of the larynx or vocal folds. Precise diagnosis of carcinoma usually requires biopsy and histological analysis. Most carcinomas of the larynx arise from the epithelium and are of the squamous cell variety. As the severity of the lesion increases, it becomes more invasive in nature as well as more extensive in size.

### STROBOSCOPY

Early carcinoma in situ can be more readily diagnosed using stroboscopy than other methods of examination. The distinguishing feature is the presence of a small lesion that has a markedly negative effect on vibratory vocal fold behavior (Sessions et al., 1989). We have found that in patients with small cancers, stroboscopy can help better define the level of invasion (Woo, Colton, Casper, & Brewer, 1991). As the cancer becomes more extensive and invasive the entire vocal fold may become fixed, showing no movement of any kind.

### PATHOPHYSIOLOGY

Cancerous lesions invade the tissue and destroy the normally behaving cells. Depending on its location and size, the tumor may affect vocal fold closure, will result in reduced horizontal excursion of the affected fold and often of the contralateral fold and restricted or absent mucosal wave.

### TREATMENT

There are several approaches to cancer treatment. These include surgery, radiation therapy, and chemotherapy. Their use depends on many factors and is determined on a case-by-case basis. Spector and Ogura (1985) have discussed some of the considerations in the diagnosis and treatment of carcinoma. Patients who undergo radiation therapy as the primary treatment mode may experience some alterations in voice during the course of the treatment (Colton, Sagerman, Chung, Young, & Reed, 1978). Depending on the extent of the lesion, a patient may still have a normal-sounding voice after radiation therapy. Voice therapy is usually not necessary or indicated.

There are a variety of surgical approaches in the treatment of laryngeal cancer, which may involve excision of the lesion, of up to half of the larynx, of supraglottal structures only, or of the entire larynx. The effect on voice production capability will depend on the extent and the nature of the surgery performed. In addition to concerns about voice, patients who have had extensive surgery may also have difficulty with swallowing. A full discussion of the problems of dysphagia and those associated with the total absence of the larynx is beyond the scope of this book. These topics are well covered in the literature.

The voice problems associated with partial laryngeal excisions will vary a great deal. Both voice problems and dysphagia will require the assistance of a speech-language pathologist. The role of the speech-language pathologist is to assist the patient in producing the best possible voice. In order to do so, the speech-language pathologist must be completely informed about the specifics of the surgical procedure. It is important to know what structures remain intact, how the anatomy is altered, and what functional skills remain relative to phonation.

Some patients with laryngeal cancer have extremely extensive disease that requires excision of not only the larynx but also of other structures essential to the production of speech, such as the tongue. The speech-language pathologist should also be involved with these patients in an effort to provide a means of communication.

## OTHER TUMORS

A variety of benign and malignant tumors may be found in the laryngeal or neck area in both children and adults. Such tumors may obstruct the airway directly, or they may occupy space and place pressure on the trachea or larynx, thereby creating airway problems indirectly. The effect on the voice will depend on the position of the tumor. These lesions require medical and/or surgical treatment. In many cases of small or benign tumors, surgery is a viable treatment option. In cases of extensive malignant tumors, radiation therapy or chemotherapy or a combined protocol may be possible treatment choices. Rarely is there need for speech therapy services unless the tumor (or surgery) has compromised vocal or speech function. Tumors that are frequent in children include cysts, hemangiomas, and lymphoangiomas; malignant neuroblastomas and lymphomas also occur. Many of these same tumors may also be found in adults.

## THE GERIATRIC VOICE

In this section, the biological and voice characteristics of the elderly will be discussed. Here, *geriatric* will refer to individuals 65 years or older. Aging is a process that results in a progressive decline of the multiple control mechanisms needed for daily life (Barry & Eathorne, 1994). All organs are affected although the change may be prevented or minimized by physical activity. There may be a large difference between the chronological age of an individual and his or her biological age. We do not all age at the same rate biologically. Individuals with identical chronological ages can be very different in their biological abilities. In his preface to the book *Geriatric Otolaryngology*, Dr. Jerome Goldstein reported on several geriatric individuals to demonstrate that even at 72, 76 or 81 years of age, an individual can be very active and biologically fit. One of his examples was an 81-year-old female power lifter who deadlifts 245 pounds, squatlifts 148 pounds, and works out daily with running, swimming, and lifting (Goldstein, 1989). Clearly, we do not all age at the same rate; we merely count the number of years from birth in the same way.

### Anatomical and Physiological Changes

Aging in the larynx affects the cartilages, connective tissue, blood supply, secretions, and muscle. Changes in the lamina propria include loss of collagenous and elastic fibers, atrophy of submucous glands, disorganization of collagen fibers, increased fibrosis, and atrophy of the muscles (Gracco & Kahane, 1989; Kahane, 1981a, 1981b, 1987). Structural changes include ossification of the thyroid cartilage and changes in the articular cartilages. Presumably, these anatomical changes will affect the vibratory characteristics of the vocal folds and the perceptual, acoustic, and physiological voice signs. Anatomical changes that may occur in the brain and spinal cord may also affect the neurological control of the vocal muscles.

### Perceptual Signs

Extensive reviews of acoustic and perceptual features of the geriatric voice have appeared in the literature (Colton, 1989; Hollien, 1987; Linville, 1987a, 1987b, 1994; Shindo & Hanson, 1990) and only a brief review will be presented here. Perceptually, listeners can identify a geriatric voice and can do so from a recorded sample with surprising accuracy. Some of the major features of the geriatric voice include hoarseness, low pitch, imprecise articulation, breathiness, and long pauses (Hartman & Danhauer, 1976). In another study (Ryan & Capadano, 1978), the important perceptual features of the geriatric voice included pitch, volume, speed, clarity, and authority. According to this study, geriatric voices sounded less clear and less flexible.

## Acoustic Signs

Acoustically, there are several features of the voice that change as a result of aging. Fundamental frequency tends to rise as a function of age in males (Benjamin, 1981; Hollien & Shipp, 1972) and fall in females (Brown, Morris, & Michel, 1989; Linville & Fisher, 1985). This has led Hollien (1987) to postulate a male-female coalescence model of voice change where, as they age, men and women become more alike, at least vocally. The model predicts that the fundamental frequency of a male voice will increase substantially as it ages whereas the female voice will show a slight downward change of fundamental frequency or no change at all.

Fundamental frequency variability is also affected by aging. Mysak (1959) reported larger values for males and Stoicheff (1981), Linville and Fisher (1985) and Morris and Brown (1994) for females. Fundamental frequency range is also reduced both in males (McGlone & Hollien, 1963; Ptacek, Sander, Maloney, & Jackson, 1966) and females (Linville, 1987b).

Fundamental frequency perturbation may be affected in aging. Orlikoff (1990) reported much higher jitter values for his old group of subjects (0.728) versus the young group (0.461). On the other hand, others (Brown, Morris, & Michel, 1989; Casper, 1983; Linville, 1987a, 1987b; Ramig & Ringel, 1983) reported no difference of jitter between young and geriatric subjects.

The intensity of an older voice may be slightly greater than a young voice (Brown, Morris, & Michel, 1989; Ryan, 1972) although the differences are small. Morris and Brown (1942) reported smaller variability of intensity for their old group (mean age = 79.4 years) versus their young group (mean age = 27.5 years). These results suggest that the geriatric have stiffer, less flexible vocal folds. Amplitude perturbation or shimmer is generally higher in the geriatric speaker (Biever & Bless, 1989; Ramig & Ringel, 1983; Ringel & Chodzko-Zajko, 1987).

## Observable Physiological Signs

Laryngoscopic changes have also been reported, including bowed vocal folds, atrophy or apparent thinning of the vocal folds, edema, and a posterior glottal gap (Honjo & Isshiki, 1980). Segre (1971) noted a yellowish discoloration of the vocal folds, atrophy of the ventricular folds, loss of normal tension, and a fissure in the middle or anterior one-third of the glottis. A sulcus has been noted in some elderly subjects (Honjo & Isshiki, 1980; Mueller, Sweeney, & Baribeau, 1984).

Stroboscopic signs studied in the elderly voice mostly have been concerned with glottal closure configuration (Biever & Bless, 1988, 1989; Linville, 1992; Södersten & Lindestad, 1990). Most young males will have complete closure of the glottis during the closed phase of the vocal fold vibratory cycle (Linville, 1992). Geriatric males appear to show a greater incidence of incomplete vocal fold closure (Honjo & Isshiki, 1980) but the data are based on a small number of subjects. In the female voice, Biever and Bless (1989) reported that 90% of their 20 geriatric subjects exhibited some kind of glottal gap. However, 80% of their group of 20 young men also exhibited some form of a glottal gap. Most of the young women with glottal gaps had a posterior chink whereas the older subjects had mid-membranous or anterior gaps in addition to a posterior chink. Linville (1992) also reported a high incidence of glottal gaps in her sample of 10 patients (79%). Most common was an anterior chink (22%) but she also reports configurations such as posterior chink (11%), anterior-posterior gap (9%), and incomplete closure (4%). Linville also reported that 86% of her group of 10 young subjects had some form of a glottal gap. It would appear that the presence of a glottal gap, at least in women, is not a significant feature of aging.

Other stroboscopic features studied in older individuals include mucosal wave, amplitude of vibration, asymmetry, and stiffness (Biever & Bless, 1989). In their study of 20 geriatric females, Biever and Bless (1989) reported that 85% showed aperiodicity of vocal fold vibration, 45–55% had some mucosal wave changes on either vocal fold, 50–55% showed changes of amplitude of vibration for either vocal fold, and between 5 and 10% of the patients showed some degree of stiffness on either vocal fold. Their young female subjects showed much smaller percentages of these signs. Thus it would appear that aging may result in physical changes that produce changes in the vibratory characteristics of the vocal folds.

## *Pathophysiology of the Geriatric Voice*

Aging affects the structures of the larynx in varied ways and at varied times during the aging process. Although there is a general trend towards a decline of function in many body systems, the decline may be ameliorated or exacerbated by other factors such as lifestyle, diet, and amount of physical activity. Similar comments may be said about the voice itself. Singers who remain active singing can produce wonderful tones well into their 70s and, in rarer cases, 80s. Concomitant with aging is the likelihood that an individual will contract some kind of disease or have some kind of accident. In our clinic, the vast majority of elderly patients with a voice disorder have had a physical or neurological problem thought to have caused the disorder (Woo, Casper, Colton, & Brewer, 1992). Aging per se may not result in vocal problems. However, geriatric individuals in poor physical condition may experience more communication problems than geriatric individuals in good physical condition. We believe that voice problems that might be attributable to aging can be minimized and perhaps even "cured" by proper attention to lifestyle, diet, and physical condition. Exercise is known to maintain or improve heart rate, blood pressure, muscle strength, bone mass as well as many other bodily functions (Lowenthal, Kirschner, Scarpace, Pollock, & Graves, 1994). A program of "vocal aerobics" may be the only "therapy" program needed for many older patients who have difficulty with their voice. Prevention of communication problems in the geriatric population may be the best course of action.

## SUMMARY

In this chapter, some organic problems that may affect the voice have been reviewed. The etiology of these problems is not related to voice use. However, their effects can drastically alter voice production. A variety of medical and surgical approaches are the primary treatment modalities. Vocal rehabilitation may be helpful in establishing the best voice the patient is capable of producing. A section on geriatric voice discusses physical changes attributable to aging that may affect phonation and stresses the need to distinguish between age-related changes and those attributable to associated disease states.

# Chapter 7

# The Voice History, Examination, and Testing

## VOICE HISTORY

The clinical skills of the practitioner are critical when working with a patient with a voice problem. The interview with the patient, the search for information, and the elicitation of the history require a combination of art and science. The art is the skill of the clinician with the interview process and in fitting together the various pieces of information. The science is the knowledge base that guides the selection of questions and informs the interpretation of responses. The two are inseparable, and there is a constant interplay between them throughout the interview and the treatment. It is not enough to know what questions to ask, if there is no skill in the asking. It is not enough to know what questions to ask, if there is no understanding of their implications or of why it is important to ask. It is not enough to know what questions to ask, and to have skill in the asking, without adequate knowledge and understanding for interpretation of the responses.

Another way to distinguish between what we have referred to as art and science is to think of them as process and content (Reiser & Schroder, 1980). All communication between people involves a process level. It is at this level of communication that many unspoken associations, silent questions, and feelings are expressed by both the patient and the professional through both verbal and nonverbal means. The content level of the interview refers to information specific to the problem.

### The Interview Process

Teaching the skill of interviewing and the art of communication with patients is woefully neglected in the training of most speech-language pathologists and physicians. Aronson (1985) states:

> Any in-depth study of voice disorders forces us to conclude that so long as clinicians obtain privileged information from patients; so long as people have voice problems because of life stress and interpersonal conflict; so long as voice disorders produce anxiety, depression, embarrassment and self-consciousness; so long as patients need a sympathetic person with whom they can discuss their distress, will speech pathologists *and physicians* [author's addition] need to consider their training incomplete until they have learned the basic skills of psychologic interviewing and counselling. (p. 271)

Aronson presents further rationale for the need for good interviewing and counseling skills and also discusses the personal characteristics clinicians must bring to the process. Although Aronson targets his discussion on the interaction of the clinician with patients whose voice problems are largely of psychological etiology, we feel the concepts are pertinent to interactions with all voice patients.

During the past decade, the field of medicine has shown an increasing awareness of the emotional components of disease processes. Furthermore, it has been recognized that effective treatment of these components occurs when there is a positive relationship between the patient and the health professional (Bernstein & Bernstein, 1985). The initial interview, usually the history-taking session, establishes the patient-clinician relationship. It is the foundation on which the success of treatment may depend (Bernstein & Bernstein, 1985; Hersen & Turner, 1985).

An interpersonal relationship by definition involves the dynamic interaction of at least two people, each of whom brings emotions, expectations, experience, and knowledge to the process. How these two sets of "baggage" match up, or fail to do so, will determine how well the process unfolds. Indeed, some studies have indicated that the breakdown in this relationship may be a major cause of malpractice suits (Blum, 1960; Rosenthal, 1978).

The clinical interview is an interaction of a particular type. Its specific purpose is to explore the nature and history of the patient's presenting symptoms. Unfortunately, it occurs within set time limits and a busy office environment. Despite these limitations, the interaction need not and must not be allowed to become rigid with preset boundaries.

Before we become clinicians, we are people who have been socialized into avoiding certain topics of conversation, not asking overly personal questions of relative strangers, and not probing when a topic appears to make our conversational partner uncomfortable. As clinicians we must recognize that clinical interviews are different from social conversations. The professional has not only the right but indeed the obligation to ask personal questions and to probe gently when areas require further exploration. A patient's indication of discomfort or avoidance may be a very important sign to the skilled clinician who knows how to probe without shutting off the flow of information. A clinician can only do this successfully by reaching a level of self-comfort in discussing sensitive areas.

## What the Patient Brings to the Process

The patient comes to an evaluation or examination with a heightened sense of anxiety. The patient brings a personal history not only of the current problem but also of previous problems, previous contacts with members of the health professions, relationships, education, social ease, personal needs, and culture. The patient's ethnic background may shape attitudes toward illness and affect interaction with professionals (Bernstein & Bernstein, 1985). The patient may also have need for support and guidance in understanding the current problem. All of these factors will fashion the patient's behavior and responses.

## What the Professional Brings to the Process

The most obvious contribution of the professional is expertise with a body of knowledge concerned with voice production. But the professional also brings a history of encounters with many patients, relationships with peers as well as with family and friends, personal needs, and the pressures of time. In the current climate of frequent litigation, the practitioner may also bring a sense of anxiety or wariness to the process, perhaps generating a defensive posture toward the patient.

Bernstein and Bernstein (1985) identify the following as the responsibilities of the professional in the interview process:

1. Assume responsibility for the conduct of the interview.
2. Avoid control and rigidity that inhibits or intimidates the patient.
3. Keep the interview in focus.
4. Maintain flexibility.
5. Remain sensitive to the patient's feelings expressed both verbally and nonverbally.
6. Do not permit expression of subjective, personal feelings.
7. Remain open and accepting of the patient even when the patient is hostile or uncooperative.

To that list we would add that the professional must be able to speak in language tailored to the individual patient—language that the patient can understand and that is neither insulting to the patient's intelligence nor patronizing in manner.

## Listening

Although we cannot fully explore all of the crucial aspects of interview skills in a single chapter, the art and skill of listening demands more discussion. A frequent request of beginning clinicians, or of those who have not developed a level of understanding of a particular area sufficient to allow them to be comfortable with it, is for a checklist of questions to ask. Indeed, forms providing such questions are readily available (Boone, 1983; Darley & Spriesterbach, 1978; Wilson, 1987; Wilson & Rice, 1977). They will, however, prove to be of little help to the inadequately trained clinician. For the trained and skilled practitioner, a form is a convenient way to organize the interview, as long as one recognizes that it is not meant to be adhered to strictly. The value of a form is directly dependent on the skill of the clinician in conducting the interview and extracting the relevant information.

Attentive and sensitive listening on the part of the professional, rather than extensive talking, is the key. Some argue that engaging in note taking during an interview is disruptive to the process of attentive listening. Furthermore, patients may be influenced to focus on specific areas if the clinician's note taking appears to indicate those as areas of importance. Others, however, feel that patients are made to feel confident about the importance of their reporting when they observe the practitioner taking notes. Whichever system is used by a given clinician, it is important that the taking of notes be done in such a way as to minimize interference with active and attentive listening.

Listening is more than hearing the spoken words. It involves observation of facial expressions, both as one's questions are heard and during the response. It involves observation of body language. It involves attention to the sound of the voice, the suprasegmentals of stress and inflection and prosody. And it involves hearing messages sometimes hidden behind the words, the well-known "listening with the third ear" (Reik, 1948), and utilizing the sixth sense of feelings or intuitions (Browne & Freeling, 1976). If the clinician is focused on self or the next question to be asked, all of this will be missed. Indeed, much information will never be elicited.

As a component of developing good listening skills, it is necessary to develop a tolerance for moments of silence. The beginning or insecure clinician tends to abhor silence, and the very busy and rushed clinician has no time for it. Moments of reflection, of allowing the patient to provide additional information or sometimes to raise a new point, can be exceedingly valuable. The silence must be a comfortable one, however, in which the clinician must nonverbally project a sense of ease and of understanding.

Listening well need not be a lengthy process. Good listening skills enable the clinician to shape and control the interview. A balance must be maintained between the patient's need to talk and the clinician's need to elicit pertinent information. The clinician learns to pick up the important cues, to follow them while always targeting the problem, to ask directed questions when indicated, and to refocus responses when necessary. Patients will usually provide all the information needed by the professional, if they can be helped to express it in their own way in an environment of understanding and acceptance.

It is difficult to learn the skill of interviewing by reading about it. Our intent here is not to exhaust the topic but rather to raise it and recognize its importance. It is so extremely important when dealing with voice patients because of the very close linkage between voice and personality and emotional states. There are readily available resources that provide skills training in listening and in interview skills. We would strongly urge that all academic courses in voice disorders incorporate such skills training as part of the curriculum. Suggested readings on interviewing may be found at the end of this chapter.

Before leaving this topic, we must not ignore the use of history questionnaires that can be completed by patients prior to their appointments. There is some value in the use of such questionnaires because they make it possible for patients to review personal medical records, to validate their impressions against those of other family members or friends, and to think about the issues raised by their answers. However, if questionnaires are taken at face value, they clearly eliminate the immensely important interview process and abort the establishment of a relationship between the patient and the clinician. If such forms are to be used, it is very important for their contents to be reviewed verbally, allowing the patient to elaborate and clarify, and opening the door for further probing by the clinician.

## Content of the Interview: The Case History

### THE PROBLEM

After initial introductions and review of identifying and demographic data, it is usually appropriate to begin the interview by asking the nature of the problem that has brought the patient for the examination. Not only is this a natural place to begin the interview, but the patient's response may hold a vast amount of information. The clinician will begin to get an impression of how aware the patient is of the problem, how articulate the person is in providing descriptive information, and what the patient's level of concern or motivation is relative to the problem. It is important to recognize that these early impressions should be recognized as just that—impressions—which need to be verified or altered as the interview progresses. Indeed, what eventually results from the interview and subsequent examination may be quite different from the concerns voiced initially. Nevertheless, it is important to have this starting point.

Some patients will provide an almost nonstop narrative in response to the very first question, whereas others will have to be prodded and asked many questions. Either type of patient will require that the clinician manage the questioning skillfully so as to obtain all the important information without being either drowned by trivia or blinded by an absence of response. It is important to ask many open-ended questions in an attempt to elicit information without putting words into the patient's mouth. For example, the open-ended request "Tell me about the problem that brought you to see me today" may bring a more complete response than "I understand you are here because you have a polyp on your vocal folds."

In response to the question concerning the nature of the problem, it is helpful to obtain the patient's description of the sound of his voice and how it differs from other voices or from his own premorbid voice. We have found that patients often are accurate in describing the problem and that their statement of the primary symptom is an important one.

It is instructive to ask what patients believe may have caused the problem or what they have been told about the problem by others they have consulted. Patients frequently indicate a lack of understanding, or perhaps a misunderstanding, of information received from the physician. It is not unusual for a patient to say, "My doctor said I have polyps or something growing in my throat, but I don't know what that means or what it has to do with my being sent to you." Other patients, of course, can quote the dates of office visits, procedures that were done, and their outcome. Despite what they have been told, or in the absence of having been given any information, patients often have their own ideas about the cause of the problem. Frequently heard comments include "It's this postnasal drip," "It's probably my sinus condition," and "I think I'm allergic." It is important for the clinician to recognize that patients frequently have difficulty giving up such ideas, even when they are unsubstantiated, and that the inability to do so may compromise the treatment program. Therefore, it will be important for these issues to be raised at the appropriate time in the process, and for the patient to be provided with information that is understandable and acceptable. The nature of the clinician-patient relationship established during the initial contact will have an important impact on this subsequent interaction and the patient's acceptance of new ideas.

## EFFECT OF THE VOICE PROBLEM

If the patient has not spontaneously commented on the effect of the voice problem on his life, it is important to ask about this as a follow-up question. Once again, this information will help the clinician understand the degree of importance the patient attaches to the problem. Voice problems may exert profound effects on people, including depression, anxiety, withdrawal, embarrassment, and self-consciousness. Indeed, a voice problem may have a profound effect on the individual's total being. On the other hand, for some the voice problem may be a minor embarrassment or have little effect on lifestyle. The severity of this reaction is not always directly proportional to the severity of the voice problem. Equally as important is information as to what effect the problem has had on family members, on work-related activities, and on coworkers or superiors; that is, on all aspects of the person's life. Some patients may express denial of a problem and a lack of personal concern. Such statements must be fully explored before they are accepted as valid. Feelings expressed by the patient in this discussion must be listened to carefully. The clinician must use skill in helping the patient to discuss feelings openly without fear of being judged or humiliated.

## DEVELOPMENTAL HISTORY OF THE PROBLEM

Very valuable information may be obtained from this section of the case history. It is important to learn as much as possible not only about the onset of the current episode but also about how it has developed. Information relative to previous episodes of voice difficulty and any prior treatment and outcome must be known. When patients suggest dissatisfaction with the outcome of previous treatment, it is well to inquire whether there is any litigation in progress or in planning. This information may sometimes be obtained in an oblique or indirect manner rather than by a direct, confrontational question. In some instances patients may have been referred by a lawyer specifically for a second opinion. This knowledge may have little impact on your assessment of the patient, but it is helpful to know it in advance, and it may have some impact on the degree to which the entire interaction is documented.

### Onset

The onset of a voice problem may be gradual or precipitous. Why is this a critical piece of information? In understanding the natural history of the development of laryngeal pathologies, we know that it is most likely that certain problems will develop over a period of time, while others may have a very sudden onset. While some patients can provide only rather vague information about the onset of the problem, others will provide the date, time, and exactly what they were doing at the very moment that the problem began. Clues to the diagnosis may be contained in each of these types of responses, as well as in the host of responses that lie between these two extremes. Patients frequently date the onset of the symptoms of a problem to another stressful occurrence in their lives. This is a natural tendency that can sometimes be misleading if accepted without full and careful exploration. Another common report is the association of an episode of laryngitis or upper respiratory infection with the onset of the current problem. This event may indeed have some bearing on the problem, but it requires verification.

Most laryngeal lesions develop over time. An exception to that would be the apparently rapid development of a polyp or vocal fold hemorrhage coinciding with a specific episode of excessively strenuous voice use. Patients have reported the sensation of a sudden, sharp pain during shouting or loud, stressful singing, with the subsequent finding of a hemorrhage or hemorrhagic polyp. We know that professional singers may show evidence of beginning nodules immediately after a performance; these usually resolve spontaneously if the voice is allowed to rest in a state of less strenuous use.

The majority of patients with laryngeal growths that affect the vibratory behavior of the vocal folds (and thus the sound of the voice) report a gradual onset of voice symptoms over a period of weeks, months, or even years. Often they describe early episodes of voice change lasting only brief periods of time, with return to what they describe as normal voice. The episodes increase in frequency and in duration over time, and the normal voice does not return. By the time they seek medical attention, the problem may have become chronic and be worsening.

Voice changes that result from vocal misuse, including increased musculoskeletal tension, also tend to run a gradual course even though observable laryngeal pathology may not be present. Indeed, it is not uncommon for patients to be totally unaware of when or how a problem developed. Small, gradual changes tend not to be noticed, and persons unaware of these minor changes show little or no concern until a more obvious change is noticed either by themselves, a friend, or a family member.

Neurologically based voice problems may have either a sudden or a gradual onset. Progressive deteriorating neurological diseases that affect the voice tend to do so in a gradual manner, while the precipitous nature of a stroke or a head injury may have an equally precipitous effect on voice production. Recurrent laryngeal nerve paralysis is not an uncommon result of severing the nerve during thyroid surgery (Johns & Rood, 1987). Obviously, the resulting voice problem will be immediately noted postoperatively. However, the history provided by patients with idiopathic recurrent laryngeal nerve paralysis is not so clear. Some patients report a slight voice change at first, with worsening of the voice symptoms over a relatively short period of time. Others report a very sudden change that neither worsens nor improves.

The voice of the adolescent male that fails to lower in pitch despite normal laryngeal growth no longer sounds exactly like it did prior to laryngeal growth, but it usually takes months, or more likely years, for it to be recognized as unusual.

Sudden, marked vocal change that can be pinpointed as to date and time, in the absence of other symptoms suggestive of an organic etiology, is often the first clue of a psychogenic dysphonia. It is important to caution, once again, that the process of differential diagnosis involves the exploration of all facets of a problem and does not allow for premature conclusions. Clues such as this must be viewed as only one piece of a puzzle, and the clinician must be careful to maintain an open mind so as not to overlook important information that might not fit a preconceived notion.

### Duration

When a voice problem has occurred in a sudden manner, its effect on the person is usually more disturbing than a gradual change, and, as a result, consultation may be sought more quickly. Nevertheless, it has been our experience that a period of months has usually elapsed from the onset of the problem to the time the person is referred for a voice evaluation. The pattern usually involves a period of consultation and treatment with the family physician, pediatrician, or other practitioner, followed by referral to an otolaryngologist. Another period of treatment may ensue, and if the problem persists, referral is made to a voice management team, to an otolaryngologist who specializes in laryngeal problems, or to a speech-language pathologist.

As noted previously, many problems have a gradual onset or may have been tolerated at a low level of dysfunction for lengthy periods of time. It is often not possible to determine how long a condition has been present. The germane question, then, is, does it matter? The answer is yes—and maybe. Obviously, if the patient's problem involves a malignant lesion, time is of the essence. The earlier a malignancy is identified, the more positive the prognosis and the less traumatic the treatment. Early identification of any organic condition is, of course, a desired goal. It is easier to obtain resolution of a small, soft, new nodule than one that has become increasingly fibrotic over time. It is also easier to change abusive habits that have not had a lengthy period to develop. Early identification of certain neurological disease processes may allow early treatment of symptoms, if possible, although such treatment may not change the course of the disease. Early diagnosis and treatment of psychogenic dysphonias may shorten the period of time during which the patient must be dysfunctional.

The clinician needs to obtain the best estimate possible of the duration of the problem. This information, put into context, will help the clinician plan a treatment protocol.

## Variability Versus Consistency

The reporting of the variability or the consistency of a voice problem is very important. It is unlikely, for example, for a person with paralysis of the recurrent laryngeal nerve to report much variability in voice production from hour to hour or day to day. Some minor worsening of symptoms might occur with extensive or strenuous voice usage. (It is important to recognize, however, that return of nerve function and thus return of normal voice may occur in cases of idiopathic paralysis. This would not constitute variability of symptoms so much as a change or improvement of voice.) We would not expect a person with a mass lesion to experience periods of normal voice. Such a patient may report improved voice for periods of time, but if questioned carefully it will become apparent that improved does not mean a return to normal voice. However, that same patient may experience worsening of symptoms associated with voice use. Another caution here is that patients who have experienced months or years of disordered or changed voice may no longer have a very clear auditory memory of how they used to sound, nor be sensitive to minor variability.

Variability in voice production can be understood in the light of certain neurological disorders. For example, patients with myasthenia gravis may experience periods of entirely normal voice production but will report a gradual worsening of voice with prolonged speaking and increased fatigue. Patients with voice disorders of psychological origin frequently report much variability in voice production. This variability, usually unpredictable, may occur throughout the day, from day to day, or for other time intervals.

Some patients report that their voices are at their worst in the morning, for the first hour or two after arising. Such report should raise the suspicion of gastroesophageal reflux disease. Such reflux frequently occurs while the person is sleeping in the prone position, allowing acidic stomach contents to actually wash up over the posterior laryngeal areas, including the arytenoids.

Variability of voice production may be situation related, use related, or related to general physical well-being. Voice-disordered patients frequently report a worsening of vocal function when under stress and when physically fatigued. Both of those states have a tendency to exacerbate any existing condition, but the clinician must not assume psychological causation based on such reports. When patients report variability in symptoms, they should routinely be asked to describe those things that seem to make the problem better and those that make it worse.

Once again, it is important to emphasize that in order to understand the implications of information received, the clinician's knowledge base must include awareness of the ways in which phonation can be affected by pathology and use factors.

## Associated Symptoms and Sensations

It is always important to ask patients about any other symptoms they may have experienced that they associate with the voice problem. These may include difficulty in swallowing, slurring of speech, loss of fluids through the nose, weight loss, excessive coughing, increased fatigue, heartburn, and the like. In addition, it is important to inquire about sensations in the neck, throat, and larynx, either accompanying phonation or at other times. Patients with patterns of vocal abuse and increased musculoskeletal tension frequently report the sensation of pain localized lateral to the larynx and a feeling of fatigue. It is not uncommon for a patient to say, "I just feel my throat is too tired to talk." Some patients with mass lesions or laryngeal irritation report the sensation of a constant lump in the throat and a need to strain to produce voice loud enough to be heard. A feeling of dryness in the mouth and throat is often reported. Reporting of many other sensations may be provided by the patient. Such reports may be helpful not only in the diagnostic process but also as useful indicators of change in response to treatment.

## Patient History

### VOICE USE

Exploration of how much a person talks and of where and how the voice is used constitutes a crucial part of the total history. An individual's job and lifestyle may not give indication of excessive or abusive voice use until it is discovered that she is or was a cheerleader, or he is the soloist in a church choir, or she performs with an amateur theater group.

There are specific concerns relative to voice use and, indeed, the entire voice history, if the patient is a professional voice user, a person whose profession is dependent upon use of a "good" voice (e.g., a singer, actor, teacher, lawyer, minister, or public speaker). Of major importance is whether or not the person has had professional voice training. It has been our experience that among the most difficult patients to treat are singers who have had no vocal training but who have had a few years of success in singing with a small group or choir, or in amateur theatrical productions. They have not recognized their abusive vocal behavior, which now has "caught up with them," often resulting in laryngeal tissue changes. It is difficult for these patients to understand or accept that what they have been doing constitutes the problem.

Vocal performers work in a variety of settings and environments and engage in many styles of performance. Some must sing above the sound of amplified music, while others perform in large areas without adequate amplification; some use a belting style, some sing rock, some perform in smoke-filled rooms, and some may be performing at night after rehearsing all day. The vocal demands of actors' scripts vary from job to job. All of these factors must be explored. Not to be forgotten, however, are the nonperformance vocal demands and voice habits of professional voice users. It is not at all uncommon for well-trained performers who have learned their art to use their voices well when singing or on stage but show little transfer of those habits to everyday speaking behavior. In addition, professional voice users are not immune to vocal abuse when engaging in noisy postperformance parties, loud talking backstage, teaching, and during other strenuous uses of the speaking voice. Sataloff (1981, 1986, 1987a, 1987b) presents a thorough discussion of the voice history to be used with professional singers, as well as samples of case history forms.

As noted earlier, any individual whose livelihood depends on the use of voice can be considered a professional voice user. Lawyers who must effectively argue cases before juries present with their own particular sets of phonatory demands and issues. These must be explored along with the individual's total patterns of voice use in and outside of a court room. Clergy often present unique problems due to the constant demands on voice use—preaching, teaching, community meetings, person-to-person interactions—and all to be done without the benefit of voice training. It is imperative that preaching style be explored thoroughly by reviewing recordings of actual preaching or obtaining a truly representative sample. The vocal demands placed on teachers is often heavy and compounded by lunchroom and recess duty, extracurricular activities, parent-teacher meetings, dusty environment (from chalk) with poor ventilation, difficult room acoustics, and the added demands on voice outside of school. All of these factors must be thoroughly explored during the initial information gathering session.

Children constitute another group for whom the voice use history must be carefully investigated. Some children may use their voices at appropriate levels and in acceptable ways much of the time, but the voice of the playground may be excessively loud, or making "weird sounds" may be a hobby. There are, of course, children who use their voices loudly and aggressively much of the time.

The voice and the manner of voice usage demonstrated in the office situation during the initial visit may not be an accurate reflection of potentially abusive voice use on the job, at the playground, or in the home. It is necessary to explore all these areas thoroughly during the interview and perhaps pursue them further during the voice evaluation.

### HEALTH

Because the voice is such an integral part of the whole person, it serves to reflect not only emotional states and personality but also physical states. We recognize the weak voice of the very ill, the lifeless voice of the pharmacologically subdued, or the tired voice of the physically exhausted. It has been said that the whole person "is considered to be greater than the sum of its parts; each part can only be understood in the context of the whole; a change in any one part will affect every other part" (Papp, 1983). It is for these reasons that the voice history must explore a patient's health history. The vital importance of the proper functioning of all body systems for the professional singer has been described by Sataloff (1981, 1986, 1987a, 1987b), who provides as one example the effect a broken leg may have in altering the singer's posture, thereby affecting abdominal support for singing.

It is most appropriate to inquire first about the patient's present health status. We are most interested in whether the patient has any neurological problems, respiratory problems, problems affecting the gastrointestinal tract, allergy-related problems, or psychiatric problems; suffers from any chronic conditions such as arthritis; has any congenital anomalies or hearing loss; or has any other current health problem. The past health history, which may be relevant to the present vocal difficulty, is also important, as is the patient's history of surgeries and hospitalizations. It is important to know the nature of surgical procedures that the patient has undergone, particularly those that may have some connection to the present difficulty, such as laryngeal, head and neck, thoracic, or cardiac surgery. For example, a history of appendectomy at 4 years of age may not be pertinent in the case of a 35-year-old patient. However, the history of cardiac surgery in that same patient should be explored to determine whether any sequelae of that surgery were directly related in time to the onset of the voice problem. What kind of sequelae may accompany such surgery? The most obvious might be hoarseness following intubation. However, recalling the course of the left recurrent laryngeal nerve, injury to that nerve might also be a possible sequela of cardiac surgery.

When exploring the surgical and hospitalization histories of a patient, it is important to learn either from the patient or from medical records whether the patient was intubated and, if so, whether it was a difficult or traumatic intubation, the duration of the intubation, and whether there is a time relationship between the procedure and the present voice problem.

Another related area to be explored is whether or not the patient has experienced any trauma, the effects of which might have an impact on the structure of the larynx or the mucosa. Some possible categories of such trauma would be blows to the neck, knife or gun wounds, automobile or other vehicular accidents, chemical ingestion or inhalation, and body burns or smoke inhalation.

A thorough history of substance use is important and takes some skill to elicit truthfully and completely. Substance abuse, that is, excessive use of alcohol or illegal drugs, is often not readily admitted. Questions about these areas must be asked in the same manner as inquiries into all other areas. The clinician must, however, be prepared to pursue vague responses or to probe further if there is reason to believe that the patient may be withholding information. It is often necessary for patients to be reassured about the confidential nature of the interaction. But patients do not seem to be reticent in divulging a history of tobacco use even when it is quite excessive.

There is widespread use of over-the-counter and prescription drugs in the treatment of illness or various physical discomforts. Because drugs work systemically, they often have an effect on all mucosa or tissues, not just that which is being targeted. For example, diuretics are used in many conditions in which release of fluids from body tissues is desired. However, it must be recognized that the laryngeal mucosa is not exempt from the diuretic action. Whereas release of excess body fluid may be very helpful to a person with certain medical conditions, the associated drying of laryngeal mucosa may have a negative effect on phonation.

Because the effect of various drugs on the laryngeal mucosa and laryngeal motor control is such an important yet relatively unreported area, additional information on it was presented in Chapter 4.

## VOCATIONAL

It is not sufficient to simply obtain a person's occupation. It is necessary to discuss the nature of the work done, the environment in which it is done, the need for an adequate voice to carry out the job requirements, interactions with coworkers and superiors, and the level of job satisfaction. In this area, as well as throughout the history taking, open-ended questions such as "Tell me about your job and the people with whom you work" may elicit more complete information than closed questions such as "Do you need to talk as part of your work?"

## SOCIAL

The focus of questioning in this area is designed to obtain information about the patient's lifestyle, family constellation, and even living arrangements. Environmental factors such as lack of adequate humidification or the use of a wood stove may have adverse effects on laryngeal tissues. People often do not recognize vocally abusive behavior that may occur in the home when yelling to the children or pets who are out in a large backyard or upstairs in another part of a house. Perhaps a hard-of-hearing person is a member of the family, requiring louder than usual voice usage. Home life is replete with examples of the need to raise the intensity level of the voice: talking above the television or music, talking above the level of others' speech in order to gain their attention, arguments. If the lifestyle includes much entertaining of large groups or frequenting of bars where extremely loud music is a constant background noise, vocal abuse may well be involved in the voice problem. Relationships with family members or "significant others" may be a source of stress or anxiety, which may be reflected in a problem with the voice.

## RECREATIONAL

Certain recreational activities may have implications for the voice. For example, the weightlifter who strains mightily while lifting, simultaneously producing harsh, grunting phonation, is placing considerable stress on the laryngeal tissues; so, too, the golfer or tennis player who phonates with each swing of the club or racket. Forceful phonation accompanying strenuous exercise of any type may constitute abusive behavior.

## PSYCHOLOGICAL

Placing this information at the end of this section should not suggest that it has the least importance. Indeed, psychological factors may be of utmost etiological importance. Furthermore, as stated previously, all disease processes carry components of emotional stress.

Throughout this chapter, and elsewhere in this book, frequent reference is made to the close link between voice and personality, voice and self-identity, voice and emotions. After our physical appearance, it is the voice that sets us apart from others and serves to identify us to others. It reports about our physical condition as well as our emotional state and well-being. How often during a phone conversation have you commented to a friend that she sounds tired or depressed or, perhaps, really happy? Because of this close linkage, the voice may also be the primary reflector of inner turmoil. The importance of recognizing stress-related voice usage and the need to explore the patient's social interactions and interpersonal relationships cannot be overstated. The skilled clinician will be alert to indications, both verbal and nonverbal, of psychological stress factors. A patient's history of previous or current involvement in counseling or psychotherapy is valuable information.

## EXAMINATION OF THE VOICE

Examination of the larynx and testing of its performance can be carried out through a variety of techniques. It is our bias that no one or two procedures are enough to provide the best and most complete information about a person's vocal functioning. Furthermore, each procedure adds to our understanding of normal voice production and of the deviations that alter the normal state. We are well aware that many assessment techniques are not immediately available to many speech-language pathologists or voice coaches, nor to all practicing otolaryngologists (Feder, 1986). However, within the past decade there has been an explosion of interest in the voice and a concomitant development of voice laboratories. These laboratories can often provide testing, examination, and diagnosis by an interdisciplinary team of voice specialists. It is therefore highly likely that full information is obtainable from sources within the community or in close geographic proximity, if it is sought. It is no longer acceptable to make diagnoses of voice disorders without adequate data. Claiming lack of immediate availability of equipment is akin to a physician failing to obtain an x-ray because he does not own radiology equipment.

### *Examination Procedures*

There are many procedures that can be used to examine the larynx and vocal folds. Some involve direct visualization of the vocal folds whereas others record some of the aerodynamic, vibratory, or acoustic events in the larynx. Direct examination of the larynx usually requires the insertion of a device to transmit light to the folds and receive the image back. This involves invasion of the airway of the patient with potential risks to both the patient and the examiner. It is important that anyone who examines patients be aware of the potential risk of infection or injury and follow universal precautions during the examination. Usually, that means that rubber gloves should be worn by the examiner when manipulating any part of the patient's anatomy where the examiner could come into contact with the patient's fluids, i.e. saliva, blood or blood products, or other fluids. Any instrument that is inserted into the patient's oral cavity or nasal cavity should be properly cleaned and disinfected after use. If the instrument touches any blood product, it must be sterilized.

Oral or nasal endoscopes used for continuous or stroboscopic light examinations need to be disinfected (Rutala, Clontz, Weber, & Hoffmann, 1991). A solution of glutaraldehyde such as found in Cidex is often used to disinfect endoscopes. This solution will not harm the components of the endoscope (unless allowed to soak for very long periods of time) and can be effective in eliminating most bacteria and viruses. Read and follow the directions on the product to determine the effective concentration and length of time the endoscope should be immersed. It is essential to be knowledgeable about guidelines for infection control that may be in use within your employment setting. Private practitioners should also have such guidelines in place and insure adherence to them by all employees.

Face masks are often used to collect information about the airflows during speech. Although these do not usually come into contact with blood or even mucus, they should be disinfected. Although glutaraldehyde solutions could be used, we are not certain about their effects on the individual components of face masks, especially the rubber seals that surround the circumference of the mask. We routinely use a diluted solution of common household bleach to disinfect all parts of our face masks. A 25:1 dilution is recommended (Rutala, 1990) and should be effective for about 30 days. However, since bleach is so inexpensive, we mix fresh solutions every week or so. Thoroughly clean all parts of the mask with a water/soap solution (Hibiclens, Stuart Pharmaceuticals) to remove any foreign matter on the mask. Immerse the masks and its parts for at least 20 minutes in the bleach solution. Rinse off and allow to dry before use. (For more information on disinfecting face masks, see Colton, 1994) If spirometry is routinely used in your clinic, you should be aware of the potential risks of transmission of airborne pathogens via the instruments used (Rutala, Rutala, Weber, & Thomann, 1991).

## INDIRECT LARYNGOSCOPY

Indirect laryngoscopy is the traditional means of examining the larynx through the use of a laryngeal mirror. This technique requires that the tongue be pulled forward as the mirror is introduced into the oropharynx and positioned in such a way as to reflect the image of the vocal folds. Pulling the tongue forward has the effect of moving the epiglottis forward, thereby allowing visualization of the laryngeal structures. The patient is then asked to produce a high pitched /ee/ sound. The choice of the /ee/ vowel enhances visualization of the larynx during phonation because its production is usually characterized by superior and anterior movement of the dorsum of the tongue and the epiglottis. The reasons for the use of a high pitch are (*a*) the vocal folds are expected to lengthen in the phonation of a high pitch, and this lengthening maneuver tends to "open" the larynx to view, and (*b*) there is usually some degree of upward vertical movement of the larynx in the production of a high pitch, which brings the structures closer for viewing.

Indirect laryngoscopy is thought of as a fairly noninvasive procedure because it does not require anesthesia or surgery, nor does it cause any pain or other trauma to the patient. It does, however, have some limitations. There are patients who have very active gag reflexes and are unable to tolerate the presence of the mirror deep in the oropharynx. Anatomical variations not infrequently make it difficult to visualize the larynx adequately with the mirror exam. It is especially difficult to visualize the larynx of a young child through indirect laryngoscopy due to the anatomical relationships of the structures, which are different from and smaller than those of the mature adult. Another limitation is the inability of the patient to speak in a normal manner in the position required for this examination, thus limiting the information available relative to laryngeal physiology. Indeed, it is possible that the unnatural positioning required and the tension created in the patient may actually alter the typical laryngeal behavior of an individual, thereby rendering a less than accurate impression of phonatory behavior.

Despite these limitations, indirect laryngoscopy continues to be a useful means of examining the larynx, especially in conjunction with other visualization techniques.

## DIRECT LARYNGOSCOPY

Direct laryngoscopy is perhaps the most invasive of the laryngeal examination procedures. It is usually a hospital-based procedure requiring that the person be anesthetized. Direct laryngoscopy permits more detailed examination of laryngeal structures, including their actual manipulation. It is required when it becomes necessary to obtain a biopsy of a lesion and in attempts to determine the extent of a lesion. Manipulation of the arytenoid cartilages may be helpful in making the distinction between a diagnosis of arytenoid ankylosis versus paralysis.

The disadvantages of direct laryngoscopy are its invasive nature, its cost, and the inability to observe laryngeal function. Prior to the relatively recent explosion of other imaging techniques, direct laryngoscopy was sometimes necessary as the only means to examine the larynx in persons for whom indirect laryngoscopy was unsuccessful.

## FLEXIBLE FIBEROPTIC LARYNGOSCOPY

The advent of fiberoptic technology has opened much of the human body to view in ways never before possible. Fiberscopes are used in many branches of medicine as diagnostic tools. A fiberscope, in simple terms, is a bundle of flexible fibers, some carrying light to the object to be examined and others carrying the image back to the viewer. The laryngeal fiberscope was introduced in the late 1960s (Sawashima & Hirose, 1981) and has become the major means for examination of the larynx.

In order to examine the larynx, the fiberscope is passed through the nasal cavity, over the soft palate, and into the oropharynx and the hypopharynx, as shown diagrammatically in Figure 7.1. Its moveable lens tip can be angled (the degree depending on the particular instrument), and the fiber bundle can be rotated to view the full larynx. The tip of the scope is usually positioned vertically, slightly above the epiglottis, but can be moved closer to the vocal folds for more detailed visualization. One of the benefits of this instrument is the flexibility possible in the positioning of the scope in the vertical dimension so as to allow visualization not only of the larynx but also of supraglottal structures and even of the velopharyngeal mechanism. Within the larynx, it is usually possible to view the anterior commissure, which is difficult to do with a mirror exam. The use of wide angle and zoom lenses also adds to visualization capabilities. The zoom lens allows for a closer look at specific laryngeal structures without discomfort to the patient, while the wide angle lens permits visualization of the entire larynx and supraglottal structures as well (depending on the vertical placement of the scope

*Figure 7.1.* Schematic of instrumentation used in a fiberoptic examination of the larynx. The procedure used during the examination is listed.

within the vocal tract). An example of a fiberoptic view of the vocal folds during respiration is seen in Figure 7.2, while Figure 7.3 shows the same larynx during phonation.

There are many advantages to this examination method. Although it may be characterized as invasive because the scope is introduced into the body, it causes only minimal discomfort as the scope is passed through the narrowest part of the nose. As the diameter of the scope has decreased in size (and will perhaps continue to do so), discomfort to the patient has decreased. The fiberscope can be used to successfully visualize laryngeal structure and function in all but a relatively few patients. It is used with all age groups including infants, and it allows visualization of the larynx in per-

*Figure 7.2.* A normal larynx during respiration. See color plate.

*Figure 7.3.* A normal larynx during phonation. See color plate.

sons with hyperactive gag reflexes and those in whom the anatomic relationships are only minimally distorted. It is possible to have the instrument coupled to a video camera, thereby allowing for visualization of an enlarged image on a television monitor during the examination and for videotaping the examination for careful subsequent review. The image can be observed simultaneously by a number of people and has been used by some as a feedback tool during therapeutic intervention (Bastian, 1987). Videotaping provides the addition of visual documentation to the traditional verbal description and can make comparison of laryngeal conditions over time, or over a course of treatment, much more reliable. A method for computer-assisted measurement of fiberoptic images has been described by Conture, Cudahy, Caruso, Schwartz, Brewer, and Casper (1981) and was demonstrated to be useful in measuring and documenting actual intrasubject change in laryngeal physiology accompanying the use of therapeutic techniques (Casper, Brewer, & Conture, 1981). Digital acquisition of flexible fiberoptic images now permits the use of digital manipulation and analysis techniques on these images (Colton, Casper, Brewer, & Conture, 1989). Kay Elemetrics offers a stroboscope that features software to perform measurements of vocal fold amplitude, glottal area, and lesion size. A major advantage of fiberoptic laryngeal examination is that the patient is able to speak, sing, whistle, play a wind instrument, or simply to sit at rest, with minimal interference created by the presence of the fiberscope. This makes it possible for the patient's phonatory and nonphonatory laryngeal and supraglottal behavior to be observed. Speech tasks tend to move the scope because of the movements of the soft palate and occasionally structures in the larynx may displace the instrument. Rarely does the presence of the endoscope result in excessive nasality.

The quality of the fiberoptic examination will be influenced by the quality of the equipment used. Casper, Brewer, and Colton (1987b) cautioned that imaging of laryngeal structures will also be affected by factors inherent in the equipment, such as the wide angle lens distortion effect, particularly at the periphery of the image, and distortions created by the angling of the scope tip. Although these effects are not of sufficient degree to deny the overall effectiveness of the instrument, they must be taken into account when interpreting observed structural or behavioral deviations. Hibi, Bless, Hirano, and Yoshida (1988) have described the distortions as systematic and have suggested a mathematical procedure that corrects for the distortions. In addition to knowledge of the capabilities of the equipment and the skill of the examiner in handling the fiberscope, it is important to consider the sample of laryngeal and supralaryngeal behavior elicited from the patient. One of the primary advantages of this technique is that it allows such a diversity of behaviors to be explored. In examining singers who are having difficulty in a particular portion of their range or in some aspect of their singing technique relative to phonatory behavior, it is possible to watch the larynx and vocal tract as they "perform." For examination of the voice-disordered patient, a complete protocol of speech and nonspeech activities, designed to elicit habitual speech behavior, flexibility of pitch adjustments, adductory nonspeech behavior, resting state, and any other behaviors of interest, must be well thought out. In order to obtain the best visualization of the larynx during speech, stimulus sentences should be heavily loaded with the /ee/ and /oo/ vowel sounds. Whistling, a nonphonatory activity, frequently provides the opportunity to observe abductory-adductory vocal fold behavior at a slower rate than occurs in speech. A suggested examination protocol can be found in the Appendix. This protocol may serve only as a starting point, after which activities designed to elicit a particular behavior of interest or to attempt to change a laryngeal gesture may be added. The person who performs this aspect of the fiberoptic examination must be skilled in "reading" the image, in understanding the physiology, and in knowing the types of vocal maneuvers that might elicit the desired changes in behavior. That person is frequently the speech-language pathologist skilled in diagnosis of phonatory function.

One of the limitations of the fiberoptic technique with a continuous light source is that vibratory behavior of the vocal folds cannot be seen. The technique does not alter the speed of movement of the structures beyond what is visible with the human eye. Thus, in a certain sense, fiberoptic examination provides a relatively gross look at phonatory behavior at the vocal fold level. It can be used to assess the valving function of the vocal folds and, of course, to visualize any pathology. It can be also used to assess vibration if it is used in conjunction with a stroboscopic light source (as described below).

Who should perform fiberoptic endoscopy? Naturally, any ENT physician should have the the necessary training and experience to perform this procedure and to be able to handle any potential problems that might arise. Speech-language pathologists in increasing numbers are receiving the training necessary to perform these procedures. ASHA has issued guidelines to be followed by speech-language pathologists who are engaged in the use of this and other imaging techniques (American Speech-Language-Hearing Association, 1992). It is incumbent on the practitioner to receive adequate training and gain supervised experience before performing this or any other procedure for the examination of the larynx.

### STROBOSCOPY

Stroboscopy is a procedure that has been used to examine the larynx since late 1800s. It has received much greater acceptance and widespread use in some European countries and in Japan than it has in the United States. That situation has changed dramatically with the introduction of new, more sophisticated equipment that is easier to use. Hirano (1981b) states that "stroboscopic examination, as a routine clinical test, is the most practical technique for examination of the vibratory pattern of the vocal folds." Stroboscopy, indeed, permits visualization of vibratory behavior in a way otherwise not possible with the human eye, and in so doing enhances understanding of the physiological basis of voice disorders. Kitzing (1985) further points up the benefits of the stroboscopic technique for early detection of neoplasms and for differential diagnosis

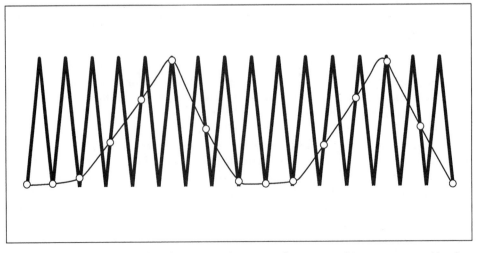

*Figure 7.4.* Basic principle of stroboscopy. When a rapidly moving object (represented by the high frequency waveform) is strobed by flashes at a lower frequency (curve with open circles), the rapidly moving object appears to move more slowly.

of laryngeal paresis and its outcome. Stroboscopy has been helpful in differentiating between functional voice problems and those caused by subtle structural abnormalities of the larynx (Bless & Brandenburg, 1983; Woo, Colton, Casper, & Brewer, 1991).

The stroboscopic light emits rapid pulses at a rate that can be set by the examiner or controlled by the fundamental frequency of the vocalization. If the frequency of the light pulse is the same as the vocal frequency, the resulting image will appear to be static and the vocal folds will seem to be at a standstill. At a frequency slightly less or greater than the frequency of vocal fold vibration (often between 1 and 2 Hz), the image is, in effect, sampled at different points in the vibratory cycle and over several successive cycles takes on the appearance of slow motion movement of the vocal folds. Each pulse of light illuminates a different point of the vibratory cycle, as schematized in Figure 7.4. These fragmented sections become fused due to the phenomenon of Talbot's law, that is, the persistence of an image on the human retina for 0.2 seconds after exposure.

Thus, stroboscopy differs from ultra-high speed photography in that it creates an optical illusion of slow motion and does not show details of each vibratory cycle, whereas high speed photography captures parts of each vibratory cycle at a very rapid rate, which appears as slow motion when the film is projected at a normal rate of 24 frames per second.

The clearest images are obtained by using a rigid endoscope, a straight tube in which the light-carrying and image-carrying fibers are encased. At the end of the scope is a prism that directs light and receives the image at various angles depending on the specific endoscope in use. Common angles are 90° and 70°. The flexible endoscope can also be used with the stroboscopic unit but does not usually provide as clear an image as the rigid scope.

At the start of the examination with the rigid endoscope, the patient is asked to protrude his or her tongue, which is held by the examiner outside the oral cavity with a gauze pad. The endoscope is then inserted into the mouth until its end is in the pharynx (but not touching the velum or posterior pharyngeal wall, which may cause gagging). The exact position of the endoscope needs to be altered slightly as the examination progresses to bring the vocal folds into view. The technique is not difficult and can be learned rather quickly. Possible dangers are gagging, bruising (if the endoscope is pushed hard against the delicate mucosa) or chipping of the teeth. Practice can increase the skill of the examiner in obtaining good examinations even with wide variations of anatomy and patient cooperation.

It is possible to carry out a stroboscopic examination using a rigid endoscope, a flexible fiberoptic laryngoscope, or both. Kitzing (1985) also describes the use of stroboscopic light in the operating microscope, combining good magnification and "superb optic resolution" while providing stereoscopic evaluation of the mucosal wave.

The method for obtaining stroboscopic images is not difficult. A microphone is placed or held on the patient's neck along the lateral aspect of the thyroid lamina in order to record the voice signal from which the fundamental frequency is extracted and used to control the rate of firing of the stroboscopic light. The rigid or flexible scope is introduced, the stroboscopic light is switched on (usually by a foot pedal), and the patient is asked to sustain phonation of the vowel /ee/. The patient needs to produce a sufficiently long sample to permit the stroboscopic unit to track the phonation and produce reliable stroboscopic light pulses. Because vocal fold vibratory behavior will vary with frequency and loudness, it is important to obtain samples of phonation produced in various ways. The following conditions should be a part of the examination: (*a*) a minimum of 2 seconds (4 seconds is better) of sustained vowel phonation at the patient's habitual pitch and loudness level; (*b*) another phonation at a higher pitch; (*c*) another phonation produced at a pitch lower than the habitual pitch level and, (*d*) production of sound at habitual pitch but at much louder than habitual loudness level. Often patients will initially produce a vowel at higher than their habitual pitch or loudness level. With coaching and practice, they will be able to produce a phonation more typical of their habitual pitch and loudness. Sometimes, additional samples of phonation may be requested such as a string of the vowel /ee/ with intervening silences, or a pitch glide. Samples of speech are not appropriate for stroboscopic examination.

### Interpretation of the Stroboscopic Image

The stroboscopic image provides information about the following areas: symmetry of movement of the vocal folds, regularity or periodicity of successive vibrations, glottal closure, amplitude (horizontal excursion) of the vocal folds, presence and adequacy of the mucosal wave, phase closure (open/closed phase), presence of any nonvibrating portions of the vocal folds, and additional observations relative to the presence of lesions and their apparent effect on the vibratory behavior. Observations of the stroboscopic image must be based on a thorough understanding of laryngeal anatomy and physiology, as well as of the changes in the mechanical characteristics of the vocal folds that result from variations in frequency and intensity. Interpretation of the observations requires understanding and knowledge of laryngeal pathologies.

### Symmetry of Vocal Fold Vibration

The judgment of symmetry refers to the timing of the opening and closing of the folds relative to each other, as well as to the extent of lateral excursion of the folds. If the folds are functioning equally, they are said to be symmetric and are mirror images of each other. When there is phase asymmetry, one fold may appear to move out of phase or the vocal folds may appear to be following one another. It is important to remember that if one fold is abducting, the other fold should be abducting also. Furthermore, in order to be symmetric in movement, they should be abducting at about the same speed.

### Aperiodicity

As noted previously, when the stroboscopic light flashes are synchronous with the fundamental frequency, the image appears to be static. Under this synchronous condition, any visible movement is evidence of irregularity of successive vocal fold vibratory cycles, or aperiodicity. Aperiodicity may be present always or the vibration of the folds may be intermittently irregular, in which case the image appears static part of the time, moving at other times. It is not necessary to stop the stroboscopic light at a specific part of the cycle in order to judge aperiodicity. The judgment can be made from the typical stroboscopic image by using the slow motion feature of the playback and observing the clarity of the image. If the image is clear, the vocal folds are reasonably periodic, if the image is fuzzy or unclear, even momentarily, the frequency of phonation is more variable. Hoarseness is usually associated with periodicity of vibratory behavior. When aperiodicity is constantly present the rapid variations in $f_0$ will interfere with the stroboscopic tracking of frequency and thus the image will not be meaningful.

### Glottal Closure Configuration

Judgments about glottal closure (the extent to which the vocal folds approximate each other) and glottal configuration during the closed phase are made during observation of phonations of normal pitch and intensity level; that is, at the patient's normal or comfortable pitch level. Bless, Hirano, and Feder (1987) have described seven categories of glottal closure that seem to encompass the possible variations (complete, anterior chink, irregular, bowed, posterior chink, hourglass, incomplete). *Complete* closure occurs when the vocal folds close completely during each vibratory cycle. *Anterior chink or gap* is a noticeable opening in the anterior portion of the vocal folds. Irregular refers to the appearance of several points of contact with openings in between along the length of the vocal folds. *Bowing* refers to a pattern in which the folds close anteriorly and posteriorly but not in the midsection. It is possible for one cord to be bowed and the other straight. *Posterior chink or gap*, as described by Bless et al. (1987), is an opening at the posterior area of the folds. We have observed variations in the size and configuration of this chink. In some it appears as a Y formation with a relatively small gap at the vocal processes. In others, it has the appearance of a V with the opening or chink tapering down as far anteriorly as two-thirds of the length of the vocal folds. *Hourglass* closure pattern looks just like an hourglass, a noticeable narrowing of opening at about the midpoint of the vocal folds. *Incomplete* closure is when no portion of the vocal folds touch each other. Although the primary judgment of closure is made during the speaking pitch and comfortable loudness condition, it is also advisable to note any changes that occur during the other conditions of voicing, particularly loud voice.

### Horizontal Excursion of the Vocal Folds

Amplitude is defined as the extent of horizontal (lateromedial) excursion of the vocal folds during vibration. Each vocal fold is rated independently for this parameter. The absolute amplitude is contingent on the size of the vocal folds; thus, it tends to be larger for adults. The amplitude of the horizontal excursion is approximately one-third the width of the visible part of the vocal fold in normal subjects (Figure 7.5). During abnormal vibration, the amplitude of movement may be less than normal or greater than normal. We rate amplitude as normal, slightly, moderately, or severely decreased or increased, or absent. It is important to remember that with increased

*Figure 7.5.* Schematic of the larynx to illustrate rating horizontal excursion of the vocal folds. The solid line between the folds illustrates no horizontal movement; the first mark along the dotted line illustrates normal horizontal excursion whereas the second mark outside of the dotted line illustrates greater movement.

loudness there will be greater lateral excursion, and with high pitch lateral excursion will be reduced. Therefore, when interpreting stroboscopic examinations, judgments of amplitude should be made during the habitual pitch, habitual loudness condition.

### *Horizontal Excursion of the Mucosal Wave*

The mucosal wave, a ripple-like wave of mucosa, originates in the subglottal area and follows the contour of the vocal fold. In stroboscopy, we see, and thus rate, only the horizontal excursion across the superior surface of the fold. It often appears as a ripple along the surface much like the ripple on the surface of a body of water. Sometimes it can be visually tracked as a light reflection traveling along the upper surface.

Normal refers to the range and size of the mucosal wave for phonation produced at habitual pitch and loudness levels. The extent of the wave varies but it normally traverses at least a third of the width of the visible part of the vocal fold. If a wave is visible on only part of the fold, the rating should be based on the overall impression of the wave travel.

### *Vocal Fold Edge*

This judgment pertains to the straightness and smoothness of the edge of each vocal fold individually. This is rated on a 4-point scale where 1 is smooth and 4 is extremely rough. This rating can be affected by the particular point in the cycle chosen for making the judgment. If the tape is advanced frame by frame through a cycle it is possible to see an edge that appears smooth on full abduction whereas on partial adduction a lesion may clearly be present. With this understanding it may be important to routinely make the judgment at a given point in the cycle. This parameter refers to the smoothness of the medial edge and should not be confused with the appearance of a bowed vocal fold which, despite the convexity of shape, nevertheless has a smooth edge.

### *Phase Closure*

Phase closure refers to the approximate proportion of time the vocal folds are open. On a 5-point scale, 3 refers to normal phase closure with an open phase of about 40–60% of the total cycle. A rating of 1 refers to a wide open phase as one might find during a whisper whereas 5 indicates hyperadduction or a condition in which the closed phase predominates. *Phase closure will depend on the loudness, effort, and pitch as well as mode of phonation.* It is important that this rating be made on a phonation that is appropriate. Phase closure can be estimated by counting the number of video frames during the open phase and the number for the entire cycle and computing an approximate open quotient. Because there can be much cycle-to-cycle variability, it is well to sample more than a single cycle. Ten to twelve open frames out of a 20-frame cycle is considered normal. Ratings made using this slow motion or stop frame counting procedure may differ from those based on an overall gestalt using regular tape playback speed.

### *Vibratory Behavior*

This is a judgment of whether or not the entire vocal fold is seen to vibrate. We rate vibratory behavior independently for each fold. It is sometimes difficult to distinguish between mucosal wave and vibratory behavior. Indeed, we probably judge vibratory behavior by the presence of mucosal wave. For a complete rating of all phonatory conditions, a 5-point rating scale can be used, i.e., 1 is always fully present, 2 is partial absence sometimes, 3 is partial absence always, 4 is complete absence sometimes, and 5 is complete absence always (totally immobile fold).

Based on our experience with judging stroboscopic images, we are aware of a number of unresolved questions with respect to this process. Among them are the following:

1. What criteria should be used in selecting the sample for judging?
2. Should judgments be made on the overall gestalt without attention to a specific sample?
3. Is it better to use slow motion to rate mucosal wave, amplitude, and phase symmetry, or is viewing at regular speed adequate?
4. How much of the length of the vocal fold must be visible to judge glottal closure, mucosal wave, vibratory behavior, and amplitude?
5. Which of the parameters that we are rating actually make a difference clinically? There is redundancy in the information obtained. What is most valuable?

## ULTRA-HIGH SPEED PHOTOGRAPHY

This technique was developed by scientists at the Bell Telephone Laboratories in 1937, and since that time many scientists have modified and used the technique to observe vocal fold vibratory events in both normal and pathological larynges (Baer, Löfqvist, & McGarr, 1983a, 1983b; Childers, Naik, Larar, Krishnamurthy, & Moore, 1983; Hirano, Kakita, Kawasaki, Gould, & Lambiase, 1981; Hirano, Yoshida, & Matsushita, 1974; Hirose, Kiritani, & Imagawa, 1991a; Metz, Whitehead, & Peterson, 1980; Moore, 1975; Moore, White, & von Leden, 1962; Rubin & LeCover, 1960; Timcke, von Leden, & Moore, 1958, 1959; von Leden, LeCover, Ringel, & Isshiki, 1966; von Leden & Moore, 1961, von Leden, Moore, & Timcke, 1960). Although this technique is capable of providing excellent information about the vibratory behavior of the vocal folds, it has not found widespread acceptance clinically for a number of reasons. It requires an expensive array of equipment, the technical expertise to operate it, and the expenditure of much time both in the examination procedure and in subsequent analysis of the films; it also involves a procedure that is difficult, if not impossible, for many patients.

The primary piece of equipment is a camera capable of taking pictures at a rate of 3000 frames per second or more. When films taken at these high speeds are viewed at a regular speed of 24 frames per second, the recorded events are seen in ultra-slow motion. The technique for obtaining high speed films (Hirano, 1981b), requires that the patient be able to position herself onto a fixed laryngeal mirror. The mirror must be positioned in such a way as to permit visualization of the vocal folds. The laryngeal mirror is used in a manner similar to indirect laryngoscopy, with the difference being that the patient must be capable of moving forward onto a fixed mirror rather than the mirror being moved into a stationary patient. An example of a high speed motion film sequence is shown in Figure 7.6.

Hirose and his colleagues (Hirose, 1988; Hirose, Kiritani, & Imagawa, 1987, 1988, 1991a, 1991b) have described a variant of high speed photography technique. Instead of recording the high speed image on film, it is captured using a digital image array that is sampled and stored in the computer. They are able to obtain images at a rate of 1000 per second and can display the image sequence immediately after capture. Furthermore, since they are dealing with a digital image to start with, they can use digital techniques to track desired aspects of vibration almost in real time. The technological problems discussed previously remain the same for this technique.

The information obtained from high speed films is glottal area over time. That is, we can determine the amount of opening of the vocal folds during the vibratory cycle.

*Figure 7.6.* Example of a high speed motion picture sequence. This plate is a single cycle of vibration produced by a female speaker sustaining the vowel /ee/ at about 275 Hz. The film was exposed at a rate of 4000 frames per second.

It is also possible to determine the vibratory movement of each vocal fold, as well as the pattern of their opening.

As valuable as the information obtained from high speed films is to our understanding of the vibratory characteristics of the vocal folds, it does not seem to be a tool appropriate for routine use in the diagnosis and treatment of voice problems.

### ULTRASOUND

Ultrasound is an imaging technique in which a high frequency current is passed through a portion of the body and partially reflected back when it strikes a change in body composition. Analysis of these reflections can be used to create an image of the part of the body of interest. It is a relatively safe procedure because the currents and frequencies used are low.

Ultrasound has been little used in the analysis of voice function. A few reports concerned with the analysis of normal voice function are available (Hamlet, 1981). Few voice clinics or laboratories possess the costly equipment and have personnel with the expertise to use it properly.

## LABORATORY TESTING

### *Acoustic Studies*

#### FUNDAMENTAL FREQUENCY

Fundamental frequency is an acoustic measure that directly reflects the vibrating rate of the vocal folds. The term "fundamental frequency" refers to the component in the vocal fold tone with the lowest frequency or to the frequency spacing between the component frequencies. The unit of measurement is Hertz (Hz).

Fundamental frequency may be measured in a variety of ways and using any of several types of speech samples. The phonatory tasks may include sustained vowel phonation, reading, and conversational speech. The simplest of these is the sustained vowel phonation, in which the patient is instructed to produce and sustain a vowel (most commonly /ah/ or /ee/) at a comfortable, natural pitch and loudness level. The advantages of using a sustained vowel are that it can usually be sustained in a steady manner and for an adequate period of time. The uncomplicated nature of the task makes it possible to obtain accurate measures with relatively simple and inexpensive equipment. The use of a reading passage or conversational speech as the phonatory task will usually introduce greater variability of fundamental frequency, thereby making extraction of fundamental frequency a slightly more complex procedure or one that requires more expensive instrumentation. There is not full agreement as to whether the speech sample used has a significant influence on the actual measured fundamental frequency (Hirano, 1981b).

There are a variety of methods available for the measurement of fundamental frequency, ranging from the very simple to the complex and elaborate. Subjective judgments can be made through a matching procedure, but such judgments are often quite incorrect. Indeed, subjective perception of fundamental frequency, particularly in persons with disordered voice, may be misleading (Murry, 1978). Objective measurement of fundamental frequency from sustained vowel production can be carried out very simply with the aid of a frequency counter and a low pass filter (available for less than $500). Without the filter, the frequency counter would attempt to count the many frequencies that a vowel contains. A low pass filter, when appropriately set, will remove the higher components of the laryngeal tone, leaving only the fundamental frequency. The output of this equipment provides objective documentation that can be used to demonstrate and chart change.

A commercially available and easy to use pitch meter or analyzer is available (Visi-Pitch, Kay Elemetrics Corp.). A sustained vowel or a speaking or reading sample using the patient's live voice or a recorded segment is fed into the instrument, and the fundamental frequency as a function of time is displayed on the screen. It is possible to control the total time to be displayed and thus to obtain a detailed fundamental frequency trace for short periods of time, or a less detailed trace of fundamental frequency over longer periods of time. This instrument can provide measures of other voice and speech parameters as well.

Computer programs, such as Computerized Speech Lab (CSL, Kay Elemetrics Corp.), CSpeech, and Dr. Speech Science for Windows (Tiger Electronics), that run on IBM or IBM-compatible computers, extract fundamental frequency from sustained vowels or longer speech samples. For the Macintosh computer, MacSpeech Lab can be used. These programs can perform many more measurements than simple frequency measurements and are relatively simple to use. An example of a fundamental frequency analysis using the CSpeech program is presented in Figure 7.7.

Three summary statistics of frequency data that are useful for comparing patients to normal speakers or to themselves over a course of treatment are mean fundamental frequency, the standard deviation of fundamental frequency (pitch sigma), and frequency range. Clinically, these measures are helpful diagnostically and as documentation of pre- and posttreatment status. Mean fundamental frequency is useful to estimate the appropriateness of frequency level for the patient's age and sex. The other two statistics help to assess and document variation of fundamental frequency during speech, or lack thereof. Speakers who are judged to be monotonic would be expected to have small standard deviations and small ranges of speaking fundamental frequency.

## PHONATIONAL RANGE

Another useful measure of the frequency characteristics of a patient's voice is phonational range, that range of frequencies from the highest to the lowest that a patient can produce. The highest and lowest frequencies are defined as the absolute limits of frequency that a patient can produce usually of short duration (approximately 1 second),

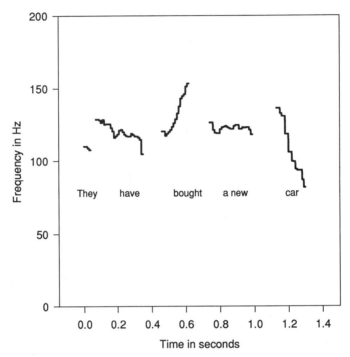

*Figure 7.7.* Fundamental frequency during the production of a sentence produced by a normal male speaker. The sentence was "They have bought a new car." The average fundamental frequency of the sentence was 120.45 Hz with a standard deviation of 12.28 Hz. The minimum fundamental frequency was 81.79 Hz, the maximum 153.32 Hz. Total time of the sentence was 1.3 seconds. Analysis was made using the CSpeech computer program.

without regard to intensity level or voice quality. Phonational range is said to reflect the physiological limits of the patient's voice. It is expressed in either Hertz or semitones and can be measured using any of the instrumentation discussed in the preceding section and also by using the phonetogram.

The absolute limits of frequency may be obtained by asking subjects to produce the highest and then the lowest sounds they can, or by using a singing scale progressing upward and downward in a stepwise fashion. Whichever technique is used, it is usually necessary to practice this task, encouraging the person to keep extending the range in both directions. The lowest and highest frequencies produced can be plotted, as shown in Figure 7.8. Kent, Kent, and Rosenbek (1987) have noted that intra- and intersubject variability on maximum performance tasks is large and may be affected by practice, motivation, or instructions. These caveats hold true for measurement of phonational range.

### VOCAL INTENSITY

Measurement of vocal intensity is useful in documenting the dynamics of the voice. Mean intensity correlates with the perception of vocal loudness, and the variability of intensity would presumably correlate with a patient's loudness variations.

Clinically, the mean intensity level of a patient's voice is usually a more meaningful measure than the absolute limits of intensity. However, the intensity range, frequently referred to as dynamic range, may be diagnostically important and helpful in documenting change. Patients whose mean intensity level is lower than expected for age (see Chapter 13 for some normative data on vocal intensity) and whose vocal in-

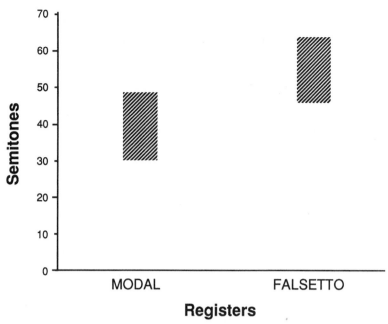

*Figure 7.8.* Mean phonational range of 35 male speakers. The modal register refers to that range of frequencies used most often during speech. Falsetto is a voice quality usually produced at high fundamental frequencies.

tensity range is markedly reduced need very careful and complete examination, including, of course, audiological assessment. The case of K. B. presented in Chapter 2 is a good example of this point. Although K. B. reported that she had been constantly admonished by teachers to speak louder, this reduction in vocal intensity was not subjected to examination until she was 13 years old. The reduced vocal intensity had been assumed by teachers and others to be a behavioral manifestation, when, in fact, it was easily explained physically by the finding of congenital unilateral vocal fold paralysis.

The procedure for establishing intensity or dynamic range requires that the person produce the very softest /ah/ possible and, at the other extreme, the very loudest /ah/. Patients should be asked to produce both of these sounds at a natural and comfortable frequency because frequency level will have an influence on intensity level (Coleman, Mabis, & Hinson, 1977; Colton, 1973). An example of plotting the highest and lowest sustainable intensity is shown in Figure 7.9.

Intensity can be measured from sustained vowels or connected speech. A simple intensity measurement device can be found on most tape recorders (e.g., the VU volume unit meter). However, this provides a very rough measure because these meters usually lack calibration in traditional intensity units (dB sound pressure level). A sound level meter that is so calibrated can be purchased at reasonable cost (Radio Shack). A digital version is also available at slightly higher cost. The patient is asked to sustain a vowel at a normal loudness level with the microphone of the sound level meter held at a given distance from the mouth, and the intensity of the phonation in decibels is read from the meter. This device is of little use, however, for measurement of vocal intensity during connected speech.

The Visi-Pitch can be used to measure and to visually display vocal intensity during connected speech. CSL and CSpeech will display the intensity of speech production

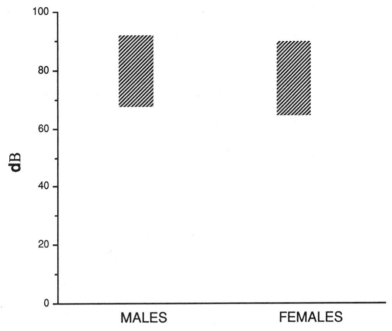

*Figure 7.9.* Example of intensity range measurement and portrayal. These data were collected on a sample of 35 older males (mean age = 56.17 years) and 27 females (mean age = 57.48 years) while they were phonating the vowel /ah/ at 40% of their modal register frequency range.

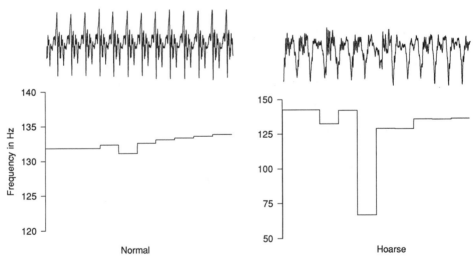

*Figure 7.10.* Example of frequency and amplitude perturbation in a sustained vowel produced by a normal (left panel) and a hoarse voice (right panel). These waveforms were produced using CSpeech.

over time. It is also possible to obtain summary statistics such as average intensity level and standard deviation from these instruments and programs. It is important that the microphone used be capable of responding to all of the frequencies present in the tone whose intensity is to be measured. All sound level meters have microphones that can respond to those frequencies expected in the speech signal, as does the Visi-Pitch. In computer programs, the sampling rate of the speech signal determines the frequencies present in the waveform and should be high enough to accurately reproduce frequencies of at least 5000 Hz (i.e., a sampling rate of 10,000 samples per second).

Another consideration when measuring vocal intensity is the distance between the speaker's lips and the microphone. The actual distance is not as important as that it be documented and consistent. Remember, sound intensity will be reduced by the square of the distance. That means a doubling of the distance will produce an intensity difference of 6 dB. The noise level of the room in which phonation is measured must also be taken into account. It is not necessary to have a sound-isolated room, although that would be ideal. It is important to have a reasonably quiet room and to know its noise characteristics. Most rooms will have a considerable amount of ambient noise below 60 Hz. Because most speech exhibits frequencies above 100 Hz, the use of a simple high pass filter will attenuate the energy below 100 Hz and permit valid measurements to be made. Many sound level meters possess a weighting function that, in effect, carries out this filtering process. The presence of heavy drapes and floor carpeting helps to reduce noise and yield usable recordings.

Once again, it must be noted that the variability of maximum performance measures may be large. Thus, caution must be used in the interpretation of measures obtained.

## PERTURBATION

Perturbation refers to the small, rapid, cycle-to-cycle changes of period and amplitude that occur during phonation. These changes reflect the slight differences of mass, tension, and biomechanical characteristics of the vocal folds, as well as the slight variations in their neural control (Baer, 1979). Perturbation correlates with perceived roughness or hoarseness in the voice (Wendahl, 1963, 1966) so that patients with voice problems manifesting roughness or hoarseness would be expected to show a large amount of both frequency and amplitude perturbation.

Perturbation must be measured from sustained vowel phonations in which the subject is instructed to produce a steady pitch level. Connected speech confounds the measure because linguistically produced frequency variations cannot be separated from frequency variations produced by the biomechanical characteristics of the vocal folds.

An example of frequency perturbation within a sustained vowel /ah/ is shown in Figure 7.10. In the left panel is shown an example of normal, sustained phonation. The acoustic waveform is shown in the upper portion of this panel and the results of a CSpeech analysis of fundamental frequency is shown in the lower portion of the panel. The average fundamental frequency is 133.02 Hz with a standard deviation of 1.0 Hz. The frequency did not vary more than 4 Hz. The percent jitter value was 0.30 and percent shimmer was 2.11. In contrast, an example of hoarse voice is shown in the panel on the right. Note the greater irregularity both in the period of the raw acoustic waveform shown at the top of the panel and in the amplitude of the phonation. The lower frequency track shows large swings of fundamental frequency in what is supposed to be a steady state sustained vowel. The mean fundamental frequency is 132.67 Hz with a standard deviation of 17.67 Hz. The largest frequency variation was about 76 Hz. The percent jitter value was 3.335 and percent shimmer was 11.82. The differences of perturbation between the normal and hoarse voice is very striking, suggesting that frequency and amplitude perturbation should be an important acoustic measurement to make on pathological voices.

Frequency perturbation, also called jitter, is obtained by measuring the period of each cycle of vibration, subtracting it from the previous or succeeding period, averaging the differences, and dividing by the average period. If the result is multiplied by 100, jitter can be expressed as a percent change of period relative to the average period. That measure is referred to as the jitter factor. There are several other formulations for computing frequency perturbation, which make comparison of data somewhat difficult (Casper, 1983). Titze (1995) recommends the use of some form of ratio measurement of jitter.

Frequency perturbation can be measured by the Visi-Pitch which reports it as a ratio measurement. These measures are helpful for comparison of intra- or intersubject data when the same measure is being used for that comparison. The computer programs CSL and CSpeech calculate frequency perturbation, and report their results in a variety of ways. For example, CSpeech reports jitter results both as the average absolute change of period in milliseconds and as percent change of frequency. It is possible to make the measurement of frequency perturbation from oscillographic recordings, but this requires much hand measurement and is a tedious and impractical task.

Amplitude perturbation, or shimmer, refers to the small cycle-to-cycle changes of the amplitude of the vocal fold signal. As was the case for the measurement of frequency perturbation, the amplitude of each glottal cycle is measured, subtracted from the previous or following period, and averaged over all differences. Shimmer is most often expressed in average change in decibels although percentage and ratio measurements may be reported and may be preferred (Titze, 1995).

Amplitude perturbation can be obtained directly from the CSpeech program, CSL, as well as from a number of other software programs. The measure of amplitude perturbation from the speech signal emitted at the lips is determined not only by the vocal folds but also by the resonance characteristics of the vocal tract. Thus, a measure of amplitude perturbation probably reflects the effect of the vocal tract on the speech signal, as well as the effect of the vocal folds.

## SPECTROGRAMS

Spectrograms reflect the properties of the source of sound (the vibratory characteristics of the vocal folds) and the resonator (the vocal tract). In order to compare spectral characteristics of a given phonation, it is important to use the same vowel. It is also necessary to have a good working knowledge of the acoustic characteristics of normal speech to properly interpret spectrograms obtained from voice patients.

Spectrograms are useful for analyzing and showing changes in the spectral characteristics of the vocal fold sound. Noise and weak sounds will exhibit characteristics that can easily be studied from a spectrogram. As shown in Figure 7.11, the spectrum of a hoarse voice (right panel) has considerable noise energy in the higher frequencies,

*Figure 7.11.* Spectrogram of a normal voice (left panel) and a hoarse voice (right panel).

whereas the normal voice on the left has little high frequency noise energy but strong low frequency periodic energy. Amplitude sections can be taken at selected points and a detailed analysis made of the spectral characteristics of the sound. Spectrograms can be stored in the patient's record for analysis and comparison with later phonatory samples.

One useful measure that can be obtained from spectrograms is harmonics-to-noise ratio (also called signal-to-noise ratio). This is a measure of the energy in the harmonics of the voice signal (i.e., the frequencies produced by the vibrating vocal folds) and the noise energy in the signal. Abnormal voices will exhibit greater noise either directly (i.e., produced at the vocal folds) or indirectly as greater perturbation (Klingholz & Martin, 1985). On a spectrogram of an abnormal voice, there would be greater noise and less energy in the harmonics of the sound. The harmonics-to-noise ratio is a convenient measure to express this relationship. For example, the normal sustained vowel shown in Figure 7.10 had a signal-to-noise ratio of 22.4 dB whereas the signal-to-noise ratio for the hoarse voice was 11.61 dB. After treatment, the spectrogram of a voice patient would exhibit greater harmonics-to-noise ratio because greater energy in the harmonic components of the sound would be expected, along with less noise energy.

An instrument commonly used to make spectrograms is made by Kay Elemetrics Corporation. Many voice clinics will not be able to afford this expensive equipment. There are, however, several computer software programs that produce acceptable spectrograms at less cost (CSL, Kay Elemetrics; RSL, CSpeech, Paul Milenkovic; DSPS Inc.; Dr. Speech Science for Windows, Tiger Electronics; MacSpeech Lab, GW Instruments). The use of these programs makes it possible to obtain spectrograms routinely on voice patients and greatly speeds the process of measurement. It is also possible to compute a harmonics-to-noise ratio via computer analysis (Kitajima, 1981; Kojima, Gould, & Lambiase, 1979; Kojima, Gould, Lambiase, & Isshiki, 1980).

## ACOUSTIC SPECTRUM

Acoustic spectrum is a plot of the energy in each of the frequencies present in a complex tone. The amplitude section from a spectrograph is an example of acoustic spectrum. It is possible to determine acoustic spectrum directly from the speech signal using special purpose spectrum analyzers or appropriate computer programs. Special purpose spectrum analyzers are very expensive but several computer programs are available that are not only less expensive but also more practical for clinical application. An example of a spectrum analysis produced by the CSpeech software program is shown in Figure 7.12. Such spectral profiles can be printed out for inclusion in a patient's file. Of course, it is important that the patient produce the same vowel or sound under similar conditions for each profile to properly interpret any spectral changes that might be obtained.

Another variant of spectrum analysis is computation of the one-third octave spectrum of the speech sample. One advantage of a one-third octave spectral analysis is that it produces a small, manageable number of distinct frequency bands. In normal speech, one expects to find energy in frequencies from 100 to 5000 Hz. In a one-third octave display, the spectrum is analyzed into 10–20 different frequency bands, depending on the frequency range desired. Furthermore, there is a well-documented and internationally accepted body of data concerning standardization of one-third octave spectra and the characteristics of the filters. Another advantage of one-third octave analysis is that it is similar, although not identical to, the way in which the ear analyzes sound. In view of this, the results of a one-third octave analysis may correlate best with perceptual measurements of voice. Unfortunately, there are few data

*Figure 7.12.* Spectral plot of a vowel produced by a normal speaker. These data were produced using CSpeech. A fourier analysis produces a plot of all of the frequencies present in the phonation. An LPC analysis is used to compute the formant frequencies of the utterance.

available on this relationship. In our judgment, the one-third octave or some variant seems to be the best choice at this time for analyzing the spectral characteristics of normal and abnormal voices.

There are several expensive one-third octave spectrum analyzers available for performing these measurements. It is also possible to extract one-third octave information from a computer-generated spectrum.

## *Physiological Studies*

### ELECTROGLOTTOGRAPHY

Electroglottography (EGG) is a technique for the measurement of vocal fold contact area based on the principle that tissue conducts current. A high frequency, low current signal is passed between the vocal folds via electrodes located on the external neck over the thyroid lamina. When the vocal folds touch, greater current flows than when they are open. There is a proportional variation of current when the vocal folds are less than maximally open or closed. Electroglottographic recordings can be used to determine when the vocal folds are closed and how fast they are closing. If carefully interpreted, it is possible to determine characteristics of the opening of the vocal folds from an electroglottographic recording.

Devices to record the electroglottographic signal are readily available. Currently these include the Voiscope and Laryngograph (Laryngograph, Ltd.), the single channel SC1 or the dual channel MC2-1 (Glottal Enterprises), and the unit from FJ Electronics. For a full discussion of the measurement technique, see Baken (1987). The electrical output of the electroglottograph can easily be converted to hard copy using an oscillograph or similar graphic recording device, or from a computer generated display.

The literature on EGG is primarily qualitative in nature, based on interpretation of the waveform. Several studies have related the shape of the EGG waveform to the underlying physiology of vocal fold vibration (Childers, Moore, Naik, Larar, & Krishnamurthy, 1983; Dromey, Stathopoulos, & Sapienza, 1992; Hicks, Larar, Moore, & Childers, 1985; Houben, Buekers, & Kingma, 1992; Kiritani, Imagawa, & Hirose, 1986; Painter, 1988; Rothenberg, 1981; Titze, 1984, 1990; Titze & Talkin, 1981). Information has also been reported on characteristic waveforms in patients with vocal pathology (Berry, Epstein, Fourcin, Freeman, & MacCurtain, 1982; Berry, Epstein, Freeman, MacCurtain, & Noscoe, 1982; Borden, Baer, & Kenney, 1985; Chevrie-Muller, Arabia-Guidet, & Pfauwadel, 1987; Childers, Alsaka, Hicks, & Moore, 1986; Colton, Brewer, & Rothenberg, 1983; Dejonckere & Lebacq, 1985; Gerratt & Hanson, 1987; Haji, Horiguchi, Baer, & Gould, 1986; Hanson, Gerratt, Karin, & Berke, 1988; Jentzsch, Unger, & Sasama, 1981; Karnell, Li, & Panje, 1991; Kaszniak, Garron, Fox, Bergen, & Huckman, 1979; Kitzing & Löfqvist, 1978; Sataloff, Spiegel, Carroll, Darby, & Rulnik, 1987; Scherer & Titze, 1987; Sorin, McClean, Ezerzer, & Meissner-Fishbein, 1987; Swenson, Zwirner, Murry, & Woodson, 1992; Trapp & Berke, 1988; Ward, 1990; Wechsler, 1976; Wirz & Anthony, 1979). There have been many attempts to quantify the electroglottograph signal (Brodie, Colton, & Swisher, 1988; Higgins & Saxman, 1993; Karnell, Li, & Panje, 1991; MacCurtain & Fourcin, 1982; Moore & Childers, 1984; Scherer & Titze, 1987; Singh & Ainsworth, 1992; Titze & Talkin, 1981; Rothenberg & Mahshie, 1988; Rasinger, Neuwirth-Riedi, & Kment, 1986; Wendler, Köppen, & Fischer, 1986; Wendler & Köppen, 1988).

EGG reflects the state of the vocal folds in a way that can be easily demonstrated and interpreted to patients. However, a limitation of the technique is that it cannot be used with all patients. Because the technique depends on vocal fold contact, the signal is considerably diminished or even absent in patients with lack of good contact, such as those with unilateral paralysis, or aphonia. It may also be difficult to obtain a clear waveform in the presence of severe hoarseness. The thick or large necks of some patients hinder transduction of the current and result in a poor EGG tracing. Manufacturers of EGGs have greatly enhanced its clinical value. For example, the MC2-1 EGG made by Glottal Enterprises uses two identical circuits and two sets of electrodes. The output of each electrode pair is compared and displayed on a meter. When the meter reading is 0, the output of the two channels is identical and the vocal folds are centered between the two electrode pairs. This simple monitoring device helps to insure the proper placement of the electrodes and an optimal EGG signal.

## PHOTOGLOTTOGRAPHY

Photoglottography is a technique designed to obtain estimates of variations of glottal area during phonation. Light is directed from above, usually from a fiberoptic light source passed through the nose. The light passes through the glottis and is detected by a light-sensitive device usually positioned over the skin of the trachea immediately beneath the vocal folds. As the vocal folds vibrate, their area of opening will vary and so will the amount of light passing through the glottis. It is a simple, relatively noninvasive device that yields a good, but not exact, approximation of glottal area. The photoglottographic technique is complementary to the EGG signal (Baer, Löfqvist, & McGarr, 1983a, 1983b).

There are several measurements that can be made from photoglottographic recordings. The first, speed quotient (SQ), is the speed of the opening phase of the vocal folds divided by the speed of their closing phase. The second, open quotient (OQ), is the time of the open phase of the vocal folds divided by the total period of vibration. This term is somewhat analogous to the term "duty cycle" used in engineering. Open quotient and speed quotient reflects efficient vocalizations although it is unclear which values are produced with maximally efficient phonations. Titze concluded that an OQ around .50 resulted in efficient vocalization (1994).

There have been a few studies relating photoglottographic results to different kinds of speech and voice production (Gerratt, Hanson, & Berke, 1988; Gerratt, Hanson, Berke, & Precoda, 1991; Gerratt, Hanson, Hunt, & Karin, 1985; Hanson, Gerratt, & Ward, 1983; Hanson, Ward, Gerratt, Berci, & Berke, 1989; Sonnesson, 1959; Vallancien, Gautheron, Pasternak, Guisez, & Paley, 1971).

There is some concern that the waveform obtained from this technique is not an entirely accurate representation of the actual glottal area waveform (Wendahl & Coleman, 1967). However, it may be useful for extracting measures such as speed or open quotient, which are known to be affected by disorders of the vocal folds (von Leden, Moore, & Timcke, 1960).

## INVERSE FILTERING

In the inverse filtering procedure, the voice signal emitted at the lips is analyzed to remove the resonant effects of the vocal tract, producing an estimate of the waveform produced at the vocal folds. According to the acoustic theory of speech production (Fant, 1970; Stevens & House, 1961), speech is the product of a sound source and a filter. That is, the sound output of the vocal folds is modified by the resonant characteristics of the vocal tract. If the resonant characteristics of the vocal tract are known, it should be possible to retrieve the characteristics of the output of the vocal folds from the orally emitted speech signal.

Inverse filtering has been performed on the acoustic sound pressure waveform (Hillman & Weinberg, 1981; Miller & Mathews, 1963; Sondi, 1975), and on the airflow waveform (Rothenberg, 1973, 1977, 1981). We have used the airflow waveform for inverse filtering of normal and voice-disordered subjects (Brodie, Colton, & Swisher, 1988; Casper, Colton, & Brewer, 1985; Colton & Brewer, 1985; Colton, Brewer, & Rothenberg, 1983). We routinely record the EGG signal simultaneously with the inverse filtered airflow signal to extract information about the vibratory characteristics of the vocal folds during the complete cycle. The techniques complement each other in that airflow will often not be present during the closed phase of the vocal folds, but the EGG provides information about vibratory characteristics of the vocal folds during that phase. Thus, with both techniques, we are able to obtain a more complete picture of vocal fold vibratory characteristics during speech.

The result of inverse filtering the oral airflow waveform is called a flow glottogram and an example is shown in Figure 7.13. Four channels are collected directly into the computer using CSpeech. These are the (a) acoustic waveform, (b) raw oral airflow waveform, (c) EGG waveform, and (d) intraoral air pressure pulses associated with the stop plosives in the utterance (not shown in Figure 7.13 but see Figure 7.14). The oral airflow waveform is inverse filtered using CGlott, a computer program separate from but complementary to CSpeech. The result is the inverse-filtered or flow glottogram shown in Figure 7.13. An explanation of the analysis of the intraoral air pressure traces may be found in the next section.

Collection of electroglottographic and inverse filtered airflow waveforms is routine in our clinic. The following measures are obtained from computer-assisted analysis of the waveform: (a) each cycle's minimum (or leakage) and ac airflows, (b) the ratio of the time of the airflow pulse relative to the total period (airflow duty cycle), (c) the ra-

*Figure 7.13.* Acoustic waveform (top trace), inverse filtered airflow (middle trace) and electroglottograph waveform (bottom trace) of a normal speaker. In this plot, vocal fold contact is indicated by a downward deflection in the electroglottogram waveform.

tio of the closing and opening slopes of the airflow pulse (airflow speed quotient), (*d*) the ratio of the open time to the total period of the electroglottographic waveform (abduction quotient), (*e*) the closing time of the electroglottogram waveform, and (*f*) lung pressure (described below). Each cycle's measurements are added to the other cycles in the data and averaged. Patient data are thus available for comparison with data collected on a small group of normal speakers.

### SUBGLOTTAL (LUNG) AIR PRESSURE

Proper interpretation of the airflow rates through the vocal folds requires knowledge about the driving pressure beneath the vocal folds, often called subglottal pressure (and sometimes by a variety of other names such as lung pressure, tracheal pressure, etc.) There are various techniques for the measurement of the air pressure beneath the vocal folds including the esophageal balloon technique and intratracheal puncture.

In the esophageal balloon technique, a small, latex balloon attached to a catheter is swallowed and positioned in the esophagus immediately behind the trachea and inferior to the cricoid cartilage. The posterior wall of the trachea is composed of smooth muscle and any pressures in the trachea will be reflected through this muscle wall into the esophagus. The balloon will reflect these pressure changes, which will be converted to a recordable voltage by a pressure transducer at the other end of the catheter. There are several potential problems and pitfalls in the use of this technique (Kunze, 1964) but, with care, reliable and accurate measurements can be made (Schutte, 1980).

The second technique used to measure subglottal pressure is a tracheal puncture. A small needle attached to a catheter is inserted through the skin/tissue between a tracheal ring, usually the second or third ring. The pressure in the trachea is recorded using a pressure transducer. With both techniques, appropriate calibration maneuvers are performed to be able to relate pressure magnitude to the level of the electrical signal.

A third way of measuring subglottal pressure is by recording the intraoral air pressure variations when stop plosives (e.g., /b/, /p/) are produced by a speaker. The theory is that the pressures produced behind the oral constrictions are the same as the pressures in the rest of the respiratory tract since the tract is a closed system. Thus, the intraoral pressure magnitudes will be similar to the subglottal air pressure magnitudes, at least during the production of the consonant. During the actual production of the vowel following the consonant, intraoral pressure will drop markedly; however, there will still be subglottal pressure since now the constriction is at the vocal folds. However, the intraoral pressures will be good estimates of the subglottal pressure during the vowel (Hixon & Smitheran, 1982; Rothenberg, 1982; Smitheran & Hixon, 1981). An illustration of the technique for obtaining subglottal air pressure estimates from intraoral air pressure traces is shown in Figure 7.14. In our sys-

*Figure 7.14.* Air pressure traces during the production of the syllable /bœp/. The line drawn between each peak represents an estimate of the subglottal air pressure during the production of the vowel.

tem, the peak pressures before and after the vowel are measured, averaged, and used to estimate the subglottal or lung pressures.

## ELECTROMYOGRAPHY

Electromyography (EMG), a technique in which electrodes are inserted into specific muscles to measure their electrical activity, is used routinely by neurologists for the study of peripheral muscle function in various neuromuscular and neurological diseases. EMG is invasive and requires expertise; precautions must be taken to safeguard the patient's well-being. For these reasons, EMG has enjoyed limited use in the diagnosis and management of voice disorders. EMG of the vocal muscles requires detailed knowledge of head and neck anatomy, along with considerable experience in manipulating needles or needle carriers within the pharynx and larynx. The muscles involved in phonation are not readily accessible. Electromyographic recording equipment is available from a variety of manufacturers and has been engineered to be medically safe. The output of the equipment, an electromyogram, is a detailed tracing of muscle activity. An example of an electromyogram is shown in Figure 7.15.

Interpretation of electromyographic recordings requires experience and practice. Onset or offset of muscle activity, the pattern of muscle activity and the overall amplitude of muscle activity are the parameters that provide the most valuable information. Electromyographic patterns of neurologically disordered patients will show greater or lesser than normal amplitudes of muscle activity, extraneous bursts of muscle activity, and slower or faster than normal muscle activation. Laryngeal electromyograms may be helpful in those patients with voice problems of suspected neurological or neuromuscular etiology. Another use for EMG is to verify excessive muscle activity prior to injection of BOTOX for symptom relief of spasmodic dysphonia. The needle used to inject the BOTOX is used as an electrode whose electrical activity is monitored aurally to assist in the placement of the toxin in muscle. An EMG study can be helpful in differentiating vocal fold paralysis from arytenoid ankylosis.

*Figure 7.15.* Electromyogram of the cricothyroid muscle in an elderly speaker during sustained vowel production (upper trace) and consonant-vowel syllable production (lower trace).

## Respiratory Studies

### AIR VOLUMES AND CAPACITIES

Many clinicians advocate the analysis of a patient's respiratory function, including studies of lung volumes, vital capacity, residual capacity, and phonation volume. Others doubt the necessity for obtaining these data and question their value provided the patient is able to maintain adequate air volumes and airflows needed for speech. There is no controversy concerning the helpfulness of this information when dealing with professional voice users, particularily singers and actors. There are, of course, research issues for which such information is important.

The wet spirometer is the most common instrument used for the analysis of respiratory volumes. This device consists of an upper and a lower canister, each with an open end. The lower canister is filled with water. The open end of the upper canister fits into the mouth of the lower so that an airtight seal is produced. The two canisters are now effectively sealed, partially filled with known volumes of air and of water. A pipe, into which the patient breathes, connects to the air within the sealed canisters. When the patient exhales, air is forced into the sealed lower canister, the upper portion of which is allowed to move to accommodate the increased air volume. A pen or other marker attached to the vertically moving drum records the movement of the drum in response to the patient's breathing. Since the relationship between the air volume change and the movement of the pen is known, it is possible to obtain the volume of air used by the patient. Common measurements obtained from voice patients include tidal volume (the volume of air in an average breath), vital capacity (the volume of air that can be maximally exhaled after maximum inhalation), and total lung capacity (the total volume of air in the lungs). Other volumes that may be measured are inspiratory reserve volume (the amount of air that can be inspired from the end-expiratory level of a tidal breath) and expiratory reserve volume (the amount of air that can be expired from the end-expiratory level of a tidal breath). Respiratory physiologists are also concerned with reserve volume and gas exchange, but such measurements are not performed routinely for voice patients.

A certain amount of air volume, flow, and pressure is required for speech. The respiratory system, however, can provide considerably more volume, flow, or pressure than is required for speech or even for singing. Only a small portion of the total available volume is normally used in speaking. Thus, it would seem unnecessary, and perhaps unproductive, to spend inordinate amounts of time gathering information about lung volumes for most voice patients. Information that may be more valuable is that concerning the control of the respiratory system during speech. It is necessary and vitally important that informed decisions be made concerning the relative contributions of respiratory versus laryngeal function to the presenting voice problem.

### RESPIRATORY MOVEMENTS

It may be important to assess control of respiratory movements in some voice patients. Assessment of the movement of the thorax and abdomen during speech may provide important information about the control exerted by a voice patient. Analysis of these movements is possible using a variety of tools, including mercury-filled strain gauges (Baken, 1987), the respiratory inductive plethysmograph (Bless, Hunker, & Weismer, 1981; Sackner, 1980; Watson, 1979), and magnetometers (Hixon, 1987). Bless et al. (1981) provide a comparison of these techniques. Although their methods vary, all of these tools are able to monitor the movements of the chest and abdominal walls using noninvasive external devices. All are available from commercial manufacturers; there is some variation in the expertise required for their operation.

A typical recording of the movements of the chest wall and abdomen is shown in Figure 7.16. Note that the rib cage (upper trace) shows a steady decrease of circumference as exhalation progresses, with irregular but decreasing changes noted in the abdominal channel. These curves can be calibrated to produce estimates of lung volume.

## NONINSTRUMENTAL TESTING

### Critical Listening and Description

Although we have presented the voice history as a separate section, in practice there can be no separation between history taking and the voice evaluation. The initial

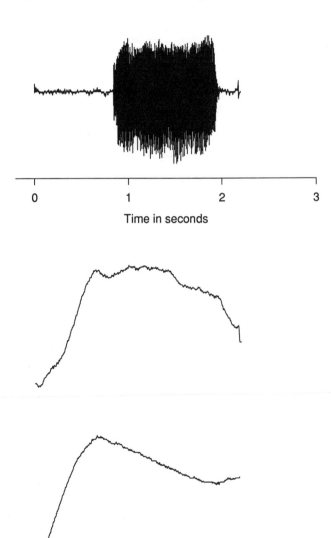

Figure 7.16. Examples of traces obtained with an inductive plethysmograph. The top trace is the acoustic signal, the middle trace reflects the circumferential changes occurring in the chest wall, and the bottom trace shows changes occurring in the abdomen. The speaker was a male who inhaled normally and produced a sustained vowel /œ/. Since we were only interested in time events, the rib cage and abdomen traces reflect voltage changes and not volume changes.

interview, during which the history is elicited, is the point at which the evaluation begins. It affords the clinician the opportunity to listen critically not only to the content of the message but also to the vocal output. Because patients are referred for voice therapy from various sources following laryngological examination, it is well for the speech-language pathologist to always have this question in mind: Are the vocal symptoms consistent with the referral diagnosis? The voice clinician's ears must always be turned on and tuned in. It is not unusual to pick up very significant clues about the presenting problem before the patient is aware that the examination is in progress.

## Case Study

A 35-year-old woman who complained of having lost her voice several weeks previously was answering all questions put to her in an aphonic whisper. During her aphonic explanation of the effect of this problem on her work, she cleared her throat. The clinician noted the entirely normal sound of the throat clearing. What information did this present?

While listening critically, the clinician should make observations about the consistency or variability in the sound of the voice and about its stability. When the voice exhibits variability or instability, it is important to be aware of the nature or pattern of that variability. For example, is the voice clear and strong initially, with gradual worsening over time? Does this happen with each sentence or two or over a more extended period of time? What is changing: quality, pitch, or loudness?

It is appropriate to make a perceptual judgment of vocal pitch, but such judgments must be made with caution and later verified with objective data. Perhaps the most important perceptual judgment to be made relative to pitch is whether or not its level is appropriate for the age and sex of the speaker. Perceptual impressions of fundamental frequency in the presence of laryngeal pathology tend to suggest lower than expected levels; however, it has been shown (Murry, 1978) that the fundamental frequency of some voice problems does not differ systematically from the norm, with the exception of reduction in phonational range in laryngeal paralysis. Another aspect of pitch to which the clinician must attend is its variability. Variations in pitch are used linguistically to mark the meaning of utterances. In the English language, pitch is expected to fall at the end of a declarative sentence and to rise to mark a question. Voices that show pitch variability are generally thought to be more "interesting" and less apt to lull the listener.

## Case Study

While taking the history from a 65-year-old man, the clinician was struck by an absence of inflection and a monotonic, flat, and unvarying delivery. Questions and statements were undifferentiated by the usual pitch changes. This observation, combined with noticeable slurring of speech, alerted the clinician to look for additional signs of neurological involvement. What would this absence of pitch variability suggest to you, and what other signs might you expect to find?

The loudness level of the patient's voice during assessment in presumably quiet surroundings should be another focus of the clinician's critical listening. The salient judgments to be made are whether the voice is too loud, too soft, or out of control. The consistency or variability of the loudness level are also important to note.

## Case Study

Another observation made about our 65-year-old patient mentioned above was the tendency for the loudness level of his voice to remain constant, with some decay at the end of an utterance. When asked to count and to alternate loud and soft voice for each successive number, the patient was able to comply with only the first three numbers, after which the loudness level became constant. Is this consistent with our previous observation, and why?

Descriptions of voice quality are most difficult to make. Many adjectives are used to describe voice quality, but they are difficult to quantify, and there is not widespread agreement on the meanings of voice quality terms. Some perceptions of quality can be checked against objective measures. For example, in the presence of hoarseness, there is the expectation of increased frequency perturbation (Coleman & Wendahl, 1967). Scaling of perceptions is perhaps the most valid approach to assigning a degree of objectivity to subjective judgments. Various types of scales will be discussed later in this chapter.

Those aspects of speech referred to as suprasegmentals may hold information about voice production or may add to other findings in the search for the diagnosis. The rate of speech is one such aspect. Excessively fast or laboriously slow rates may be suggestive of neurological involvement or may simply be a reflection of personality. Persons who tend to talk very rapidly often tend also to stretch vocalization to the last bit of air they can squeeze out. This style of speech is often characterized by increased tension in the respiratory and laryngeal systems. Prosody of speech may be disturbed by vocal behavior, as is the case with spasmodic dysphonia. If the clinician is aware of a disturbance of prosody, it is important to determine the nature of that disturbance and to describe it as accurately as possible.

Attention must be paid to any unusual vocal characteristics, such as stridor, grunts, and vocal tics. Of particular importance is the observation of stridor, inspiratory and/or expiratory noise. The presence of stridor suggests obstruction somewhere in the airway, subglottally, glottally, or supraglottally. It may be a sign of a laryngeal web, an obstructing lesion, severe inflammation, or abductor vocal fold paralysis. In infants inspiratory stridor is usually symptomatic of laryngomalacia. Yet another cause of stridor may be fixation or ankylosis of the cricoarytenoid joints as a consequence of rheumatoid arthritis.

## Case Study

J. W., a 41-year-old nurse, presented for a voice evaluation with a 10-year history of vocal difficulty and shortness of breath. She denied concern about her voice quality, which she claimed was unchanged. She believed that her vocal pitch was perhaps slightly higher than it had been but not significantly enough to be of concern. Perceptually, we were in agreement with these judgments. Her main vocal complaint was the inability to complete a whole sentence on one breath. J. W. has continued to work during this 10-year period but admitted to shortness of breath in climbing stairs or during other physical exertion. Throughout this history taking, the examiner was aware not only of her obvious shortness of breath and the disruption in the prosody of speech caused by frequent interruptions in order to renew breath supply but also of her characteristic thrusting forward of the mandible during inspiration and of audible inspiratory stridor. J. W. was immediately referred for laryngological examination, which revealed abductor vocal fold paralysis, probably as a consequence of a viral infection.

Vocal tics are characterized by sudden, unexpected, and involuntary vocalizations. They are usually thought to be a symptom of a neurological disorder. Other unusual vocal manifestations that may suggest a neurological etiology include grunts, barking sounds, and echolalia.

## Critical Observations and Descriptions

It is very important that the clinician maintain eye contact with the patient and be in visual contact so as to be able to make observations of behavior that may not be audible. This requires that note taking be kept to a minimum, freeing the clinician to take full advantage of all diagnostic clues. After completion of the examination, the clinician should describe all observations made.

Watch facial expression and body language. Do they match the words being spoken? How do they change in response to questions? Is the person comfortable, anxious, tense, fidgety? Is eye contact made and maintained? Are there extraneous facial or body movements? Is there tremor of the head, the hands, the jaw? Can you observe signs of neck, face, or laryngeal tension or strain? What is the emotional affect being projected? Does the person make adequate use of mouth opening and lip movement?

We suggest that observations of respiratory behavior be made during the period of eliciting the history and prior to asking the patient to engage in any specific vocal or respiratory tasks. It is important to observe respiratory behavior both during speech and at rest. Does the person have sufficient air supply to complete sentences? Does the person habitually speak until the air supply is exhausted? Does the person release exhalation prior to voice onset, or do you observe a holding of the breath in anticipation of speaking with an abrupt, sharp voice onset? Where do you observe the greatest amount of respiratory activity when the person is speaking, and when at rest? Is it clavicular, midthoracic, or abdominal/diaphragmatic?

## Diagnostic Therapy

The procedures used in this part of the evaluation cannot be rigidly specified because they often depend on the symptoms presented by the patient and the observations made by the clinician up to this point. The objectives of this part of the evaluation are to explore the patient's response to different ways of producing voice, to attempt to elicit an improved voice, to test the patient's ability to manipulate parameters such as pitch, loudness, and resonance, and to test the limits of the voice. Sometimes this involves making sounds and noises that create some self-consciousness. Patients with psychogenic voice disorders often appear frightened and threatened when asked to produce "different" sounds, perhaps because they are uncertain of their ability to maintain control over such phonations. Each step of this process must be carried out with sensitivity and encouragement. It is also essential that the clinician demonstrate the task being required of the patient. If the patient is being asked to produce a grunt, it will ease self-consciousness if the clinician models the grunt as the patient is to do it.

The following are some diagnostic therapy tasks that might be useful.

### PRODUCTION OF REFLEXIVE SOUNDS

These include coughing, laughing, clearing the throat, and the vocalized pause "uh-huh." The clinician's ears should have been tuned in to hear these sounds if they occurred spontaneously during the interview. It is interesting then to compare the quality of the sound produced spontaneously with that elicited during this task. The rationale for using this task is to determine the quality of the phonation produced in a non-speech task. It is most important to judge whether this elicited quality differs from the voice heard in speech in quality, pitch, or loudness. It is often necessary to work with the patient on these tasks until you are satisfied that the best sound that person is capable of, or is willing to produce, has been heard.

### ALTERING PITCH

Before attempting to obtain a phonational range, it is helpful to work with patients on the concept and on their ability to change pitch upward and downward. Some patients are unable to succeed on this task for reasons having to do with the nature of their problem. Others seem unable to carry it out due to difficulty in discriminating pitch changes and difficulty in matching pitches. It is important to try, during this diagnostic therapy period, to determine which of these is operative. It is helpful to engage in this activity as a practice for the actual testing of phonational range that may be carried out later. When patients exhibit difficulty in either matching a pitch or spontaneously altering pitch, we have found it useful to have them imitate animal sounds, such as the high-pitched meow of a kitten, the squeal of a mouse, or the howl of a wolf. Once again it is important to emphasize that such activities often create feelings of self-consciousness, which must be allayed by the clinician. One of the most effective methods of accomplishing this is through humor as the clinician models the desired sounds. The rationale for this activity is to test one of the limits of the voice, to explore whether the patient is capable of copying a model presented by the clinician, and to determine whether there is an overall improvement in the clarity of the sound at any point in the range. (Caution: This is not a search for an optimal pitch, which we do not believe is a viable concept, but rather an attempt to understand the physiology responsible for the vocal behavior.)

### SUSTAINING STEADY, PROLONGED PHONATION

As in the previous activity, it is helpful to allow the patient some practice on this task prior to the taking of measurements. An increased level of tension is often generated in patients when they know an activity is being timed, and it is not unusual to find that they perform better in a more relaxed activity. The vowel of choice is usually /ah/. It is important for the clinician to observe carefully how the patient prepares to carry out this task and how natural or strained the phonation is, as well as noting the steadiness and length of the phonation. The rationale for this activity is to observe the patient's ability to control phonation and respiration. Vocal tremor, if present, will become more obvious on this task than during connected speech. The patient may be asked to produce such a phonation at various pitch levels as a means of continuing to explore vocal capacity.

### ALTERING VOCAL LOUDNESS

It is usually not difficult to elicit a very quiet sound, but people are often quite reticent to produce the loudest phonation of which they are capable while seated in a quiet office. Therefore, it may be necessary to pursue increments of loudness in steps, with the clinician providing the model. Clearly, if the patient has been referred with the diagnosis of a vocal fold lesion, inflammation, or edema, this activity should not be carried out. Some persons who have habituated very loud voice use find it difficult to lower the loudness level and ask with incredulity whether they can be heard. The rationale for this activity is to further test the limits of voice production and explore the patient's ability to manipulate isolated vocal parameters and match a model.

## PHONATION WITH EFFORTFUL GLOTTAL CLOSURE

It is essential that this activity be used wisely and only with those patients for whom the activity itself will not be harmful. There are a variety of techniques that elicit effortful closure of the glottis: grunting, isometric pushing together of the palms of the hands held chest height, isometric pulling apart of linked hands held chest height, lifting a very heavy object, and attempting to raise a chair while seated on it. The person is required to phonate while tension is maintained during the activity. The rationale for the use of such a stressful phonatory act is to attempt to force vocal fold adduction and elicit a nonspeech sound that is difficult to control voluntarily. It is an activity that we have found helpful in eliciting a lowered pitch level in young boys who present with puberphonia and an improved voice in some patients with psychogenic dysphonias. Use of this procedure in therapy is discussed in Chapter 9. The intent here is to use the technique as an exploratory measure as part of the total assessment.

## "PLACING THE VOICE"

This is often referred to as placing the voice in the mask, or voice focus. As a diagnostic task, it constitutes one of the methods used in the search for the best voice a patient can produce. This technique is discussed more completely in Chapter 9.

## *Noninstrumental Objective Measurements*

### MAXIMUM PHONATION TIME

An individual's ability to sustain phonation provides some information about the control of respiratory function, glottal efficiency, and laryngeal control. When respiratory function is compromised, there will be either reduction in the amount of air available to support phonation or a problem in the control of the airflow. If the problem is at the laryngeal level, glottal resistance to airflow may be reduced due to inadequate glottal closure, or increased due to obstruction or hyperadduction. Certain problems affecting motor control of phonation may not inhibit or restrict maximum phonation time but may affect the quality of the phonation. The task is designed to test the limits of function and as such may uncover weaknesses that are not apparent at lower levels of function. Thus, for example, in the case of an individual with essential tremor, a vocal tremor may become increasingly obvious as phonation is sustained, although it may have escaped notice during speech.

The patient should be instructed to take a deep breath and sustain the vowel /ah/ for as long as possible. This should be done at a pitch and loudness level that are comfortable for the patient. A stopwatch should be used to obtain the measure, and patients should be asked to repeat the task at least three times (Hirano, 1981b), with the greatest duration being adopted as the maximum phonation time. Kent et al. (1987) caution, however, that the database for this, as well as many other maximum performance measures of speech production, may not be adequate for confident clinical use. Although Stone (1983) and others (Finnegan, 1984, 1985; Lewis, Casteel, & McMahon, 1982; Neiman & Edeson, 1981) have reported instability of the maximum phonation time measure over as many as 15 trials, Bless and Hirano (1982) found that three trials were adequate if subjects were given adequate instruction and practice in the task. Corroboration of this can be found in the report that coaching and instruction led to a mean increase in maximum phonation time of 5.2 seconds for a group of 3rd-grade girls (Reich, Mason, & Polen, 1986). The available normative values for sustained phonation may be found in Chapter 13.

The ability to sustain phonation is developmental and increases from childhood to adulthood. It is logical that this should be the case in view of the physical growth of the body and increased lung capacity. Significant differences in maximum phonation time exist between the sexes, but that difference does not begin to appear until puberty, when growth spurts between the sexes differ in degree (Hirano, 1981b). There is an overall reduction of pulmonary function with aging, as well as a lessening of laryngeal efficiency (Kent, Kent, & Rosenbek, 1987), resulting in a decrement in maximum phonation time in the geriatric population.

### S/Z RATIO

As noted previously, both respiratory and laryngeal factors play some role in determining maximum phonation time. However, the measure of maximum phonation time does not provide sufficient information to differentiate between deficits in respiratory support versus laryngeal inefficiency. Boone (1977) introduced the s/z ratio as an expansion on the measurement of maximum phonation time. The underlying theoretical construct suggests that individuals with normal larynges should be able to sustain vocalization (i.e., /z/) for a period of time equal to that of sustained expiratory airflow without vocalization (i.e., /s/), resulting in a ratio that approximates 1. If the respiratory system is compromised and the laryngeal system is intact, there should be an equal reduction in expiratory airflow for the voiceless /s/ and the voiced /z/ components of the task, which again would yield a ratio approximating 1. However, reduced vibratory efficiency of the abnormal larynx should result in air wastage, with reduction in the ability to sustain phonation but without a reduction in duration of expiratory airflow in the absence of phonation. Thus, the s/z ratio would be greater than 1 in the presence of laryngeal abnormality. Eckel and Boone (1981), in a study of dysphonic adults with and without laryngeal pathology, obtained results that support this notion. Ninety-five percent of patients with vocal fold margin pathology studied by Eckel and Boone had s/z ratios above 1.4, while the ratios for both the normal control group and those patients with dysphonia without pathology approximated 1.

Two studies have been reported investigating the use of the s/z ratio with children, and the results have not supported the previous research. In a study of 16 children with vocal nodules, Rastatter and Hyman (1982) report s/z ratios of 1, similar to expectations in the normal population. Similar findings are reported by Hufnagle and Hufnagle (1988) in a larger study of 123 dysphonic children, of whom 69 had vocal fold nodules. Based on the results of these studies, it would appear that the s/z ratio is not sensitive to the presence of vocal fold pathology in children, nor does it separate dysphonic children (with or without pathology) from normals. Although the reason for the difference between adults and children on this measure is not entirely clear, it is theorized that the size and stiffness of the pathology may have been greater in the adult subjects than in children, all of whom in the Hufnagle and Hufnagle study were reported to have had small to moderate size nodules that were soft in consistency. Measures of maximum duration of production of both /s/ and /z/ have been reported by Tait, Michel, and Carpenter (1980) for 53 children aged 5, 7, and 9 years with normal voices. Their results are shown in Figure 7.17. As one might expect, the older children had longer maximum phonations than the younger children, reflecting perhaps greater lung capacity or greater phonatory control. The maximum duration times for both /s/ and /z/ reported by Rastatter and Hyman (1982) and by Hufnagle and Hufnagle for their subjects who had vocal fold nodules or were dysphonic were lower than those reported by Tait et al. for their normal subjects.

The procedure for measuring the s/z ratio is very straightforward. The patient is instructed to take a deep breath and then sustain an /s/ for as long as possible. The examiner should model the task, although it is not necessary to sustain the model maximally. The task should be repeated at least twice by the patient, with the longest

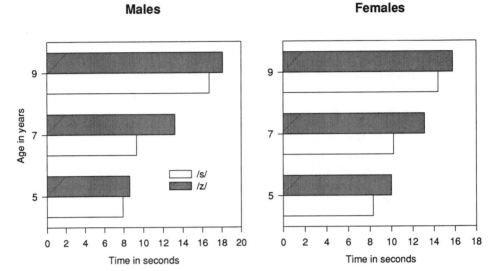

**Males**                                        **Females**

*Figure 7.17.* Maximum duration of phonation in sustained vowels produced by male and female children age 5, 7, and 9 years.

duration taken as the score. The same procedure is carried out for sustaining the /z/. It is best to use a stopwatch in obtaining these measures. The ratio is obtained by dividing the maximal /s/ value by the maximal /z/ value. Available normative s/z ratio data are presented in Chapter 13.

Although this measure has been demonstrated to have some validity for adults, the cautions discussed relative to maximum phonation time measures also apply here. The s/z ratio should be used primarily as a screening measure or as one test among many others. A diagnosis of pathology should never be made based on the result of this procedure alone. However, it may alert a clinician to the need for medical examination, if that has not been done, or conversely, it may raise questions about a diagnosis of pathology if the results are not consistent. The validity of this measure for children is still open to question, and thus it should be used in that population with even greater caution.

The apparent simplicity of this measure may be somewhat deceiving. Clinically we have found that it is necessary to teach this task to patients and to allow them adequate practice before taking formal measures (Chapter 13).

### SCALING

Perceptual judgments of various aspects of voice, quality in particular, are usually described as being subjective and with the implication that such judgments are not valid. However, perceptions can be quantified using well-established techniques of psychophysics and the procedure of scaling. The simplest type of quantification of qualitative or categorical variables is at the level of the nominal scale. The fundamental principle of nominal scales is equivalence; that is, all observations placed within the same category are considered to be equal. For example, voice qualities can be assigned names such as harsh, breathy, hoarse, or strident, which constitute categories. The perceptual judgment task may be to place voice samples within categories along that scale. No judgments are made or implied as to quantity or severity of the quality perceived. This is simply, as the name of the scale implies, a naming task.

However, we are usually interested in more than naming. Perhaps we want to make judgments about the degree of a quality that is present. Using our group of subjects who were nominally scaled as having hoarse voice quality, we can now engage in rank ordering them according to severity, using an ordinal scale. In this scale, numbers are used to express order of magnitude of the perception. The rank order means that higher numbers have a greater amount of a feature than lower numbers. Thus, the voice quality given a rank order of 1 has been judged to have less hoarseness than that with a rank order of 15. Ranks do not tell us how much of a feature is present or how much difference there is between ranks or even if the differences between ranks are equal. The only information we have is that at a given rank there is less or more of a feature than at the ranks above or below.

Interval scales are very common in voice quality scaling because we can use them to determine how much of a feature is present in one quality compared to another. The refinement over an ordinal scale is that the distance between adjacent points on the scale has meaning, and a given interval between measures has the same meaning any-where along the scale. Common examples of this type of scale are degrees of temper-ature and calendar years. In the latter we know that as much time elapsed between 1790 and 1800 as between 1970 and 1980. The interval scale thus has a defined unit of measure. However, it does not necessarily have a defined beginning or a meaningful zero point.

The ratio scale has all the properties of the interval scale, with the added benefit of an absolute zero. Such a scale makes it possible to talk meaningfully about ratios. Ex-amples of this type of scale are measures of length.

A visual analog scale simply presents a continuum between two anchor points, such as an undifferentiated 5-inch line-scale along which a mark is made representing the quantity of a feature judged to be present. Such a scale does not use any verbal de-scriptors along it and is reported by some to produce more reliable and valid judg-ments because it permits finer discriminations to be made (Kempster, 1984). For scor-ing purposes the 5-inch line in the example above could be converted into a 100-point rating scale.

The most complex scaling method is referred to as multidimensional scaling, a method for identifying the perceptual attributes of complex stimuli such as voice qual-ity (Kempster, 1984; Schiffman, Reynolds, & Young, 1981). Algorithms of multidi-mensional scales represent stimuli as points on a spatial map. The difference between points is then a reflection of the judged similarity or dissimilarity of the stimuli. The closer the points, the greater the similarity of the feature being judged.

### Scaling of Pitch

Perceptual judgments of voice quality are often confounded by other perceptual at-tributes of the voice sample and may not always be related to a simple acoustic corre-late. For example, let us examine the perception of pitch. Wolfe and Ratusnik (1988) have shown that listeners will rate the pitch of rough vowels much lower than the pitch of normally produced vowels. Consequently, vowels produced by a patient with a hoarse voice may be expected to be perceived as lower in pitch than their measured fundamental frequencies would predict. Furthermore, Wolfe and Ratusnik reported that the pitch matches they obtained were related to the acoustic measures of noise energy level and jitter ratio rather than to fundamental frequency. Thus, it appears that with respect to pitch, other abnormal perceptual (e.g., roughness, hoarseness) or acoustic (e.g., jitter, noise level, spectrum) attributes may result in inaccurate judg-ment. This may account for some of the discrepancies that have been noted between perceptual pitch judgments of abnormal voices and the measured acoustic correlate of fundamental frequency. Wilson, Wellen, and Kimbarow (1983) suspect that there is a skill in discriminating pitch differences in the speaking voice that is not easily developed. Their judges, described as trained and untrained, performed at chance level on a pitch discrimination task until there was at least a 20–29 Hz difference present between paired voice samples.

Another factor affecting the reliability and validity of perceptual judgments is the experience of the listener. Many studies in which perceptual judgments were reported used experienced listeners or listeners with extensive exposure to normal and abnormal voice qualities. How much experience is needed to produce reliable judgments is somewhat unclear. Bassich and Ludlow (1986) conducted a study using 4 judges who required 16 half-hour training sessions before reaching 80% agreement with one another. Perhaps the lack of training or experience may account for the lack of difference between groups of trained and untrained listeners in distinguishing pitch differences between pairs of children's voices in the Wilson et al. (1983) study. The trained group consisted of 10 graduate students in speech-language pathology, of which only 4 had had previous experience in working with patients with voice disorders.

It would seem highly unlikely that graduate students with only a brief exposure to voice disorders (usually a single academic course and perhaps an actual patient in clinic) would be able to reliably and accurately rate attributes of the voice such as pitch, loudness, and tremor. In a study reported by Colton and Estill (1981) concerned with the identification of four distinct voice qualities, the group of 6 speech-language pathologists performed slightly worse than the group of 15 "naive" listeners (66% versus 68%). Singers and individuals who played a musical instrument performed somewhat better than these two groups (73% for singers, 75% for instrumentalists). Although the differences between the groups were not large, these results suggest that experience in music may help a listener to make judgments concerned with voice quality attributes. At the very least, musicians may attend better to the nonlinguistic aspects of the speaker's utterance.

It is clear that perceptual judgments of vocal pitch are sufficiently unreliable to cast doubt on their use in planning treatment strategies. Determinations of the appropriateness of pitch level should be made on the measurement of its acoustic correlate, fundamental frequency, for which normative values appropriate for age and sex are available for comparison. Whenever measurable acoustic correlates of vocal attributes are available, their use is encouraged in preference to reliance on the perceptual feature.

### Scaling Vocal Effort

The effort a patient uses to vocalize may be important to assess in the exploration of a voice problem. Many patients report that at the end of a day of prolonged talking, they feel vocally fatigued. They may also report that they need to expend more energy in talking than they did prior to onset of their vocal problem. It is difficult for the clinician to know how to assess such reports and what value to give them. However, there is a way for such "feelings" to be measured, and such measures can be helpful therapeutically and in assessing the efficacy of treatment and of specific treatment techniques.

How does the clinician quantify the vocal effort a patient uses during phonation? Simply by asking the patient to produce a vocalization and afterward asking that patient to assign it a number that represents the amount of effort used. It has been shown that subjects can scale their own effort levels with this simple procedure (Colton & Brown, 1973; Irwin & Mills, 1965; Lane, Catania, & Stevens, 1961; Wright & Colton, 1972a, 1972b). Wright and Colton (1972a, 1972b) asked speakers to produce the vowel /ah/ at their minimum, most comfortable, and maximum effort levels. The fundamental frequency and the sound pressure level of each phonation was measured during each vocalization. The subjects were then asked to assign a number that represented the amount of effort used. They could use any number they wished, with the understanding that greater effort levels would be associated with higher numbers. This procedure is often referred to in the psychophysical literature as the method of magnitude estimation. Median results for the group are shown in Figure 7.18. The left panel shows vocal effort in assigned numbers versus SPL in decibels. In the right panel, vocal effort is compared to fundamental frequency. The solid lines connect minimum, most comfortable, and maximum effort levels. The data points between these three effort levels (squares) were generated by asking the subject to produce a phonation whose effort was halfway between minimum and most comfortable or most comfortable and maximum. Each of these intervals then was bisected again to produce the estimates of vocal effort shown in this figure. Note how consistent the subjects were in producing and rating their effort levels, especially for effort versus SPL. The data points for magnitude production (shown by circles) were obtained by providing a number to the subject and asking him to produce a phonation with an effort level representative of the number supplied. These data are very similar to the data obtained in the magnitude estimate phase of the experiment. The vocal effort/fundamental frequency data show somewhat more variability between magnitude production and estimation than the vocal effort/SPL data. It is abundantly clear, however, that individuals can rate the effort they use to produce voice and that variations of vocal effort are manifested acoustically by variation of SPL and fundamental frequency.

Figure 7.18. Vocal effort/sound pressure level and vocal effort/fundamental frequency relationships for five normal speakers.

The data of Figure 7.18 clearly show that an increase of vocal effort is accompanied by an increase of both intensity and frequency. Colton and Brown (1973) have shown that speakers also exhibit systematic increases of intraoral air pressure with an increase of vocal effort. In simple consonant-vowel syllables, intraoral air pressure can be a good estimate of the pressures driving the vocal folds (Hixon & Smitheran, 1982; Rothenberg, 1982; Smitheran & Hixon, 1981). Thus, it is not unreasonable to suspect that the magnitude of subglottal air pressure, accompanied by the consequent tension of the vocal folds, contributes to the judgments of vocal effort.

Verdolini-Marston and her colleagues (Verdolini-Marston, Burke, Lessac, Glaze, & Caldwell, 1995) reported using vocal effort scaling in their study of the effectiveness of two kinds of therapy for vocal nodules. Prior to therapy, five subjects who received the confidential voice therapy protocol have a mean rated effort level of 115 (a judgment of comfortable level of effort while talking was assigned the number 100) whereas the 3 subjects who received the resonant voice therapy protocol have a mean rated effort level of 142. After a two-week, concentrated period of voice therapy, the confidential therapy group reported a mean effort level of 90; the resonant therapy group an effort level of 105. These measures were obtained two weeks after therapy had ended and both therapy groups had a mean effort level of 97. These results suggest that monitoring vocal effort may reflect the physiological changes that occur as a result of therapy and may monitor the vocal usage by patients with voice disorders.

Listeners can also rate vocal effort from recorded samples of speech (Brandt, Ruder, & Shipp, 1969; Lane, Catania, & Stevens, 1961; Moll & Peterson, 1969; Warren, 1962), but the ratings are not simply ratings of the vocal loudness (Brandt, Ruder, & Shipp, 1969). Listeners apparently use the increase of energy in the higher frequencies as cues for their judgments of vocal effort as well as the greater sound pressure levels that accompany increased effort levels. They may also internalize what they hear and relate their judgments to their own perceived efforts. It is important to understand that increased tension in the adducted vocal folds results in greater subglottal air pressure and also results in the production of increased energy in the higher frequencies. Thus, listeners and speakers appear to use similar cues; only the speaker has access to the significant physiological variable, air pressure, whereas the listener must depend solely on its acoustic manifestation, increased high frequency energy.

The concept of vocal effort, as well as its measurement, has implications for the management of voice problems, for monitoring progress, and for assessing treatment efficacy (see Chapter 9).

## Voice Sample Recording

One of the easiest and simplest ways of testing a subject is to obtain a voice recording. Even if no further analysis of the recording is performed, the recording itself can be invaluable. Recording makes repeated listening possible, allowing the voice clinician further opportunities to learn about the person's voice characteristics. A voice recording during the initial assessment provides a baseline record of the voice prior to intervention. This documentation can be helpful for demonstrating progress or change as a result of treatment and for judging the efficacy of treatment. A baseline recording is highly important when medical-legal issues arise. It is surprising, therefore, that so little attention is generally given to the techniques and equipment needed for producing good-quality recordings. The material presented in the following sections is based both on personal experience and on discussions by Izdebski (1981, 1983).

## TAPE RECORDERS

There are several kinds of voice recorders that can be used to make audio recordings of patient vocalizations: (*a*) reel-to-reel, (*b*) cassette, (*c*) videotape recorders, (*d*) DAT recorders and (*e*) minidisc recorders. The reel-to-reel models have an excellent frequency response and a wide dynamic range but are not often found in most voice clinics. Manufacturers of reel-to-reel units include Nigra, Ampex, and Revox. Cassette recorders are much more popular and offer the conveniences of portability and use of cassette tapes. Although inexpensive cassette recorders are available, they rarely have good frequency response or adequate dynamic range, do not produce good recordings, have high tape instability (wow and flutter), and are prone to breakdown. These inexpensive recorders are not recommended for clinical use. There are many cassette recorders costing $200–600 that have good to excellent characteristics and are easy to use. We include videotape recorders in this category because many of the medium-priced models, as well as the higher priced ones, have excellent frequency and dynamic ranges in the audio range, very low tape instability, and can store considerable data. Furthermore, many can record and reproduce in stereo.

Two additional recording devices have become available in recent years whose price and performance warrant consideration for routine and even critical clinical use. The DAT recorder is very similar to a cassette recorder except that the analog voice signal is digitized and recorded on tape. The cassette is about the size of a microcassette (the kind used in dictating equipment) but depending on the tape quantity and the recording speed, up to 4 hours of high quality signal can be recorded. At the fastest speed presently available, the quality rivals that heard on compact discs (CDs). DAT recorders are made by Sony, JVC, and Aiwa, among others. We use two models of Sony DATs. The first, the model TCD-D3, is about the size of a Walkman, operates from batteries or an ac line source, and is capable of recording with a sampling rate of 44.1 kHz (CD quality). At this rate, we can record up to 2 hours. Our second unit is a larger unit, the Sony DTC-700. Both units feature the ability to label each recording with a number permitting more rapid retrieval of a desired recordings. Prices vary a great deal and may be less for new units or units produced by other manufacturers.

Minidisc recorders use a small disc about the size of the 3½ disc used in many computer systems. The recorder can record about 60–70 minutes of vocalization with CD quality. Sony makes a minidisc recorder that is about the size of a Walkman. Although perceptually, the recordings sound excellent, the frequency response may be limited because of circuitry used to pack the samples on the small disc. Thus, a minidisc recorder may not be suitable for critical clinical applications but is suitable if the intent is only to collect audio recordings for listening purposes. Beware of minidisc players that can play prerecorded minidiscs but have no record capability.

In addition to good recording equipment, it is also important to use high quality tape. High quality tape has a number of advantages: (*a*) It is strong enough to withstand the starting and stopping required when many speech samples are recorded and played back, and (*b*) less of the oxide particles in the tape will rub off to affect the recording and playback heads and interfere with the motor and wheels that transport the tape. Tapes are available in 30–120 minute lengths. It is best to avoid the 120-minute tapes because the tape is very thin and can break easily. Cassette tapes made by TDK, Maxell, Sony, Nakamichi, 3M, or similar manufacturers are of good quality. Tapes may also differ in type, for example, standard tape, chromium dioxide tape (a high bias tape), or metal tape (also a high bias tape). Most tape recorders are able to play back all of these types of tape. Metal tape tends to have the best response characteristics, but at considerably greater cost. Many of the good to excellent cassette recorders will have metal tape recording/reproducing capability.

Videotapes also come in various time lengths, usually ranging between 2 and 6 hours (VHS format). When using the tape to obtain good audio recordings, it is best to use the highest speed settings (2 hours).

DAT tapes are made by several manufacturers including Sony, JVC, and Maxell. They are available in 30, 60, and 120 minute lengths. These tapes are considerably more expensive than standard cassette tapes but are of superior quality. Mini discs usually can record up to 70 minutes of information and are similar in price to DAT tapes.

## MICROPHONES

Microphones should be selected on the basis of low distortion, low sensitivity, wide frequency response (50–16,000 Hz), directionality, stability, and cost. Good-quality microphones can be purchased for relatively low cost ($50–100). A good source for microphones is Radio Shack. Many new microphones are of the electret type, which contain a small battery and pickup element that has very good frequency and dynamic response characteristics. There are also condenser and dynamic microphones that have excellent characteristics at moderate cost. A pressure zone microphone, a relatively new type of microphone that permits recording large groups with good fidelity, is also worthy of consideration.

## ENVIRONMENT

Recordings should be made in a quiet room, away from noisy corridors and windows that face onto busy streets. The room need not be completely sound proof, however. Carpeted floors and walls and windows hung with fabric coverings serve to reduce noise level significantly. Of course, special acoustic absorbing panels can be installed, which will produce a very quiet room. The clinician should measure the noise levels within the room to make sure they are acceptable (less than 50 dB at the low frequencies) and periodically check these levels to ensure that the noise present is predominantly low frequency.

## TASKS

It is important to chose a variety of tasks for the patient to carry out that will sample the full range of the patient's vocal capabilities. Sustained vowels are useful for subsequent measurement of fundamental frequency, perturbation, and spectra. Syllables and sentences should be used to sample the patient's voice under more speech-like conditions and yet yield data that can be compared at different time periods. Testing of vocal limits, that is, phonational (frequency) range and dynamic (intensity) range, can also be recorded. We usually include a standard reading passage, the Rainbow Passage (Fairbanks, 1960), and a sample of conversational speech as part of our recording protocol. Of course, it is important to also record any special or unusual characteristics of a patient's vocal behavior. The speech tasks from the protocol for fiberoptic examination in the Appendix may be used for any audio recording.

## SPECIAL TESTING

### *Psychiatric*

The link between personality and voice cannot be overemphasized. It is expressed in a multitude of ways by all speakers. Second only to our appearance, the voice serves as our identity, as a means of identification even in the absence of the visual presence. It serves as our emotional escape valve as we laugh, cry, scream in fear, or shout in rage. It speaks of our well-being, of our energy level, of our emotional state. We use it to cajole, to seduce, to energize, to subdue, to question, to arouse, to soothe, to scorn, to demand, to plead; in short, to give special meaning to our words. And we are called upon to use our voices to impart information, to express opinions, to defend our property, our rights, ourselves, to intercede for others, to influence others, and simply to interact with others. Our voices are a road between people, the road on which the words we speak travel. Is it any wonder, then, that the road is sometimes subject to bumps and irregularities, that it becomes altered due to excessive tensions and stresses? In some cases these changes are minor, requiring only that someone understand the situation and arrive at a way to resolve it. However, other problems require extensive repairs and require specific types of expertise if they are to be attended to properly.

The analogies are obvious. For some people, excess tensions are felt most keenly in the laryngeal area. The effect of these tensions may take time to gradually become apparent and bothersome, or they may reach a significant level rather quickly. There is a continuum of effect, from the very mild hoarseness that tends to come on at the end of the day to the constant and all-pervasive lack of voice. However, that continuum should not be equated with the depth of the problem. The degree of the dysphonic symptoms is not necessarily correlated with the "severity" of the problem.

Clinically, patients with voice disorders of psychological origin constitute a fascinating group of people, for many of whom almost magical return of voice is not infrequent. Skill, understanding, and patience are required, but the reward for the speech-language pathologist is an immediate gratification that comes rarely in the practice of the profession. Specific procedures for the treatment of these kinds of problems will be discussed in Chapter 9.

For a significant number of patients, however, the basic problems are much deeper. The patient is unable to give up the symptom, or unable to do so permanently. In such cases, there is a clear need for referral for psychiatric or psychological consult or counseling. Indeed, such a referral is also often necessary and helpful for those persons who, with our help, may be able to abandon their symptoms, but for whom there continue to be problems that need attention.

## Case Study

R. W., an overweight and not very attractive 16-year-old, was referred for voice therapy with a diagnosis of dysphonia in the presence of a normal-appearing larynx. It was very difficult to engage R. W. in conversation. He responded to all questions in as few words as possible. He made only fleeting eye contact. The dysphonia was in its third month, and he had been out of school for that entire period on doctor's orders. Prior to this referral, he had already been on a regimen of voice rest and through several courses of pharmacological treatment, with no change in symptoms. R. W.'s voice sounded very strained and tense. Hoarseness was present. Working very slowly, with constant encouragement and praise, we were able to elicit a normal voice quality. R. W. refused to recognize this change at first, but slowly became willing to use the good voice more frequently. Within a few therapy sessions R. W. had full return of normal voice and was ready to return to school.

During the therapy sessions the need for R. W. to see a psychiatrist or psychologist was raised both with him and his mother. With return of normal voice a direct referral for such additional treatment was made. A month later R. W. returned. His voice had worsened, with a full recurrence of earlier symptoms. Our referral for psychiatric follow-up had not been carried out. R. W. was seen again for several sessions of voice therapy, during which he continued to be very closed in all respects. Once again voice was restored and once again referral for psychiatric consultation was made even more strongly. Two months later R. W.'s mother wished to schedule another appointment as once again the symptoms had recurred. She was advised that it was not appropriate to continue voice treatment, because it was clear that numerous other problems were present and particularly in view of the lack of follow-up on our referral for psychiatric consultation.

---

It is often necessary to move slowly when referral for counseling or psychiatric examination is being considered. A sense of trust must be built between the clinician and the patient. The clinician must be sufficiently attuned to the patient's needs to be able to approach the referral in the manner that will be most likely to be accepted. Referrals made too abruptly may be totally rejected by the patient, who may also reject the person making the referral. When that occurs, the patient may be lost to follow-up or treatment of any kind for some period of time. This is what we were hoping to avoid in R. W.'s case. Unfortunately, even our best efforts sometimes do not bring about the desired result.

It is vitally important to consider all possible etiologies of a presenting problem before adopting the diagnosis of psychogenic voice disorder. There are a number of neurological disease processes whose early symptoms may be very similar to those presented by patients with emotionally based problems. Furthermore, the presenting symptoms and signs of psychogenic dysphonia sometimes may be similar to those of spasmodic dysphonia or musculoskeletal tension/hyperfunctional dysphonia. These patients present with minimal visible laryngeal changes, if any and with symptoms that may be mystifying and histories that may be confounding.

## *Neurological*

---

### *Case Study*

---

J. R., a 37-year-old woman with intermittent dysphonia, had been examined and treated by several otolaryngologists over a period of months with no change in her vocal status. She was then referred for a trial of voice therapy. J. R. reported a rather troubled social history involving a very difficult recent divorce preceded by a number of years in an abusive marriage during which she had suffered attempted strangulation and blows to the neck. She and her 7-year-old son were now living with a friend as she was trying to put her life in order. Her voice symptoms began during the course of the divorce process. She described a "gravelly" quality that came on gradually with any extended period of talking but that cleared when she was able to rest and be silent for a while. She denied any other physical symptoms.

The history thus far seemed to suggest a classic voice disorder of psychological etiology. During the initial evaluation, however, the clinician was impressed with this patient's attitude, forthrightness, and overall affect. Furthermore, we noted the gradual worsening of voice as the evaluation progressed, which J. R. attributed in part to having engaged in much conversation during a lengthy car trip from her home to our office. Trials of diagnostic therapy procedures were totally ineffective in eliciting improved voice quality. J. R. was subsequently referred for neurological examination and a diagnosis of myasthenia gravis was made.

---

Referral for neurological examination is usually well accepted by patients. It should be considered when laryngeal findings are either negative or suggestive of disordered coordination of laryngeal function, when the voice symptoms are neither consistent with nor explained by the history, when changes in vocal output cannot be altered by behavioral approaches and whenever there is a family history of neurological problems. Similarly, patients usually respond well when referred for further medical examinations, as might be indicated when gastroesophageal reflux is suspected as a key factor in the voice problem.

## Imaging

The past decade has seen major growth and development of increasingly sophisticated imaging technology: computed axial tomography (CT scan), ultrasound, magnetic resonance imaging (MRI), and positive emission tomography (PET), to name a few. Although these techniques are being widely used to determine the location and extent of disease, data relevant to phonatory behavior are only beginning to appear. Baer and others (Baer, Gore, Boyce, & Nye, 1987; Baer, Gore, Gracco, & Nye, 1991; Lufkin & Hanafee, 1985; Stark, Moss, Gamsu, Clark, & Gooding, 1984) have applied the technique of MRI to the study of normal neck anatomy and the physiology of the vocal tract during speech acts. Leboldus and his colleagues (Leboldus, Savoury, Carr, & Nicholson, 1986) showed how MRI imaging could be applied to the diagnosis and treatment of ENT problems. Others (Shaefer, Freeman, Finitzo, Close, & Cannito, 1985; Swenson, Zwirner, Murry, & Woodson, 1992) have used MRI to study brain dysfunction in patients with spasmodic dysphonia. There is considerable promise of MRI and CAT images to the study of normal and disordered speech and voice. At this time the primary use of these techniques for the study of laryngeal function is in the realm of research. Clinical use is more limited, due in part to limitations of the equipment, limited equipment availability, and the cost of the procedures.

### SUMMARY

The voice history is a critical part of the diagnostic process not only for the information obtained but also because of the relationship that is established between the clinician and the patient during the information gathering. The first section of this chapter was devoted to a discussion of the skill involved in the interview process. The content of the interview was presented in some detail and included the following sections: the problem and its effects, the developmental history of the problem, its onset and duration, the variable or consistent nature of the problem and associated symptoms, the patient's health history, and vocational, social, and recreational histories.

The array of techniques used in the examination and testing of the voice have been described in the second and third sections of this chapter. Examination of the larynx can be carried out through both direct and indirect methods. Technological advances have substantially increased our ability to visualize not only the structure of the larynx and supraglottal vocal tract but also the dynamic physiology of both phonatory and nonphonatory behavior. The examination procedures described include indirect laryngoscopy, direct laryngoscopy, flexible fiberoptic laryngoscopy, stroboscopy, ultra-high speed photography, and ultrasound. Advantages and disadvantages of each are discussed.

Laboratory testing procedures provide documentable and measurable evidence of vocal function. These techniques sometimes provide indirect evidence about the functional status of the larynx. They include acoustic measures of fundamental frequency and its variability, functional limits of the voice relative to frequency and intensity, periodicity and stability of the voice as evidenced by measures of perturbation, and visual evidence of the acoustic components of the voice as displayed in a spectrogram or an acoustic spectrum. Physiological studies provide further evidence and information about the larynx and the voice. These include electroglottography, photoglottography, inverse filtering of airflow, and electromyography. Testing of respiratory function is another aspect of physiological function that can add to the total data pool in selected cases.

We have also included various forms of noninstrumental evaluation of the voice, usually carried out by the speech-language pathologist but useful to all who examine and work with the voice-disordered patient. These noninstrumental methods include critical listening, observation, and description. Formalization of the kinds of observations that should be made, both auditory and visual, will help to focus the examiner's careful attention to the variety of clues that can be obtained about vocal function through this approach. The clinical trial involved in a diagnostic therapy approach allows the examiner to test hypotheses and extend the observations.

Objective measurements that can be made without the benefit of any equipment more sophisticated than a stopwatch are also discussed. Although fairly simple to obtain, these measurements can be extremely useful in establishing baseline measures of vocal function and subsequently to chart progress or assess the results of treatment. Within this section we have also discussed the need for suitable audio recordings and the types of equipment that are appropriate to address this need.

The final section of this chapter dealt briefly with the need for referral for additional testing. Such testing may include psychiatric or psychological consultation, neurological examination, medical assessment for associated problems, and special imaging techniques.

## SUGGESTED READINGS

Bernstein, L., Bernstein, R. S. (1985). Interviewing, a guide for health professionals (4th ed.). Norwalk, CT: Appleton-Century-Crofts.

Hersen, M., Turner, S. M. (1985). Diagnostic interviewing, New York: Plenum Press.

Levinson, D. (1987). A guide to the clinical interview. Philadelphia: WB Saunders.

Maple, F. F. (1985). Dynamic interviewing, an introduction to counseling. Beverly Hills, CA: Sage Publications.

# Chapter 8

# Surgical and Medical Management of Voice Disorders

There are three general approaches to the management of voice problems, no one of which necessarily excludes the others. These approaches are (*a*) surgical, (*b*) medical, and (*c*) behavioral.

The first two will be discussed in this chapter; the behavioral approach will be discussed in Chapter 9. Although these approaches are being presented separately, it is often the case that ideal treatment requires the use of combined treatment modalities. For example, the patient who has sustained traumatic laryngeal damage in an automobile accident may first be a surgical candidate. However, after surgery and healing, this patient may well benefit from vocal rehabilitation to reestablish the best possible voice production.

Surgery is considered the more radical treatment approach because of the need to cut into tissues to remove body parts or abnormal growths, or to physically alter or augment the shape or position of structures. A review of surgical techniques that are currently being used in the management of laryngeal problems with a phonatory component is presented in the first section of this chapter. The medical approach to the treatment of voice disorders refers to techniques that are not invasive or do not involve surgical ablation, reconstruction, or alteration; these will be discussed in the second section.

## SURGICAL MANAGEMENT

### Concept of Phonosurgery

Phonosurgery refers to a collection of surgical techniques that have as their aim the improvement of voice. Some phonosurgery techniques have long been in practice. Among these are the removal of benign masses of the vocal folds, including nodules and polyps; vocal fold mediofixation and/or intrafold injection for unilateral vocal fold paralysis; and glottal reconstruction following partial laryngectomy.

Recently, however, there has been renewed interest and marked growth in phonosurgery for many other laryngeal conditions and voice disorders. There are three good reasons for this renewed interest. The first relates to a change in the focus of surgery from an emphasis on procedures designed to eradicate or ablate to those in which the goal is to conserve, reconstruct, or improve function. The second, probably concomitant reason is the recent development of surgical techniques and instruments that permit more refined surgeries. The third is the growth of information on the anatomy, physiology, and pathologies of voice, which is now being seen in clinical applications.

The term "phonosurgery" was first used by Hans von Leden in two articles (von Leden, Poyle, Goff, & Miller, 1969; von Leden, Yanagihara, & Werner-Kukuk, 1967) discussing some surgical approaches for voice improvement. The 1970s saw marked progress in technique and growth in the use of phonosurgical procedures, primarily in Japan (Hirano, 1975; Isshiki, 1977; Saito, 1977). Since the 1980s, phonosurgery has found rapid acceptance in many countries around the world.

There are five major groups of phonosurgery: (*a*) removal of pathological tissue; (*b*) surgical correction of the position, shape, and/or tension of the vocal fold(s); (*c*) surgery to alter or restore laryngeal neuromuscular function; (*d*) surgical reconstruction for partial loss and/or deformity of the larynx; and (*e*) surgical reconstruction for loss of the entire larynx. Each group, except for (*e*), will be described in the following sections. This final group will not be included because total laryngectomy and related issues are beyond the scope of this book.

## Surgical Removal of Pathological Tissue of the Phonatory Organ

The development of endolaryngeal microsurgery in the 1960s (Saito, Ogino, Ishikura, Niino, & Fukuda, 1966; Tucker, 1985) opened up new avenues for phonosurgery. The operating microscope permits visualization of lesions in ways not previously possible in the living patient. It allows safe and precise removal of pathological tissue, with greater ease. Jako (1972) and Strong and Jako (1972) developed the use of the $CO_2$ laser in combination with the operating microscope. The use of this combined technique for removing laryngeal lesions has become widespread.

In removing vocal fold pathologies, extreme care must be taken to avoid invading normal vocal fold tissue beyond the minimum required. Normal vocal folds have a unique and delicate layered structure, as described in Chapter 3. Once this structure is destroyed, complete surgical reconstruction is usually extremely difficult, if not impossible.

### VOCAL FOLD NODULES

The need for surgical excision of vocal fold nodules is limited because almost all nodules in children disappear spontaneously by the end of adolescence, and most nodules can be successfully treated with voice therapy. In children, surgery is indicated only in extreme cases in which the effects of the voice abnormality on the child are serious and voice therapy has not been effective. Surgical removal of nodules in adults may be indicated when voice therapy has not been effective.

When nodules are surgically removed, only the excessive tissue should be ablated. The postsurgical result should be a vocal fold with a minimal surgical wound (Fig. 8.1). Note how the small, delicate forceps are used to grasp and then cut the nodule on the left vocal fold. It is important to cut only the nodule and not extend the cut into the deeper layers of the lamina propria. Otherwise, healing will be slower, and scar tissue may develop that will interfere with normal vocal fold vibration.

### VOCAL FOLD POLYP

Fresh and small polyps are subjected to surgical treatment when they have not responded to voice therapy. For large and/or old polyps, surgery followed by voice therapy is the protocol of choice.

In surgery, only excessive mass should be removed; care should be taken not to excise healthy tissue. Again, the result should be a normal contour of the vocal fold with a minimal wound (Fig. 8.2). In this procedure, a fine knife is used to excise the upper attachments of the polyps. Then, forceps are used to grasp and cut the remaining attachments of the polyp.

### REINKE'S EDEMA

The surgical approach is indicated in almost all cases of Reinke's edema. Cigarette smoking, highly implicated as an etiological factor, should be stopped prior to surgery. Surgery should then be followed by voice therapy.

The most important principle in surgery for Reinke's edema is to preserve the mucosa at the vocal fold edge. If the mucosa is removed at the edge, stiff scar tissue may form, resulting in dysphonia. The surgical procedure involves the removal of the edematous mucosa of the upper surface of the vocal fold first (Fig. 8.3B and C). The fluid contents of the vocal fold are then sucked and pressed out of the wound (Fig. 8.3D and E). Redundant mucosa, if any, is removed (Fig. 8.3F and G).

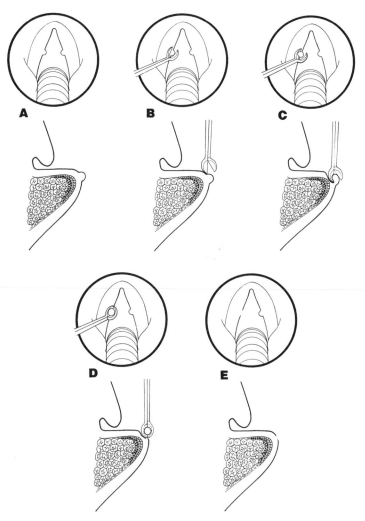

*Figure 8.1.* Surgery for vocal fold nodules.

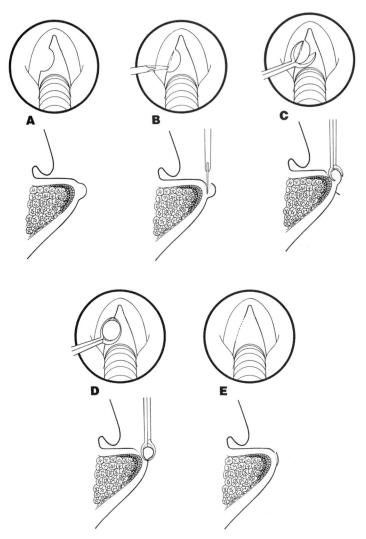

*Figure 8.2.* Surgery for vocal fold polyps.

### EPIDERMOID CYST

A surgical approach is indicated in all cases of epidermoid cysts. As was discussed in Chapter 4, small cysts are occasionally misdiagnosed as nodules or even completely overlooked under examination with regular light. Stroboscopy, especially when conducted with a fiberscope located close to the vocal fold, is useful in detecting such small cysts.

The ideal surgical technique is one that enucleates the cyst. A mucosal incision is made along the lateral margin or above the cyst (Fig. 8.4B). The cyst is carefully elevated from the neighboring structures and removed (Fig. 8.4C and D). A straight line incision on the upper surface of the vocal fold is the result (Fig. 8.4E).

### NONSPECIFIC GRANULOMA

Almost all nonspecific granulomas of the larynx are caused by either endotracheal intubation (intubation granuloma), or gastroesophageal reflux (see Chapter 6). They are usually located on the lateral aspect of the posterior glottis, under which the arytenoid

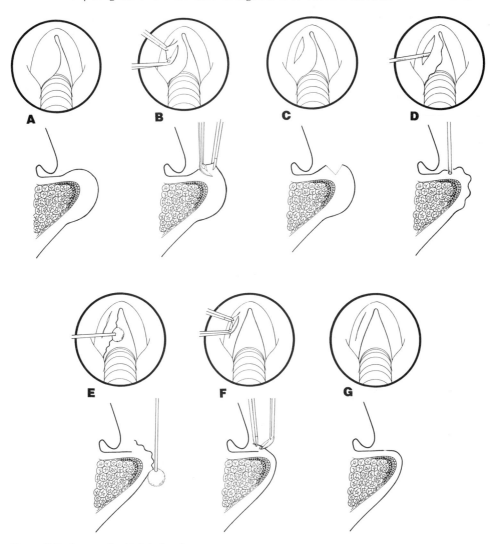

*Figure 8.3.* Surgery for Reinke's edema.

cartilage lies. Granulomas should first be treated with nonsurgical modalities, including vocal hygiene programs, and antireflux therapy. When nonsurgical modalities do not prove effective or the granulomas are very large, causing respiratory distress, they need to be treated surgically.

Surgery is best conducted under general anesthesia with Venturi ventilation. (Venturi ventilation is a technique where a fine jet of gas oxygen, nitrogen, or appropriate combination is directed into the trachea, replacing the usual endotracheal tube.) The major portion of the granuloma is first removed with the use of scissors and forceps, leaving the base (Fig. 8.5A and B). A laser is used to remove any material from the base (Fig. 8.5C and D). Care should be taken not to injure the arytenoid perichondrium.

## EPITHELIAL HYPERPLASIA AND DYSPLASIA

Cessation of smoking occasionally results in the disappearance of hyperplastic and dysplastic epithelium. Immediate surgery can be delayed with discontinuation of

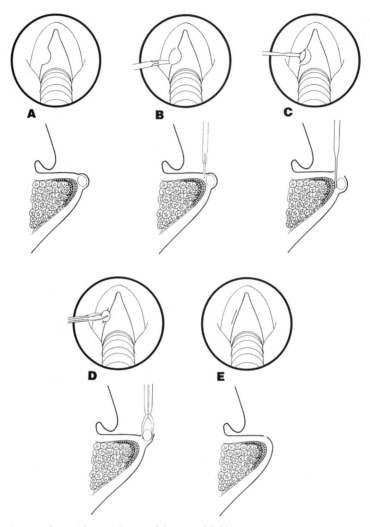

*Figure 8.4.* Surgery for epidermoid cyst of the vocal fold.

smoking and periodic follow-up. If surgery is undertaken, it should be followed by cessation of smoking.

The surgical procedure requires that a specimen be taken first for histological examination (Fig. 8.6B). Inclusion of the basement membrane in the specimen is essential for correct diagnosis. The remaining lesion is shaved using a $CO_2$ laser (Fig. 8.6C and D). This is continued until normal tissue of the Reinke's space is reached. Preoperative injection of local anesthetic with epinephrine into the Reinke's space makes it easier to perform a precise removal of pathologies. The specimen is serially sectioned perpendicular to the basement membrane and studied histologically. Clinically, it is occasionally difficult to differentiate very early carcinoma from hyperplasia and dysplasia. If the histological study reveals early invasive carcinoma, further laser surgery, as described later, or radiotherapy is indicated.

### BENIGN NEOPLASMS

The most frequent benign neoplasm of the larynx is papilloma. Hemangioma, fibroma, and other types of benign neoplasms are seen much less frequently. Most be-

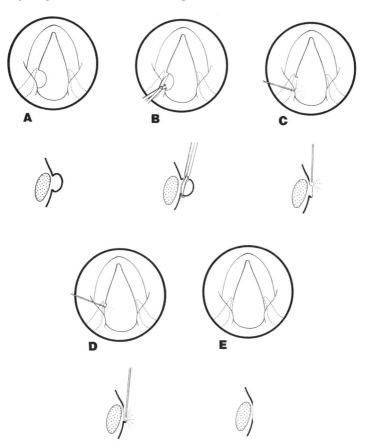

*Figure 8.5.* Surgery for granuloma.

nign neoplasms can be removed by means of a $CO_2$ laser although conventional microsurgical techniques are often routinely used (Fig. 8.7).

### GLOTTAL CARCINOMA

Glottal carcinoma confined to the membranous vocal fold (T1 classification) is a good candidate for laser excision. Treatment should be associated with discontinuation of smoking. The extent of the carcinomatous lesion is estimated by means of preoperative stroboscopy and Toluidine blue-staining under an operating microscope.

An excisional biopsy is conducted by means of a $CO_2$ laser (Fig. 8.8). A part of the thyroarytenoid muscle is frequently removed. The surgical specimen is subjected to a serial section study. When histological studies reveal that cancer cells are located close to the margins of the specimens, radiotherapy, or additional surgery is indicated.

## Surgical Correction of the Position, Shape, and/or Tension of the Vocal Fold

The surgical techniques in this group are used to medialize, lateralize, tense, or slacken the vocal fold, usually without direct surgical intervention to the vocal fold.

### VOCAL FOLD MEDIALIZATION

Two major groups of techniques are now in use to medialize the vocal fold edge: intrafold injection and medialization surgery.

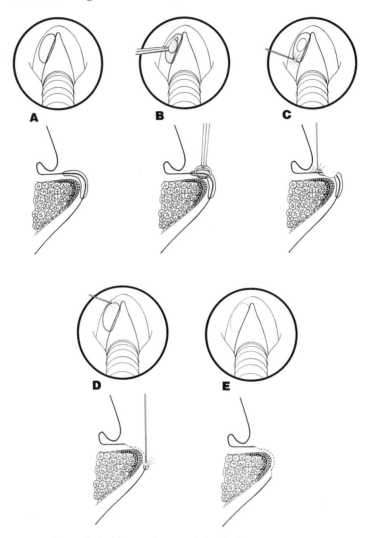

*Figure 8.6.* Surgery for epithelial hyperplasia and dysplasia.

### Intrafold Injection

Intrafold injection is indicated most frequently to correct an incompetent glottis (i.e., the inability to close the glottis resulting from unilateral vocal fold paralysis). It is occasionally performed to correct or fill in a glottal gap accompanied by sulcus vocalis, or one caused by trauma or surgery.

Four types of injection material have been used: Teflon, silicone, fat, and collagen. (Teflon is no longer available in the United States for this purpose.) There are three techniques for intrafold injection: transoral injection using an indirect laryngeal mirror (Fig. 8.9), transoral injection under a direct laryngoscope (Fig. 8.10), and transcutaneous injection through the cricothyroid space (Fig. 8.11).

When injection is conducted transorally using a laryngeal mirror, the mucosa of the pharynx and larynx is anesthetized with lidocaine solution. Injection is performed while the patient sits with the mouth open and the tongue pulled forward. A curved laryngeal needle is used to administer the substance into the fold, and its effect is monitored visually and auditorily as the injection proceeds.

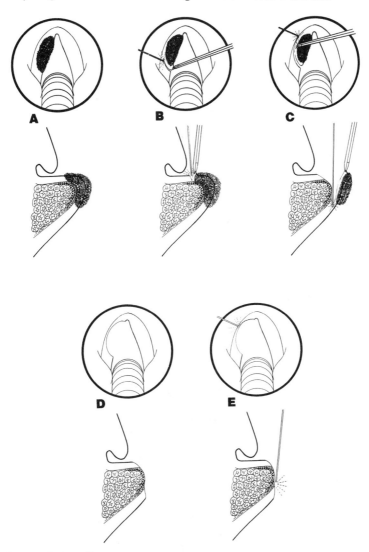

*Figure 8.7.* Surgery for papilloma.

Injection under a direct laryngoscope is performed with local mucosal anesthesia and/or neuroleptanalgesia without endotracheal intubation. (Neuroleptanalgesia is a technique in which the patient is administered a drug that effectively abolishes memory of the procedure.) The internal branches of the bilateral superior laryngeal nerves are also anesthetized. The patient is placed in a supine position. The larynx is exposed with the use of a direct laryngoscope and viewed under an operating microscope. Injection is performed by means of a specially designed injection set such as the Arnold-Beuening Teflon injection set, the Nagashima silicone injection set, or the Collagen Corporation set. The effect of the injection is monitored visually and auditorily. Injection under general anesthesia with endotracheal intubation is not recommended because the effect cannot be monitored during the procedure. It is employed only for those patients who cannot undergo the procedure using local anesthesia or neuroleptanalgesia.

For transcutaneous injection, the nasal, pharyngeal, and laryngeal mucosa is anesthetized with lidocaine. The patient assumes a supine position with the anterior neck stretched. A fiberscope is inserted through the nose down to the larynx. It is coupled

*Figure 8.8.* Surgery for early glottal carcinoma.

*Figure 8.9.* Technique for intrafold injection using an indirect laryngeal mirror.

to a video camera, and the fiberscopic image of the larynx is viewed on a television monitor screen. Local anesthesia is administered through the cervical skin at the cricothyroid space. The needle for intrafold injection is inserted into the larynx through the cricothyroid space. Its location is monitored by moving it back and forth medially as it proceeds. The effect of injection is monitored visually and auditorily during the procedure.

*Figure 8.10.* Intrafold injection under a direct laryngoscope.

Ventricular fold

Vocal fold

Thyroid cartilage

Injection material

Cricoid cartilage

Needle

C

*Figure 8.11.* Transcutaneous intrafold injection. **A,** An entire view during the procedure. **B,** A view of the patient's neck. **C,** Schematic presentation of the technique.

For unilateral vocal fold paralysis, Teflon or silicone is injected in the lateral portion of the thyroarytenoid muscle and/or in the space between the thyroid lamina and the thyroarytenoid muscle (Fig. 8.12). It must not be injected in or near the mucosa of the vocal fold (Fig. 8.12A). Intramucosal Teflon or silicone stiffens the mucosa, resulting in a marked disturbance of vibration and subsequent dysphonia. Collagen, however, may be injected near the mucosa because its consistency is close to that of mucosal tissue. Fat is injected in the thyroarytenoid muscle.

In patients with sulcus vocalis, Teflon, silicone, or fat is injected in the middle of the thyroarytenoid muscle. The effect of intrafold injection for sulcus vocalis is limited because injection does not correct the sulcus itself but only reduces the glottal gap.

### Medialization Surgery

There are many techniques to surgically medialize the vocal fold edge. They can be classified into three major types: (*a*) surgical augmentation, (*b*) medial shift of the thyroid cartilage, and (*c*) rotation of the arytenoid cartilage. Indications for the use of the first two techniques are basically the same as discussed for intrafold injection. The third type of medialization procedure is reserved almost exclusively for cases of unilateral vocal fold paralysis where there is a large posterior gap. It may also be used in conjunction with a thyroplasty (surgical augmentation).

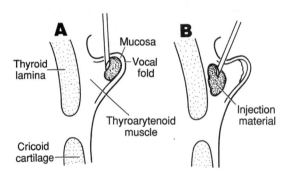

*Figure 8.12.* Location of the intrafold injection. **A,** Incorrect placement. **B,** Correct placement.

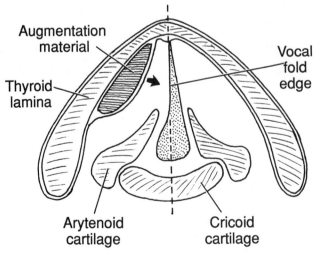

*Figure 8.13.* Schematic presentation of principle of surgical augmentation developed by Meurman (1952) and modified by others.

**Surgical Augmentation.** This procedure is often referred to as Thyroplasty Type I. The basic principle of augmentation is to insert the material to be used medial to the thyroid cartilage at the level of the vocal folds, thus pushing the vocal folds medially (Hiroto, 1976; Kleinsasser, 1987; Meurman, 1952; Sawashima, Totsuka, Kobayashi, & Hirose, 1968) (Fig. 8.13). A silicone block or autograft cartilage is commonly employed as the augmentation material. For a cartilage autograft, the upper part of the thyroid cartilage, nasal septum cartilage, or rib cartilage is used.

The surgery is performed under local anesthesia. A horizontal skin incision is made in the midportion of the anterior neck, and the thyroid cartilage is exposed on the paralytic side. The site of the augmentation implant can be reached with several different techniques (Fig. 8.14). In Figure 8.14A, a perichondrium incision is made along the superior edge of the thyroid cartilage whereas in Figure 8.14B a cartilage incision is made along the midline. In Figure 8.14C the site is reached via an anteroinferior approach by removing the medioinferior portion of the thyroid cartilage. In Figure 8.14D a block of cartilage is removed from the thyroid in order to reach the site for material implantation.

The augmentation material is located lateral to the vocal fold. The upper surface of the vocal fold is normally situated at the midlevel of the anterior angle of the thyroid cartilage. The posterior end of the membranous vocal fold is usually located at the anteroposterior midpoint of the thyroid lamina. Therefore, the augmentation material should be placed in the lower and anterior quadrant of the thyroid lamina. The size and location of the material are adjusted by auditorily monitoring the patient's voice during the procedure. Simultaneous visual monitoring with the use of a fiberscope is also useful. Once the material is located in the right place, it is sutured to the thyroid cartilage in order to prevent postsurgical migration.

**Medial Shift of the Thyroid Cartilage.** The basic principle of this technique is to medialize part of the thyroid cartilage at the level of the vocal fold, pushing the vocal fold edge to the midline (Beck & Richstein, 1982; Isshiki, 1977; Koufman, 1986) (Fig. 8.15)

The surgery is conducted under local anesthesia. Following exposure of the thyroid lamina, a quadrangular cartilage specimen to be medialized is designed, as shown in Figure 8.16A. The upper edge is placed horizontally at the midlevel of the anterior angle of the thyroid lamina. The lower edge is located parallel to the upper edge but at a distance that is one-quarter the height of the anterior thyroid lamina.

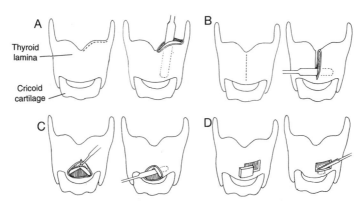

*Figure 8.14.* Approaches to site of implant. **A,** Superior approach. **B,** Anterior approach. **C,** Anteroinferior approach. **D,** Window technique.

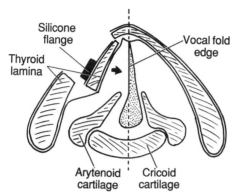

*Figure 8.15.* Schematic presentation of the principle of medial shift of thyroid cartilage, developed by Payr and modified by others.

*Figure 8.16.* **A,** Design of cartilage specimen to be medialized. **B,** Stabilization of the shifted specimen with the use of a silicone flange developed by Isshiki and modified by others.

The anterior edge is positioned 5 mm from the anterior angle, and the posterior edge is located slightly posterior to the anteroposterior midpoint of the thyroid lamina.

The quadrangle is cut through the cartilage and shifted medially. The best location of the medialized specimen is determined by auditory monitoring of the voice. A combination of visual monitoring using a fiberscope and auditory monitoring is useful. The medialized segment is then fixed into place by placing a silicone flange through the window (Fig. 8.16B).

**Rotation of Arytenoid Cartilage (Arytenoid Adduction).** The basic principle of this technique is to rotate the arytenoid cartilage by traction of the muscular process in the direction of the adductor muscles, adducting the tip of the vocal process to the midline (Furukawa, 1967; Isshiki, 1977) (Fig. 8.17).

The surgery is conducted under local anesthesia. Following a horizontal cervical skin incision, the posterior edge of the thyroid lamina is exposed on the affected side by sectioning the thyropharyngeal muscle. The cricothyroid joint is dislocated, and the thyroid edge is retracted anteromedially. A quadrangular window is made at the posterior portion of the thyroid lamina by cutting the cartilage (Fig 8.17B, C). The muscular process of the arytenoid cartilage is then exposed. It is pulled anteromedioinferiorly with a nylon thread, while the patient phonates. When the best voice is obtained, the thread is sutured to the thyroid cartilage. Medialization of the vocal process can also be monitored visually by means of a fiberscope.

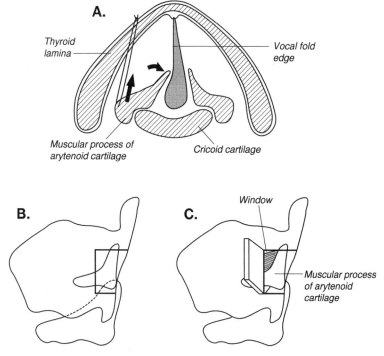

**A.**

Thyroid lamina

Vocal fold edge

Muscular process of arytenoid cartilage

Cricoid cartilage

**B.**

**C.**

Window

Muscular process of arytenoid cartilage

*Figure 8.17.* Schematic presentation of the principle of rotation of the arytenoid cartilage, as developed by Isshiki.

## VOCAL FOLD LATERALIZATION

Vocal fold lateralization is indicated in the treatment of bilateral vocal fold paralysis and in bilateral ankylosis of the cricoarytenoid joints when the vocal folds are located at or near the midline, causing dyspnea. Its purpose is to improve not the voice but the airway. It usually makes the voice worse, to a greater or lesser extent. However, when conservation of voice is part of the surgical plan, a phonosurgical approach can often help to minimize effects on the voice.

There are two major types of techniques to lateralize the vocal fold: laterofixation of the vocal fold and arytenoidectomy.

### Laterofixation of the Vocal Fold

The basic principle of laterofixation is to displace the vocal process of the arytenoid cartilage laterally, thereby widening the glottis (Fig. 8.18).

Patients requiring this surgery have usually undergone tracheostomy for relief of dyspnea. An endotracheal tube is inserted through the tracheostoma, and general anesthesia is given. Following skin incision, the arytenoid cartilage is exposed, using the same technique as that for rotation of the arytenoid cartilage. The arytenoid cartilage is dislocated from the cricoarytenoid joint, and its major portion is removed, leaving only the vocal process. The vocal process is pulled laterally with a nylon thread. The effect of lateralization is monitored with the use of a fiberscope. When the glottis is sufficiently opened, the thread is sutured to the thyroid cartilage.

### Arytenoidectomy

The basic principle of arytenoidectomy is to remove the arytenoid cartilage, thereby widening the posterior glottis (Fig. 8.19). The posterior glottis, or the

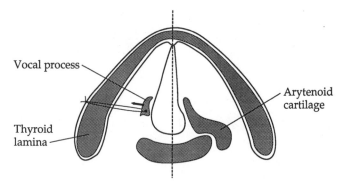

*Figure 8.18.* Schematic presentation of the principle of laterofixation of the vocal folds.

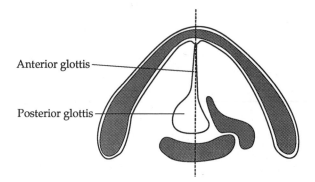

*Figure 8.19.* Schematic presentation of the principle of arytenoidectomy.

*Figure 8.20.* Schematic presentation of the principle of cricothyroid approximation, as developed by Isshiki.

intercartilaginous portion of the glottis, accounts for approximately 60% of the entire glottal area (Hirano, Kurita, Kyokawa, & Sato, 1986). Therefore, a widening of the posterior glottis is very effective in improving the adequacy of the airway. The anterior glottis is widened to a much lesser extent by arytenoidectomy than the posterior glottis. This is helpful in preserving the best possible voice.

The surgery is conducted with the use of endolaryngeal microsurgery technique under general anesthesia. The $CO_2$ laser is very useful in this procedure because its use minimizes bleeding. The entire arytenoid cartilage is removed, along with the posterior macula flava and the posterior end of the thyroarytenoid muscle.

Thyroid
cartilage

Tantalum
shim

Cricoid
cartilage

*Figure 8.21.* Schematic presentation of the principle of anterior commissure advancement, as developed by LeJeune, Guice, and Samuels (1983) and Tucker (1985).

## Vocal Fold Tensing Surgery

The major purpose of vocal fold tensing surgery is to raise the vocal pitch. Indications for such surgery may include (*a*) excessively low pitch in females caused by a protein anabolic steroid or an androgen, or by pregnancy; (*b*) the low vocal pitch of the "sex-transferred" female; and (*c*) senile, flaccid vocal folds. Surgical techniques to tense the vocal folds have been developed during the past decade by Isshiki (1977), LeJeune, Guice, and Samuels (1983) and Tucker (1985). Data regarding the long-term functional results of vocal fold tensing are not yet available. There are two major surgical techniques to accomplish vocal fold tensing: cricothyroid approximation and anterior commissure advancement.

### CRICOTHYROID APPROXIMATION

The basic principle of cricothyroid approximation is to create a permanent approximation of the cricoid arch to the thyroid cartilage anteriorly, simulating the function of the cricothyroid muscle (Isshiki, 1977) (Fig. 8.20). Recall that contraction of the cricothyroid muscle results in the approximation of the cartilages and that in so doing the vocal folds are lengthened and tensed. Both the decreased mass of the folds and the increased tension under which they are held result in a faster vibratory rate, and thus a higher pitch is produced.

The surgery is best conducted under local anesthesia so that the pitch of the voice can be monitored during the procedure. However, if the patient is unable to tolerate the procedure, general anesthesia is given. Following horizontal cervical skin incision, the thyroid and cricoid cartilages are exposed. They are approximated anteriorly by means of nylon sutures (Fig. 8.20). Stretching of the vocal fold can be visually monitored with the use of a fiberscope.

### ANTERIOR COMMISSURE ADVANCEMENT

The basic principle of anterior commissure advancement is to stretch the vocal folds by advancing the anterior commissure anteriorly relative to the arytenoid cartilages (LeJeune, Guice, & Samuels, 1983; Tucker, 1985).

The surgery may best be performed under local anesthesia, but general anesthesia is employed when the patient cannot tolerate the procedure. Following a horizontal cervical skin incision, the thyroid cartilage is exposed. A vertical cartilage flap is made in the midportion of the thyroid cartilage. The flap may be inferiorly based, superiorly based, or sectioned both superiorly and inferiorly. The flap is advanced anteriorly and stabilized in place by inserting a shim of tantalum posterior to the flap (Fig. 8.21).

When local anesthesia is employed, changes in vocal pitch are auditorily monitored during surgery. Vocal fold stretching can be visually monitored by means of a fiber-scope.

## Vocal Fold Slackening Surgery

The major purpose of vocal fold slackening surgery is to reduce the tension of the vocal folds (Isshiki, 1977). This is the reverse of the vocal fold tensing procedure described above. The indications for this procedure are not yet well established, and its use is in the experimental stage.

In order to slacken the vocal folds, it is necessary to move the anterior commissure closer to the arytenoid cartilage. The surgery may best be performed under local anesthesia because auditory monitoring of voice change is available during surgery. When the patient cannot tolerate the procedure, general anesthesia may be used. The thyroid cartilage is exposed in the same way as for anterior commissure advancement. A vertical cartilage flap is made in the midportion of the thyroid cartilage and pushed back (Fig. 8.22).

## Surgery for Sulcus Vocalis

There are no existing surgical techniques for sulcus vocalis which assure a recovery of normal voice. Some techniques have been reported to improve the voice to some extent in some patients but these techniques are unable to recover normal voice.

### SULCUSECTOMY

Sulcusectomy (Hirano, 1975), is conducted with the endolaryngeal microsurgery technique under general anesthesia. A mucosal incision is made along the upper edge of the sulcus. The stiff tissue around the sulcus is elevated from the underlying normal tissue and removed (Figure 8.23). The mucosa superior and inferior to the surgical wound is approximated as far as possible and held in place by means of fibrin glue.

Woo and his colleagues (1995) reported on endoscopic microsuture repair of various vocal fold defects such as sulcus vocalis, and various other vocal fold defects such as severe polypoid degeneration, fusiform polyps, cysts, and keratosis. Following appropriate surgical excision of the lesion, a fine microsuture is placed to aid in closure of the defect and to provide secure mechanical coupling of the mucosa as healing progresses. Whereas 12 of the vocal folds in the patients studied exhibited an adynamic

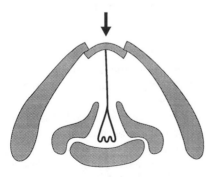

*Figure 8.22.* Schematic presentation of the principle of anterior commissure pushback, as developed by Isshiki.

segment preoperatively, this was seen in only one vocal fold following surgery in which a microsuture was placed. It would appear that this surgical procedure, when used with the appropriate patient, can be successful in restoring normal vibratory function.

### SLICING MUCOSA TECHNIQUE

Another surgical technique described by Pontes, Mara, and Oscar (1989) is a mucosal slicing technique. This surgery is performed under general anesthesia by means of endolaryngeal microsurgery technique. Following mucosal incision superior to the sulcus, the superficial layer of the lamina propria around the sulcus is elevated from the vocal ligament. The elevated mucosa is vertically sectioned or sliced at several locations and placed back on the ligament (Figure 8.24).

### INTRAFOLD INJECTION AND MEDIALIZATION SURGERY

Intrafold injection and medialization surgery are procedures sometimes used with patients with sulcus vocalis and were discussed earlier in this chapter under "Vocal Fold Medialization."

## Surgery to Alter Laryngeal Neuromuscular Function

### NEUROMUSCULAR SURGERY FOR VOCAL FOLD PARALYSIS

The ideal treatment for vocal fold paralysis would be to restore normal innervation of all laryngeal muscles. This is, however, not possible in cases of axonotmesis and neurotmesis. That the recurrent laryngeal nerve contains both adductor and

*Figure 8.23.* Histological picture of sulcus vocalis.

*Figure 8.24.* Schematic of direct vocal fold mucosa surgery. **A,** vocal fold frontal view. **B,** vocal fold medial view. **Panel 1,** schematic of sulcus vocalis (SV). **Panel 2,** cranial incision (CI). **Panel 3,** detachment of the mucosa (DM). **Panel 4,** positioning of the mucosa slices (PMS).

abductor fibers creates one of the major problems in the neurosurgical treatment of vocal fold paralysis. Simple nerve anastomosis or nerve graft of the recurrent laryngeal nerve causes misdirected reinnervation, as shown in Figure 8.25. Some neurons that originally innervated one of the adductor muscles now may innervate the abductor muscles, while some neurons that were originally for abductor innervation now act to innervate the adductor muscles, causing a disturbance in vocal fold mobility (Hiroto, Hirano, & Tomita, 1968; Siribodhi, Sundmaker, Atkins, & Bonner, 1963).

Many experimental and clinical attempts have been made to avoid the problems resulting from misdirection of regenerated nerve fibers. Some of them will be described in the following paragraphs.

The procedures that are most frequently in use employ a nerve-muscle pedicle (Fig. 8.26) obtained from the ansa hypoglossi nerve that innervates the omohyoid, sternothyroid, and sternohyoid muscles (Tucker, 1978; Tucker & Rusnov, 1981). One of the muscles (along with its nerve) is chosen as the donor. In cases of bilateral abductor paralysis in which the vocal folds are fixed near the midline, causing dyspnea, the nerve-muscle pedicle is implanted into the posterior cricoarytenoid (PCA) muscle, whose primary function is to abduct the vocal folds. For unilateral paralysis, the nerve-muscle pedicle is implanted into the lateral cricoarytenoid (LCA) muscle. This surgery has had limited success.

Other surgical approaches for bilateral paralysis have been reported and include anastomosis of the split phrenic nerve to the PCA or to the nerve branch innervating the PCA (Crumley, 1983) and anastomosis of the split vagus nerve to the nerve branch of the PCA (Miehlke & Arnold, 1982).

## RECURRENT LARYNGEAL NERVE SECTION
## FOR SPASMODIC DYSPHONIA

Since 1976 when Dedo first reported unilateral section of the recurrent laryngeal nerve (RLN) for spasmodic dysphonia (Dedo, 1976), the procedure and its various modifications have been carried out by many laryngologists. The immediate postsurgical results have been reported to be highly successful and appreciated by many patients (Barton, 1979; Dedo, 1976; Dedo & Izdebski, 1981; Wilson, Oldring, & Mueller, 1980) but the long-term results appear to be conflicting (Aronson &

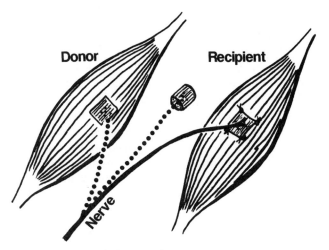

*Figure 8.25.* Schematic presentation of misdirected reinnervation in the recurrent laryngeal nerve.

*Figure 8.26.* Nerve-muscle pedicle procedure.

DeSanto, 1981, 1983; Chevrie-Muller, Arabia-Guidet, & Pfauwadel, 1987; Fritzell, Feuer, Haglund, Knutsson, & Schiratzki, 1982; Wilson, Oldring, & Mueller, 1980). While some surgeons continue to perform the procedure, others have abandoned it due to the too frequent return of symptoms in time despite continued paralysis of the vocal fold caused by the sectioning procedure. Furthermore, the effectiveness of BoTox injection has provided a treatment modality, albeit temporary in effectiveness, which spares the recurrent laryngeal nerve (see discussion later in this chapter under "Medical Management."

## *Surgical Reconstruction for Partial Loss and/or Deformity of the Larynx*

### OVERVIEW

The surgical procedures that fall into this category vary vastly. They can be classified into four major groups: (*a*) surgical reconstruction following partial laryngectomy, (*b*) surgical repair for trauma of the larynx, (*c*) surgery for cicatricial stenosis of the larynx, and (*d*) surgery for congenital deformities of the larynx. Many of the patients who require surgical reconstruction exhibit problems in breathing and/or swallowing, as well as voice disorders. All of these problems must be taken into consideration when surgical treatment is undertaken. It is therefore imperative that phonosurgeons have a thorough understanding of the physiology and pathophysiology of breathing and swallowing, as well as of phonation.

Because the focus of this book is on phonation, the only specific condition to be addressed in this section will be phonosurgery for anterior glottal web, where voice is the major concern.

ANTERIOR GLOTTAL WEB

Anterior glottal web forms as a congenital malformation or is caused by trauma, including surgical trauma. There are two major surgical techniques for its removal: endolaryngeal surgery and surgery under thyrotomy.

### Endolaryngeal Surgery

Thin and/or small webs are successfully treated with the endolaryngeal approach. The surgery is conducted under general anesthesia. The vocal folds are exposed under a direct laryngoscope and viewed with an operating microscope. The web is sectioned at the midline or partly removed. A $CO_2$ laser is useful for this purpose (Fig. 8.27A). After removal of the web, a silicone plate is placed in the glottis to prevent postsurgical reunion of the vocal folds. To do this, a tiny horizontal skin incision is first made in front of the thyroid cartilage. A hypodermic needle threaded with a piece of nylon thread is inserted through the incision into the laryngeal cavity, above the thyroid cartilage (Fig. 8.27B). The nylon thread is pulled out of the patient's mouth through the laryngoscope. A second piece of nylon thread is inserted in the same way but below the thyroid cartilage and is pulled out through the laryngoscope. The two pieces of nylon thread are sutured to a silicone plate at the outside of the mouth (Fig. 8.27C). The silicone plate is placed in the glottis through the laryngoscope as the two pieces of nylon thread are pulled through the skin incision. The nylon thread is sutured in front of the thyroid cartilage (Fig. 8.27D). The skin incision is closed. A schematic su-

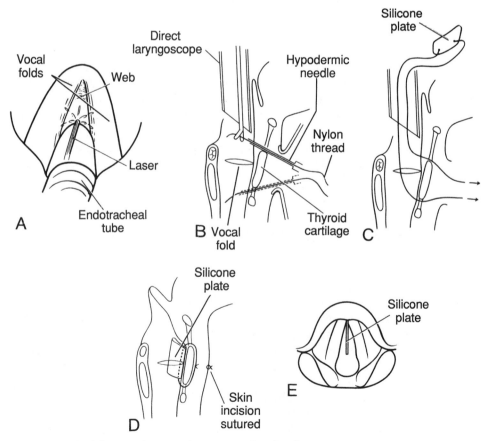

*Figure 8.27.* Endolaryngeal surgery for anterior glottal web.

perior view of the glottis immediately after surgery is shown in Figure 8.27E. The silicone plate is removed endolaryngeally 2–4 weeks after surgery.

### *Thyrotomy*

Surgery under thyrotomy is indicated for thick and extensive webs. The surgery is usually conducted under general anesthesia. Following a vertical or horizontal cervical skin incision, the thyroid cartilage is exposed and sectioned vertically at the midline. When marked scar tissue exists in the web, it is carefully removed; the covering epithelium is preserved. The wound at the sectioned web is sutured and closed (Fig. 8.28). The larynx and the wound are closed in layers.

## *Evaluation of Results of Surgery*

Results of surgical treatments are evaluated both subjectively and objectively by means of varying techniques described in Chapter 7. Some examples are shown in Figures 8.29–8.33. The effects of surgical corrections for glottic incompetence are best manifested in an increase in maximum phonation time and a decrease in airflow during phonation (Figs. 8.29 and 8.30). Improvements of voice quality related to hoarseness are objectively demonstrated in a decrease in pitch perturbation, amplitude perturbation, and noise energy of the voice signal as well as increased intensity of phonation (Figs. 8.31–8.33).

## MEDICAL MANAGEMENT

### *Edema, Inflammation, Irritation of the Vocal Folds*

Through differential diagnostic examination, acute laryngeal problems in which the vocal folds and laryngeal structures demonstrate redness, swelling, or the appearance of irritation may be determined to be the result of infection, allergy, drainage from the nose, reaction to noxious agents, gastroesophageal reflux, or directly related to recent episodes of abuse. Clearly, the diagnosis will determine the treatment. In the presence of infection, the use of antibiotic drugs is common and should be accompanied by a reduction in voice usage for the period of time that the acute symptoms are present. When an allergic reaction appears to be the cause of the tissue changes that are being

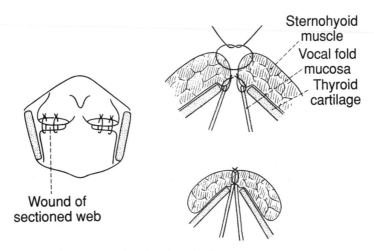

*Figure 8.28.* Surgery for anterior glottal web under thyrotomy.

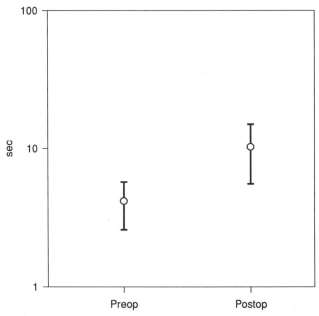

*Figure 8.29.* Preoperative and postoperative values (mean and standard deviation) of the maximum phonation time (in seconds) in 219 patients with unilateral vocal fold paralysis treated with transcutaneous intrafold silicone injection.

mirrored in the voice, it is important to determine the source of that reaction. Elimination or avoidance of the allergenic agents or desensitization of the body's reaction should restore the tissues to a healthy condition and eliminate the voice problem. Both the identification of and treatment for allergies can, of course, be a rather long process. As long as the vocal folds appear to be edematous or inflamed, the voice must be used sparingly in both amount and loudness dimensions. Some detective work might be involved in determining whether exposure to noxious agents is responsible for the observed irritation of the mucosa.

It is well recognized that the smoke of tobacco or illegal inhaled substances is irritating to laryngeal mucosa. The obvious treatment is cessation of the behavior. Because physical addiction may be involved, the person's ability to abandon the habit may be very limited. Many patients need much support, encouragement, and special assistance through a variety of treatment programs in order to stop smoking or using drugs. The doctor's recommendation, although carrying much weight, is often insufficient and should be followed with concrete offers of help or specific referral to sources of such help.

It is now recognized that a nonsmoker's exposure to tobacco smoke may be sufficient to cause eye, nose, throat, and respiratory tract irritation (U.S. Department of Health and Human Services, 1986) and indeed, increase the risk of cancer. Professional voice users, singers and actors in particular, may often find it necessary to perform in environments heavy with tobacco smoke. There are no known antidotes to the irritant effects of tobacco smoke, but other methods of relieving irritation may be attempted. However, it must be made clear to the patient that continued use of the voice in the presence of edematous or inflamed vocal folds creates increased risk for further and perhaps more lasting damage to the tissues and the voice. Passive smoking (involuntary exposure to cigarette smoke) may also take place in the home and the workplace. Recognition of this effect may lead to appropriate environmental adjustments.

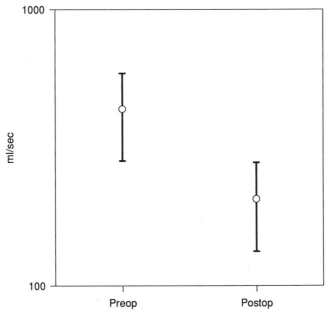

*Figure 8.30.* Preoperative and postoperative values (mean and standard deviation) of the mean airflow rate during phonation with a comfortable duration (in ml/sec) in 219 patients with unilateral vocal fold paralysis treated with transcutaneous intrafold silicone injection.

It is also possible that a person may have experienced exposure to other noxious agents. Relief from such exposure should result in resolution of the irritation, although there is not a great deal of information about such effects. Inhalation of certain gases can result in burns of and trauma to the mucosa of the respiratory tract (see Chapter 6).

Another environmental factor that may have an irritating effect on laryngeal mucosa is very dry air. Both heating and cooling systems in houses, public buildings, and airplanes often provide insufficient humidification. Breathing this air may result in dehydration of the vocal folds, increasing their stiffness and disrupting normal vibratory behavior (Brewer, Brodnitz, Gould, et al., 1979). The obvious treatment for this situation consists of environmental manipulation, increasing the humidification of the air, rather than direct treatment of the condition itself. In the case of airplane travel, it is especially important for the professional voice user to be counseled against use of the voice in performance too soon after extensive flights.

The suspicion of gastroesophageal reflux as the etiology of mucosal irritation is raised when that irritation most obviously affects the posterior portions of the larynx, when the history reveals that the voice symptoms are at their worst first thing in the morning, and when the symptoms include an acidic taste in the mouth, heartburn, frequent burping, and the like. Patients with this condition should receive a thorough work-up. Treatment will include a combination of environmental adjustments, such as elevation of the head of the bed at least 6 inches (not the use of additional pillows) and dietary constraints. The latter includes the admonition to avoid spicy foods (especially before retiring), alcohol, coffee, tea, cola drinks, and tobacco. Antacids in liquid form (Gelusil, Maalox, or similar antacids) can be used 30-40 minutes after meals and before bedtime. Other pharmacological management may consist of use of the drugs ranitidine hydrochloride (Zantac), omeprazole (Prilosec) or cisapride (Propulsid).

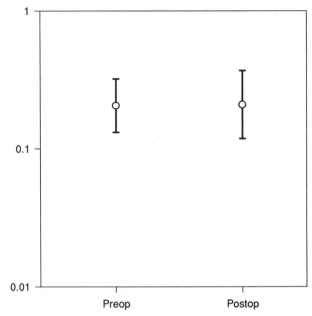

*Figure 8.31.* Preoperative and postoperative values (mean and standard deviation) of the pitch perturbation quotient in 52 patients with vocal fold polyp treated with endolaryngeal microsurgery.

Some upper respiratory infections result in vigorous coughing and excessively thick mucus while some patients present with a dry, unproductive cough. Demulcents coat the irritated or dry membranes, soothing them (Harris, 1992). Sedation may also relieve coughing and can be achieved by using antitussives. There are two major groups of antitussives: opiate-based antitussives and antihistamine suppressants. Although these drugs may be effective in controlling the cough, both kinds tend to dry the mucosa producing an undesirable condition for voice production.

Excessively thick mucus may also affect voice production and incline the patient to frequent throat clearing. Increased water intake and improved humidification of the environment may be effective. Guaifenesin, the active ingredient in drugs such as Humibid, Robitussin, and Tussin may be helpful in reducing the viscosity of secretions. It loosens phlegm and mucus in the lungs and helps to relieve a dry, nonproductive cough.

Allergies may affect the membranes of the respiratory tract including the vocal folds. Excessive histamine production results in constriction of the bronchial smooth muscle, mucosal edema, and excessive mucus. Antihistamines and bronchodilators are used to treat these conditions. Insomnia, nervousness, and tremor may be a undesirable side effects of these drugs (Harris, 1992). Inflammation of the vocal folds may be treated using glucocorticoid steroids. However, use of these drugs should be limited to short term as continued use may produce undesirable side effects.

Drugs may also be used to control vagal effects resulting from "stage fright" or jitters prior to a performance. Beta blockers are occasionally used to help the performer in these specific situations. Harris (1992) believes that there is little benefit of these drugs to most vocal performers and likens their use to the ingestion of alcohol prior to a performance. Their use is not recommended. Anabolic steroids, sometimes used by athletes to enhance performance, may be used by vocal performers for the same purpose. Such usage could result in damage to the liver and cardiovascular

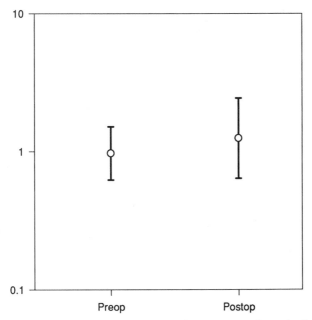

*Figure 8.32.* Preoperative and postoperative values (mean and standard deviation) of the amplitude perturbation quotient in 52 patients with vocal fold polyp treated with endolaryngeal microsurgery.

system as well as producing psychological changes. There is no place for their use in those who depend on their voice for their livelihood.

## Chronic Changes

Conditions that result in chronic changes in laryngeal tissue frequently require combined treatment protocols. In many instances, surgical intervention may be necessary, followed by a period of voice therapy. Other situations call for medical management through drugs and environmental changes, perhaps combined with voice therapy. And for some, a trial course of voice therapy may be the first treatment option, to be followed by other courses of treatment only if necessary. Patients with chronic changes of laryngeal tissue must be monitored closely, often for many years.

## Neurological Conditions

### SPASMODIC DYSPHONIA

Because we believe spasmodic dysphonia to be a type of dystonia of neurological origin, and because its treatment is primarily medical (BoTox injection), it seems most appropriate that the discussion of its treatment be in this section. In the discussion of surgical interventions earlier in this chapter we reported on severing the recurrent laryngeal nerve as an approach to the treatment of spasmodic dysphonia. A small percentage of patients who have been treated surgically have indeed had long-lasting success, although a large number have experienced recurrence of symptoms. Resection of the recurrent laryngeal nerve is a technique that is still being used by a few otolaryngologists.

Traditional behavioral voice therapy is also being used to treat spasmodic dysphonia by a few clinicians but scarce substantiating efficacy data exist. Differentiating

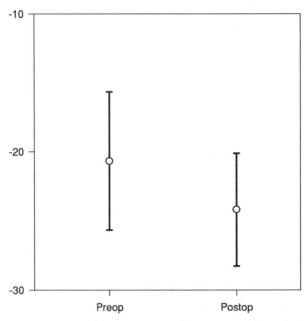

*Figure 8.33.* Preoperative and postoperative values (mean and standard deviation) of the normalized noise energy in the frequency range 0 to 4 kHz in 52 patients with vocal fold polyp treated with endolaryngeal microsurgery.

spasmodic dysphonia from muscular tension dysphonia or psychogenic dysphonia becomes exceedingly critical when determining treatment choices. Often a course of voice therapy should be undertaken as a diagnostic tool. (For additional information about voice therapy for spasmodic dysphonia, see Chapter 9.)

Injection of minute quantities of botulinum toxin into muscles produces a temporary weakening or paralysis of the muscle through denervation. New sprouting of motor nerve bundles results in gradual dissipation of the effect and the recurrence of symptoms. Thus, BoTox injection (one name given to the injectable toxin) is a treatment, but not a cure. Injections are performed percutaneously via a hypodermic needle that is connected to an EMG unit for auditory feedback of muscle activity, which confirms correct needle placement. Some otolaryngologists perform the injection transorally.

The typical post-treatment course of a successful injection is a 3–7 day period of weak and breathy speech that may not become apparent until several days after the injection. The voice gradually strengthens and is without spasmodic disruptions. The patient usually reports increased ease of talking, increased intelligibility, and a release from the strain of phonation. This period of good voice may last for weeks or months with gradual return of the spasmodic symptoms. Patients are urged to return for another injection before the symptoms return to their former severity level.

For adductor spasmodic dysphonia, the BoTox is injected into the thyroarytenoid muscle. Although injections can be given unilaterally or bilaterally, the latter approach is more commonly used. Ludlow (1995) suggests that bilateral injections be given in dosages of 2.5 units/side and in a single location, whereas 5.0 units be given in each of three locations (total of 15 units) for unilateral injections. Typically, patients require reinjection every 3–6 months, although we have known some patients who have experienced longer periods of vocal relief.

Treatment of patients with abductor spasmodic dysphonia with BoTox injection is much more difficult. There are reports of the BoTox being injected into the posterior cricoarytenoid muscle (Blitzer, Brin, Stewart, Aviv, & Fahn, 1992; Rontal, Rontal, Rolnick, Merson, Silverman, & Truong, 1991) or into the cricothyroid muscle (Ludlow, Naunton, Terada, & Anderson, 1991). Technically, the injection into the posterior cricoarytenoid muscle is much more difficult than into the thyroarytenoid muscle. The success of BoTox injection in cases of abductor spasmodic dysphonia is not as predictable as with the adductor type.

Inter-treatment predictability, dosage, placements of injections, and patient selection are still areas in need of greater documentation and research. We have found that locating the appropriate site for injection becomes more difficult in patients who have had numerous previous injections. This may be from the scarring and fibrosis of repeated needle insertions. Patients with multiple dystonias affecting the head and neck may experience less than optimal response to laryngeal injection alone. When tremor is present in addition to the spasmodic symptoms, the response to BoTox injection may also be limited. If tremor alone is present, this treatment is usually not recommended. The apparent long-term effects of BoTox injections are minimal but one must remember that the treatment is still relatively new and thus does not have a history of more than 8–10 years of use.

## OTHER NEUROLOGICAL DISEASES

Pharmacological management is sometimes available for the relief or control of symptoms in certain neurological disturbances. For example, pyridostigmine (Mestinon) is used to control the symptoms of muscle weakness in myasthenia gravis (Ravits, 1988). Levodopa (Larodopa or Dopar) or carbidopa-levodopa (Sinemet, Aldomet) is used in the management of Parkinson's disease (Merritt, 1979). These drugs have beneficial effects in reducing some of the abnormal characteristics of the disease (Larson, Ramig, & Scherer, 1994), but they have not been found to improve the voice and speech. There are numerous other drugs used in similar ways in the treatment of the many progressively debilitating neurological diseases, but their effects on voice and speech have not been well studied.

## SUMMARY

In the first section of this chapter, a review of phonosurgical techniques currently in use for the treatment of voice problems was presented. Phonosurgical techniques are divided into four categories: (*a*) removal of pathological tissue; (*b*) correction of the position, shape, and/or tension of the vocal folds; (*c*) surgery to restore laryngeal neuromuscular function; and (*d*) reconstruction for a partial loss or deformity of the larynx. A brief description of the techniques currently used by otolaryngologists was given in order to aid the reader in understanding the advantages and disadvantages of the techniques.

In the second section of this chapter, some of the techniques used in the medical management of voice problems were reviewed. Many of these techniques involve the use of drugs for the relief of symptoms, as well as for treating the original cause(s) of the voice problem. Allergies are often implicated as a cause of voice problems. Other medical techniques include counseling and simple behavioral modification techniques to encourage the patient to change habits (smoking, drinking), lifestyle, or the environment.

# Chapter 9

# Vocal Rehabilitation

## GOAL OF VOICE THERAPY

The specific goal of voice therapy will vary from patient to patient. Nevertheless, in general, the goal of voice therapy is to restore the best voice possible, a voice that will be functional for purposes of employment and general communication. The patient must be the final arbiter of what constitutes acceptable voice. However, it is important for both the patient and the clinician to recognize that restoring voice to the way it previously sounded or to some idealized goal may not be possible. When irreversible alterations have occurred in laryngeal structure or physiology, the voice may never return to what it once had been. This realization is particularly traumatic for persons who have relied heavily on their vocal skills for their livelihood or as their primary source of pleasure.

## CONCEPT OF NORMAL VOICE

An accepted definition of normal voice does not exist. There are no established standards, and no boundaries of accepted norms have been set. Attempting to set such standards might be likened to defining what constitutes normal appearance. Voice, like appearance, comes in so many varieties. Cultural, environmental, and individual factors contribute to the determination of what is designated normal. And voice, again like appearance, does not remain constant. It changes throughout the lifespan; it changes in reaction to emotion; it changes in response to environment; it reflects the state of health of the body and of the mind. It would be extremely difficult, if not impossible, to have a single definition that would encompass all of the ways that a normal voice can sound. Normal is not a single state but rather exists on a continuum.

Some normative data have been gathered about specific acoustic vocal parameters (see Chapter 13). Usually these data provide ranges within which voices that have been judged as normal have been found to fall. Often even these data are suspect, since investigators remind us that both intra- and intersubject variability may be very large (Kent, Kent, & Rosenbek, 1987). It is perhaps easier to attempt to define the abnormal. The voice that is so reduced in volume that normal-hearing listeners have difficulty hearing it is abnormal. The voice that is so different in pitch level as to be incongruent with the age or sex of the speaker may be judged to be abnormal. The voice that lacks the flexibility to alter pitch or loudness or that has a quality that calls attention to itself in an unpleasant manner or that is so loud that we are aware of it whether we choose to be or not suggests something outside our internalized norms.

The lack of a definition of normal voice creates problems in setting therapeutic goals and in describing abnormality and its degree of severity. There is no complete and objective template against which to measure and compare it. This is one of the major obstacles in clinical research confounding collection of objective, quantifiable data. If a voice improves, how can we measure that improvement? What can we compare it to? Which of the vocal attributes have contributed to its improvement? How much better is it? Is it normal? Is it normal for that patient?

This last question raises another aspect of the concept of normalcy of voice; that is, how did a particular patient's voice sound before it became disordered? It is usually the case that the only voice known to the clinician and available for any measurement is the disordered voice. This can create problems if at a given point during therapy the clinician judges a patient's voice to be quite acceptable but the patient continues to be unhappy, claiming it is different from the remembered normal voice. Or the opposite may occur if the clinician continues to seek a better voice when the patient reports that the voice being produced sounds right and normal.

## THE UNDERLYING BASES OF VOCAL REHABILITATION

Voice therapy must be rooted in and derived from an understanding of laryngeal anatomy and phonatory physiology. It is necessary to understand what is wrong in order to know how to fix it. When there is a hole in a bucket, it is important to understand the effect of that hole, not only to know that the hole is there. That understanding may lead to more than a single approach to fixing the problem. And it may be very important to understand how the hole developed in order to prevent it from recurring despite its having been fixed once.

Accurate diagnosis is critical to treatment planning. The diagnosis should provide the voice therapist with the information necessary to plan a course of treatment. However, patients are often referred for voice therapy with minimal diagnostic information. When that is the case, requests should be directed to the otolaryngologist for as detailed information as is available. Voice symptoms and signs in combination with information derived from a complete history and voice assessment must be compatible with the referral diagnosis. Communication between the speech-language pathologist and the referring laryngologist will be helpful in clarifying terminology and observations, as well as in developing a treatment plan.

The relationship between the person and the voice must be understood and incorporated into the therapy program. This is true whether or not the voice problem is psychogenic in etiology. Emotionality, stress, and anxiety may be components of many voice problems, both in terms of their etiologies and the reactions they engender. Individual reactions to voice problems may very well determine the response to treatment and the patient's ability to follow a therapy plan.

Freed from constraints imposed by organic lesions, stress factors, or abusive habits, the larynx will usually function well. Thus, it is often possible to eliminate the constraint through voice therapy and thereby to correct the voice problem. It is not always necessary to teach patients every aspect of voice production, as if they had never done it correctly before.

## GUIDELINES FOR VOICE THERAPY

A simplified explanation of normal vocal physiology and of the patient's specific deviance from it can be critical. For most patients, the idea of voice therapy is an unfamiliar one. They do not understand how, after many years of speaking without difficulty, they can now be speaking improperly. They have little appreciation for the connection between various vocal behaviors and their own particular problem. What they really would like is for the doctor to prescribe some type of medication that, taken three times a day, would cure the problem. Instead, they learn that they must assume some responsibility for dealing with the problem. In order to do so, they must begin by gaining some knowledge. Without an understanding of the nature of the problem, the patient's approach to therapy will often be highly skeptical.

Throughout therapy it is important to encourage the patient to verbalize perceptions of how the voice sounds and feels. This provides information for the clinician, but more important, it sensitizes the patient to the voice and increases self-awareness. It encourages a process of self-discovery that is exciting and motivating for the patient as changes are perceived. For the clinician, the patient's verbalizations provide information about how the patient views the problem, how tuned in to the problem the patient is, and perhaps help to shape the therapy plan.

The use of both auditory and visual feedback during therapy can be extremely helpful. Auditory feedback can be provided by the judicious use of tape recording using good-quality equipment. Visual feedback may take a variety of forms, including the use of instruments such as the Visi-Pitch (Kay Elemetrics Corp.). This type of instrumentation, as well as other computer software, permits visualization of a waveform model and of the patient's attempt to match that model. Visual feedback may also involve the use of the fiberoptic laryngoscope connected to a videotape recorder and monitor during the therapy process (Bastian, 1985, 1987). The patient is taught to identify certain desirable or undesirable laryngeal behaviors and has the benefit of the visual image to assist in shaping laryngeal activity. Spectrograms, electroglottograms, and other printouts of acoustic or physiological data can be used for demonstration and explanation but do not lend themselves as easily to direct therapeutic use. Biofeedback using surface electrodes over laryngeal muscles has been reported with inconclusive results (Prosek, Montgomery, Walden, & Schwartz, 1978; Stemple, Weiler, Whitehead, & Komray, 1980). Because this method, as currently used, is incapable of differentiating between the activity of those muscles that need to be active and those that should be relaxed, and because we have no data to specify how much activity is normal and how much is hyperfunctional for any given muscle during phonation, the meaning of electromyographic biofeedback is uncertain.

Another form of feedback is the use of instruments that monitor a behavior and supply a signal when a preset level of that behavior has been surpassed. For example, the Voice Intensity Controller (VIC), described by Holbrook, Rolnick, and Bailey (1974), is a small unit capable of being worn by a patient to monitor vocal intensity. A small throat microphone is affixed to the neck, an earphone is worn in the ear, and the unit fits into a pocket. The permissible intensity is preset. When that level is exceeded, a tone is emitted in the earphone. The use of this feedback device has been found to be very effective in modifying vocal loudness in a short period of time (Holbrook et al., 1974). However, these instruments are often difficult to obtain and are costly. Another device to monitor loudness is available from LinguiSystems. An inexpensive sound level meter can be purchased at Radio Shack (Cat. No. 33-2055). Visual feedback is provided by the Voice Light and Voice Intensity Indicator, available from Wintronix, (P.O. Box 514, Blue Springs, MO 64014).

Therapy should move gradually from one step or activity to the next. It is important to give the patient adequate time to practice a technique and to master it. Familiarity with a technique and a sense of having learned it provides a sense of accomplishment for the patient. Furthermore, if the behavior is but one phase of a progression, the patient needs to have a solid foundation on which to build. There is a fine line here between overdoing a good thing and moving on too quickly. To help make this transition, it is wise to begin to introduce a new technique while continuing to incorporate practice on those already learned. It is also important to give a technique a chance to work. The clinician must not allow the patient's anxiety and desire for instant results to affect clinical judgment. In the initial stages of therapy, it is often necessary to experiment with techniques and approaches. The patient should be made aware of this process in order to avoid feelings of uncertainty and confusion.

The clinician should always model therapy tasks for the patient. We often ask patients to produce sounds or engage in activities that might seem strange to them. Moreover, we ask them to do so in the presence of another person, the clinician. This raises the patient's level of self-consciousness significantly. In order to minimize such feelings, as well as to demonstrate clearly what the patient is being asked to do, the clinician must demonstrate therapeutic tasks. When a task is demonstrated, it must be done just as it is wished the patient do it. If the request is for the patient to produce the loudest "hey" possible, it will not do to have the clinician model it quietly. Because it is often difficult to verbally explain or describe a vocal behavior, modeling it takes on greater importance. A demonstration, like the proverbial picture, is worth a thousand words.

It is helpful to tape record therapy sessions in whole or in part. Doing so provides a record of the patient's voice and the therapy session. Memory for voice is very fleeting, and both the clinician and the patient may readily forget what the voice sounded like at a given point. When therapy seems to be taking longer than the patient expected, or when it appears that little progress has been made, the playing of an earlier tape recording may be very helpful in providing some perspective. Another valuable use for tape recorded sessions is as home practice material. Patients often report that without the clinician's model or their own from a previous time, they are not sure that they are practicing correctly. The tape recorded session provides the structure they need.

Patients must be carefully instructed in what to practice, for how long and how often. It is helpful to have the patient demonstrate the exercise or activity to be practiced before leaving the therapy session. Because talking is an activity that is so pervasive yet so rarely attended to by most speakers, we have found it effective to recommend frequent practice sessions of limited duration. This approach seems to help the patient focus on the voice frequently. Furthermore, there is usually some follow-up or generalization of practice for a period of time immediately after it has been done. Frequent practice periods capitalize on this "overflow effect" because it occurs more frequently.

The prognostic statement made at the initiation of a program of vocal rehabilitation must be viewed as an educated guess about the outcome of therapy. It must be realistic but must not be etched in stone. It should be modified appropriately as therapy progresses. The variety of factors that will enter into the development of a prognostic statement will be discussed later in this chapter.

Not all patients are appropriate candidates for a voice therapy approach, for reasons other than the nature of the pathology present. A patient must recognize that a problem is present, and must be willing to undertake a therapy program and to follow the regimen. Some find it extremely difficult to abandon abusive habits because of lifestyle, employment, or personality factors. Even when explicitly directed to do so, smokers may be unable to stop or even to significantly reduce this habit. The irritation created by continued smoking may be sufficient to maintain a condition and sabotage any positive effects that can be brought about through changed phonatory behavior. The therapeutic process is a complex one, and patient behavior may unwittingly pose a major hindrance to progress. Despite apparent cooperation, the patient may be exhibiting a variety of behaviors described by McFarlane, Fujiki, and Brinton (1984) as exemplifying the "reluctant client."

## PROGNOSTIC CONSIDERATIONS

Many factors enter into the consideration of a prognosis. Because voice therapy requires full patient participation, it is often difficult to predict its anticipated outcome. In determining whether a patient is an appropriate candidate for a voice therapy approach and arriving at a prognosis, the clinician should consider the following factors. First, the patient must recognize that there is a problem. People possess internal references about how they should feel, what is normal for them, and what they should sound like. A voice that sounds abnormal to us may not sound particularly deviant to the person with the voice. Similarly, although aware that the voice is not normal, the person may not find it objectionable or in need of "fixing." Second, the patient must be willing to follow a therapy plan including regular practice periods as required. This is difficult for those seeking the quick cure for which they do not have to assume responsibility. Third, there must be a willingness to give up abusive habits and to alter or eliminate some voice use, at least temporarily. This is easier said than done for most people. Changing manner and amount of talking involves changes in lifestyle, in everyday habits, and even, it may seem, personality. Fourth, psychiatric problems, if present, may interfere with the ability to modify vocal behavior. A voice problem may be a manifestation of a psychiatric problem. Amelioration of the voice problem may be possible temporarily, but it will not deal with the problem (recall the case of R. W. in Chapter 7). Fifth, the patient's voice disorder must be amenable to change through a voice therapy approach. For some voice problems, surgical or medical management may be the first or sole step. For other patients, the nature of the disorder may preclude any real possibility of success through voice therapy. The patient and the speech-language pathologist must be able to recognize the limitations of voice therapy. Sixth, appropriateness of the patient's expectations must be considered. If a person has an essentially normal voice but wishes to sound like another person, voice therapy is not indicated. Seventh, it is necessary to give full consideration to the patient's laryngeal condition and general health status. Some patients are insistent upon attaining full return of premorbid voice. The nature of the disorder and the resultant laryngeal changes may be such that this expectation may be unrealistic. The vocal folds may be damaged to the extent that normal phonation is not possible. Patients may have other health problems that may limit their ability to participate in voice therapy or may place constraints on their ability to control phonatory behavior. Finally, the speech-language pathologist must have an adequate understanding of the problem, feel competent in handling it, and be able to establish a good relationship with the patient.

## VOICE THERAPY IN THE MANAGEMENT OF CHANGES IN LARYNGEAL TISSUE OR STRUCTURE

Vocal rehabilitation may play a primary role, as either the sole treatment modality of choice or simultaneously with other treatment, or a secondary role, as a follow-up treatment after a primary approach has been carried out.

### *When Is Voice Therapy Alone Appropriate?*

It is unfortunate that there is a paucity of hard data to support a position on this question. Theoretical constructs and clinical experience are the primary bases on which therapeutic judgments are made.

Perhaps the most agreement exists about the treatment of vocal fold nodules. Prominent authorities in the treatment of voice, in the fields of both otolaryngology and speech-language pathology, generally agree that the initial treatment of choice for symptomatic vocal nodules in adults is voice therapy (Aronson, 1990; Bastian, 1986; Boone & McFarlane, 1988; Gould, 1987; Sataloff, 1987a, 1987b, 1987c; Vaughan, 1982; see also Chapter 8 of this book). The option for surgical intervention is not compromised or eliminated by the more conservative approach of at least a 6–8 week period of voice therapy. Some authorities make a distinction between early nodules, which appear to be soft and reddish, and nodules that have been present for months or years and are large, hard, and white. Voice therapy as the initial treatment is recommended for the former, and surgical removal followed by a period of voice therapy is most commonly recommended for the latter (Arnold, 1980; Boone & McFarlane, 1988; Case, 1984). Sataloff (1987b) states that even nodules that appear to be large and fibrotic may disappear, regress, or become asymptomatic through a course of voice therapy. Other authors suggest that decisions regarding choice of treatment have to be made on an individual basis but that vocal reeducation must be part of any treatment protocol (Moore, Hicks, & Abbott, 1985). Once again, it should be remembered that a trial period of voice therapy does not in any way compromise the option for surgical removal. Prater and Swift (1984) point out that voice therapy is more cost-effective than surgery, results in less time lost from work, and is nontraumatic. Furthermore, the learning that takes place during the therapy program will serve to eliminate vocal abuse and will be readily transferable to postoperative voice use should surgery become necessary. It is agreed that vocal nodules may well recur if vocal abuse is not eliminated through a vocal rehabilitation program.

Less agreement exists about the need for and value of any treatment for vocal nodules in children. Vaughan (1982) and Hirano (as he discusses in Chapter 8 of this book) report that vocal nodules in children resolve spontaneously in early adolescence and therefore usually require no treatment. Hirano, however, recognizes that the vocal symptoms resulting from vocal nodules can potentially create significant emotional problems for a child, in which case voice therapy is advocated. Surgical removal of vocal nodules in children is contraindicated (Arnold, 1980; Ballenger, 1985; DeWeese & Saunders, 1982). Most speech-language pathologists believe that youngsters with aberrant voices due to vocal nodules can be effectively helped to eliminate vocally abusive behaviors and thereby the nodules themselves (Boone & McFarlane, 1988; Johnson, 1983; Teter, 1976; Wilson, 1987) and that such treatment should not be withheld. The psychosocial effects of aberrant voice on a young child can be quite significant.

The controversy about the role of the speech-language pathologist in the treatment of voice disorders in children has been discussed by Sander (1989) (against) and Kahane and Mayo (1989) (for). While Sander claims that young children experience resolution of voice problems at puberty without the benefit of any treatment, Kahane and Mayo cite reports that adult vocal deviations are frequently traceable to patterns set in childhood (Cooper, 1973; Pahn, 1966) and, further, that the incidence of voice disorders in school children in the middle school grades (6th through 9th grades) may be higher than has previously been reported (Warr-Leeper, McShea, & Leeper, 1979). Kahane and Mayo present a compelling argument for the development of prevention programs and cite the positive result of such a program reported by Nilson and Schneiderman (1983).

Vocal fold polyps are often thought to be the result of vocal abuse, sometimes caused by a single or intense period of trauma during which small blood vessels rupture. They are also thought by some to be amenable to a voice therapy approach, particularly the sessile, or broad-based, polyps. Just as with vocal nodules, opinions about the preferred mode of treatment are mixed, but also, as is the case with nodules, little is lost when a period of voice therapy is the initial treatment provided.

## When Should Voice Therapy Be Combined with Other Treatment?

Contact ulcers and granulomas had been thought to result from a specific type of vocally abusive phonation. However, various studies provide additional insight into the underlying pathophysiology of contact ulcers (Cherry & Margulies, 1968; Chodosh, 1977; Delahunty, 1972; Delahunty & Cherry, 1968; Ward, Zwitman, Hanson, & Berci, 1980). Ward and Berci (1982b) cite the chronic irritation caused by hiatal hernia and by gastroesophageal reflux as the basic problem, which in turn causes chronic coughing and harsh and frequent throat clearing. It is these abusive behaviors, coughing and throat clearing, that were thought to initiate contact ulcer and granuloma formation. Response to medical treatment as reported by Hallewell and Cole (1970) was very successful in 21 of 22 cases. Chronic nonspecific laryngitis, pharyngitis, and pachydermia laryngis are included in the family of problems with this underlying pathophysiology. Voice therapy is appropriate as one part of the treatment regimen in order to eliminate laryngeally abusive behaviors. However, appropriate medical evaluation of and treatment for possible gastroesophageal reflux disease also need to be part of the total treatment protocol. Surgical and/or medical treatment without the other components of care is frequently unsuccessful in the long term, as the condition recurs.

Koufman et al. emphasize the potentially destructive nature of gastroesophageal reflux disease (GERD) on the larynx, leading to problems that may be very serious, including cancer (Koufman, 1991; Koufman, Wiener, Wu, & Castell, 1988). These authors question the viability of using traditional diagnostic radiologic techniques to assess GERD stating that "barium esophagagography has both poor specificity and sensitivity, and its reliability is questionable" (Koufman, 1995; Koufman, Wiener, Wu, & Castell, 1988). They advocate the use of 24-hour pH probe monitoring of the esophagus and pharynx as a more reliable means for detecting when reflux is occurring. Although 69% of the patients had no reflux-like symptoms, Koufman et al. found that 75% had abnormal pH studies. Most had reflux as determined by the pH probe at night but many (71%) had reflux while upright. When treated with a standard antireflux regimen (i.e., medication, dietary restrictions, head elevation during sleep, and behavioral adjustments), about 66% of the patients had resolution of their symptoms. In a much larger study, Koufman (1991) reported on 225 patients with suspected GERD. Eighty-eight percent of the patients underwent a 24-hr pH monitoring study with 62% of those demonstrating abnormal studies. Of these 30% demonstrated reflux into the pharynx. Abnormal pH probe findings were reported for 71% of the patients with carcinoma, 78% of those with stenosis, 60% of those with reflux laryngitis, 58% of those with complaints of a lump in the throat (globus), 45% with dysphagia, and 52% of patients with a chronic cough. Thus, reflux may be associated with a variety of problems affecting the larynx, not all of which produce voice symptoms.

Polypoid changes of the vocal folds (Reinke's edema) are highly related to long-term, excessive smoking and to age (Hirano, Kurita, Matsuo, & Nagata, 1980). Although a component of vocal abuse may also be present and may aggravate the condition, these lesions are generally not caused by abuse and not responsive to voice therapy. However, many patients will benefit from a course of voice therapy following surgical excision of the lesion.

There are numerous other laryngeal lesions that are not caused by vocal abuse and that require medical and surgical intervention. However, vocally abusive habits may result as the patient attempts to compensate for a poorly functioning mechanism. Those habits may persist beyond resolution of the pathology, and a period of voice therapy may be required. A specific group of patients that would be included in this category are those with papillomas, requiring frequent surgical removal over a period of years. The condition of the mucosal cover of the vocal folds following numerous surgeries will be a most important factor in determining the quality of voice that will be possible.

## Goals of Voice Therapy

When voice therapy is undertaken as the treatment modality of choice in the presence of mucosal and voice changes, the primary goals are, of course, to restore the mucosa to a healthy condition and to regain clear and full vocal function. Subgoals include identification and elimination of all abusive behaviors through the reduction of laryngeal tensions, institution of a vocal hygiene program, environmental manipulation, easy voice production, and establishment of improved vocal habits. Other goals may include identification of patient needs that require other forms of attention and appropriate referral.

When voice therapy is an adjunct or secondary treatment modality, the goals will depend largely on the laryngeal status of the patient. The primary goal may be to restore healthy function and return of good voice, or it may be to help the patient find the best voice of which she is capable. The limits on that voice may be imposed by permanent changes in the mucosa or the structural integrity of the larynx. Subgoals, in addition to those noted above, may include helping the patient to accept a changed voice, exploration of the adequacy of the voice for all necessary speaking situations, and suggesting environmental adjustments as necessary.

## Nature of Therapeutic Intervention

Vocal rehabilitation must address a variety of factors. Patients are often called upon to make changes in the manner in which they produce voice, the various ways in which they use voice (e.g., singing, lecturing, etc.), and the environments in which they may use voice. These changes are all very closely linked to how individuals see themselves and how they interact with others. Recognition of the highly sensitive nature of the therapeutic process and the impact that it may have on the patient cannot be overemphasized.

## VOICE THERAPY IN THE MANAGEMENT OF MISUSE AND ABUSE PROBLEMS

### When Is Voice Therapy Alone Appropriate?

Voice therapy is almost always the treatment modality of choice for voice problems stemming from behaviors that have been identified as misuse or abuse of the laryngeal mechanism. However, it has been our experience that these patients, who may have negative laryngological examinations or minimal signs of laryngeal irritation, frequently receive up to 3 months or more of medical treatment prior to referral to a speech-language pathologist for voice evaluation. It is not uncommon for patients in these categories to be treated with antibiotics, antihistamines, decongestants, tranquilizers, and even corticosteroids, or to be sent home with some fairly nonspecific advice about relaxing or reducing voice use. Due to the effects on laryngeal mucosa of some medications, the actual voice symptoms may worsen over the course of the treatment, rather than improve (see Chapter 4). Recognition of the problem is critical to obtaining effective treatment.

Some patients may not be appropriate candidates for a voice therapy approach due to social/emotional problems beyond the scope of practice of the speech-language pathologist. However, it is within the speech-language pathologist's expertise to recognize such conditions and to make recommendations for or to arrange appropriate referral. Patients who do not recognize that a problem exists or who are incapable or unwilling to change habits or lifestyle will be poor candidates for therapy.

## Goals of Voice Therapy

The primary therapeutic goals are to identify and eliminate behaviors that constitute misuse or abuse and to replace them with acceptable patterns of voice production. Full return of normal voice is anticipated, especially when there is no evidence of mucosal tissue change. Subgoals in the treatment of vocal abuse and misuse might include reduction of laryngeal tensions, decrease of vocal loudness, decrease in amount of talking, adjusting environmental factors, and others. For those voice problems that appear to be psychogenic in nature, a goal of therapy may be to help the patient understand the dynamics that initiated and sustained the voice problem.

## Nature of Therapeutic Intervention

As stated in the previous section, therapy directed toward the elimination of vocally abusive behavior requires that the patient change habits of voice production. Those habits, even if not of very long standing, nevertheless may be quite tenacious. In addition to altering the way in which voice is produced, it may be necessary for the patient to make some sacrifices in the ways the voice is used. The changes that need to be made may be imposed by the therapy process, rather than as limitations caused by the problem itself. For example, the patient who enjoys singing in a church choir may need to forego that activity at least temporarily. The college professor who has never used amplification despite having to lecture to very large classes in large rooms with poor acoustics may need to do so. These are difficult changes for people to make. The therapeutic process may involve discussion of personal and interpersonal concerns that require understanding, the ability to listen well, and a nonjudgmental attitude. It is also essential for the clinician to be able to provide support and encouragement in helping a patient to accept a changed or restored voice.

## Voice Therapy in the Management of Neurological Problems

Voice problems are but one of the dysarthric components of disability that may accompany certain neuromuscular disorders. With the possible exceptions of unilateral vocal fold paralysis (usually peripheral nerve damage) and spasmodic dysphonia (etiology still questioned), it is unusual for the voice disorder to be the primary disability. It is possible that the earliest symptoms of a neurological condition may be exhibited in changes or aberrations of phonation. However, in progressively debilitating neuromuscular diseases, the worsening of motor behavior and increased limitations in many areas of function may become relatively more handi-capping to the person. The speech-language pathologist may well be involved with these patients in working on phonatory problems and also the related disabilities of dysarthria (articulation and resonation), apraxia, aphasia, and dysphagia, as they exist. A therapy protocol focusing on the voice has been developed and shown to be effective for patients with Parkinson's disease and the Parkinson plus syndrome (Countryman, Ramig, & Pawlas, 1994; Ramig, Bonitati, Lemke, & Horii, 1994; Ramig & Scherer, 1992). (See "Voice Therapy Techniques" later in this chapter for further discussion.)

There is still some controversy concerning the role of voice therapy in the man-agement of unilateral vocal fold paralysis. Data to support the efficacy of vocal reha-bilitation are limited. When the etiology of the paralysis is idiopathic, the literature suggests that either spontaneous recovery or increased compensatory movement of the healthy fold occurs (Tucker, 1980). The major portion of such recovery is believed to take place within 6 months of onset, although there are reports of recovery for up to a year post onset (Ward & Berci, 1982a). When voice therapy is undertaken during that time period, to what can we attribute improved vocal function—to the therapy or to spontaneous recovery of function, or perhaps to a combination of the two? We do not have the data to answer this question. Several phonosurgical ap-proaches designed to improve vocal function are available. Injection of Teflon (as described by Dr. Hirano in Chapter 8), has in the past been effective in many individ-uals who have failed to show spontaneous recovery of vocal fold function and/or voice (Hammarberg, Fritzell, & Schiratzki, 1984; Lewy, 1993; Reich & Lerman, 1978; Tucker, 1980). However, problems of over-injection and concern about long term stability of the injected material and its positioning have also been present (Rubin, 1965) although some believe that with care these problems can be minimized (Dedo, 1988, 1992). Other surgical techniques for medializing the edges of the paralyzed vo-cal fold (see Chapter 8) appear to have gained in popularity, with the augmentation approach, often called thyroplasty (Type I), being used most frequently. Recently, in-jection of autologous fat (Jiang, Titze, Wexler, & Gray, 1994; Wexler, Jiang, Gray, & Titze, 1989) has been tried with good reports of success (Ford, Bless, & Loftus, 1992; Ford, Martin, & Warner, 1984).

Our own studies of medical, surgical, and voice therapy treatment of patients with a unilateral vocal fold paralysis have shown that both approaches can be effective in improving the voice. Thirty-nine patients were studied, all with unilateral vocal paral-ysis or paresis. Twenty-one patients received surgical treatment (either Teflon injec-tion or thyroplasty) and 18 received voice therapy as their major treatment. Both treatment groups showed improvement in voice quality and changes in several mea-sures of vocal fold function. These measurements are shown in Figure 9.1. Note that the surgery patients tended to have higher pretreatment mean, peak, and leakage air-flow rates suggesting greater severity of glottal incompetence than the therapy group. Leakage flow reflects glottal incompetence and both treatment approaches reduced the magnitude of leakage flow. Not shown in the figure are open quotient data for both groups. For patients in the surgery group, the open quotient was much greater prior to treatment than after treatment (0.67 versus 0.54, males and females pooled). For patients in the therapy group, the open quotient was also greater prior to treat-ment than after treatment (0.61 versus 0.56). These results mean that the vocal folds were open a greater proportion of the time during the cycle prior to treatment for both groups but those who underwent surgery had preoperative open quotients larger than those patients who received therapy. After surgery, the open quotient decreased, suggesting greater vocal fold adduction.

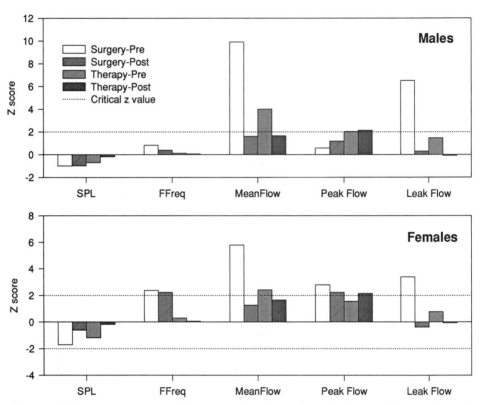

*Figure 9.1.* Z scores for a group of patients with unilateral vocal fold paralysis on selected voice measurements made prior to and after treatment. There were 15 males and 6 females in the surgery group and 6 males and 12 females in the therapy group. The dotted line represents the critical value of Z to exceed normal limits at the 0.05 level. Normal data were obtained from Holmberg, Hillman and Perkell (1988) for 25 males and 20 females producing phonations at normal loudness and frequency levels.

The issue of voice therapy procedures recommended for treatment of unilateral vocal fold paralysis will be discussed later in the section ("Unresolved Issues and Myths").

Another area of continued controversy is that of spasmodic dysphonia. Controversy continues about the etiology of this puzzling condition, as well as about its treatment. Historically, the strain/struggle voice of the patient with spasmodic dysphonia was first thought to be entirely psychologically based (Arnold, 1959). This view has been modified at least to the extent that most authors now believe that more than a single etiology may exist but that a neurological basis for the disorder exists in most cases. The need for very thorough differential diagnosis is also well accepted in order to differentiate spasmodic dysphonia from other neurogenically based disorders and from those of psychogenic origin. A trial of voice therapy is often recommended to determine whether relief can be obtained through that approach. Indeed, a trial of voice therapy is often diagnostically useful. Although voice therapy is generally not an effective treatment modality for significantly modifying the symptoms of true spasmodic dysphonia, it has been shown to increase the interval between BoTox injections (Murry & Woodson, 1995). Furthermore, voice therapy can be helpful in educating patients about the disorder: what they can expect and how to manage the variable vocal function they will experience.

## Goals of Voice Therapy

Voice therapy can offer no cures when neuromotor disability is involved. However, through voice therapy, patients may be able to learn to produce the best voice possible and to exert a degree of voluntary control over the production of voice that may allow them to remain communicatively functional in occupational and social settings (Ramig et al., 1994; Rosenfield, 1987). The speech-language pathologist can also be helpful in assessing the effects of medications on the patient's voice and speech production. If functional verbal communication is not a viable option, voice therapy becomes inappropriate, and the goal then must be to provide the patient with a means of nonverbal communication. Teaching how to optimize voice production and communicate within the limits imposed by the disability can be most productive.

## Nature of Therapeutic Intervention

The manner in which voice is produced may receive very direct attention, particularly in cases of vocal fold paralysis and sometimes of spasmodic dysphonia. Very direct work on loudness, pitch range, flexibility, and vocal stamina is the hallmark of voice therapy with parkinsonian patients (see "Voice Therapy Techniques" later in this chapter). Attention may be directed to suprasegmental factors such as utilizing breath groups, prosody, rate, and marking for stress and inflection, in work with other neurologically based disorders. Patients may have adopted particular patterns of voice use in an attempt to compensate for alterations in control of the voice. Some of these compensatory behaviors may be helpful, while others may not. Adjustment in communication patterns and behaviors are often imposed on the individual by the nature of the disability. For example, the inability to increase loudness will restrict the environments in which the person can communicate effectively. In some instances, manipulation of environmental factors may be of some assistance. Hanson and Metter (1980) describe the use of a small, wearable, delayed auditory feedback (DAF) device in the treatment of a patient with progressive supranuclear palsy and severe hypokinetic dysarthria. They report that the patient, who was noted to have weak vocal intensity, demonstrated an increase of vocal intensity with the introduction of 100 milliseconds of DAF in both reading and counting aloud conditions, and that this increase was maintained in follow-up testing after a 3-month period of daily use of the device. Desired changes were also noted in a reduction of speech rate and increased speech intelligibility.

The therapeutic process may be difficult for neurologically impaired patients with progressive disorders and also for their voice clinicians because of the constraints of the underlying disorder and the gradual but inexorable deterioration in the patient's condition. It is incumbent on the clinician to recognize the limitations of the therapeutic approach and not to promise what cannot be delivered but to make every effort to help the patient arrive at the best means of communication possible for as long as possible.

## THERAPY FOR SPECIAL VOICE PROBLEMS

A number of voice problems that do not readily fit the above categories but that may appropriately require a period of vocal rehabilitation will be covered in this section.

## The Transsexual Voice

The voice problem most immediately associated with a gender reassignment is that of inappropriate pitch. In the case of change from a female to male, this problem is usually resolved through the use of male hormones, which cause an increase in laryngeal mass and thus lower fundamental frequency. However, no drugs are available to reduce the mass of the vocal folds, so that a male to female change is not accompanied by elevation of pitch secondary to hormone therapy. The incongruity of a masculine voice in a woman can present a significant psychological barrier. Therapeutic attempts to elevate speaking fundamental frequency should be undertaken with care, recognizing the physiological limits of the larynx. The use of breathy phonation can be helpful in giving the illusion of a higher pitch without the risk of inviting laryngeal trauma.

However, in addition to differences in pitch between the male and female voice, there are differences in other speech patterns, habits, and mannerisms. This has been demonstrated experimentally by Coleman (1971, 1973, 1976) who found that female voices are still recognized as female even when the pitch difference between male and female voice is removed. Some of the difference between male and female voice lies in vowel quality, in that the relative sizes of the oral and pharyngeal cavities are different in the two sexes. Other differences include those of stress, inflection, timing, and even choice and use of words and conversational style. Changes in these areas will go far in feminizing a voice even in the presence of a low speaking fundamental frequency. The actress Lauren Bacall presents a good model of someone whose voice is low in pitch and yet whose style is entirely feminine. A program of voice therapy designed to make the man-to-woman change should include careful study of this and other models of feminine low pitched speech. The goal of therapy should be to make those changes that will be effective in changing the overall image, rather than to work on artificial changes, such as pitch change, that may never become natural and that in fact may court laryngeal problems.

The pitch of the voice is only one of many aspects of communication that differentiates and distinguishes the sexes. Because we do not advocate artificial elevation of pitch that can be potentially damaging, we recommend that some of the following areas be targeted for change.

1. slight increase in breathiness of voice
2. using the concept of vocal effort, a lighter and softer voice may be encouraged by reducing vocal effort
3. increased use of pitch variability rather than loudness to mark inflection, stress, and alter rhythm of speech
4. target nonphonatory areas, such as conversational topics, conversational style, pragmatic aspects of communication

## Voice Problems Due to Endocrine Disorders or Hormone Imbalance

### HYPOTHYROIDISM

Hypothyroidism is a condition that can occur at any age. The symptoms may develop gradually over a lengthy period of time. As a result, their effect may not be recognized until a critical level of symptomatology has been reached. Change in the voice may be one such symptom. Typically, the voice of the patient with hypothyroidism is hoarse and has gradually lowered in pitch due to increased mass (edema) of the vocal folds. Therefore, the diagnostician must be alert to this as a possible diagnosis when vocal fold edema is noted and does not appear to be related to factors of vocal abuse. Referral for testing should be pursued, and voice therapy is not indicated.

## VIRILIZATION

This term is used to refer to the increase in size and mass of the vocal folds that occurs in women as the result of excessive secretion of the androgenic hormones or due to ingestion of androgen-containing hormones in treatment for menopausal symptoms or other problems. Damste (1967) described these changes and also showed them to be frequently irreversible. Voice therapy is contraindicated.

## MENSTRUATION, PREGNANCY, AND BIRTH CONTROL PILL USE

Most of the voice-related negative effects of hormonal changes associated with the menstrual cycle occur in the pre- or early menstrual days. Excess loading of the vocal folds with fluid changes their mass and thus may affect vibratory behavior. This is usually not problematic for the average speaker but may present a problem for the professional singer. Submucosal hemorrhages in the larynx are not uncommon. Diuretics should be avoided because they do not free the protein-bound submucosal fluid (Sataloff, 1987b). Voice therapy is never indicated, but the clinician should be aware of the possibility of some subtle voice changes in female patients during these time periods.

Pregnancy may also result in change in the voice. During pregnancy the woman's endocrinological state undergoes great change. If a change in voice occurs, it is usually irreversible (Sataloff, 1987b). There are no drugs available to counteract the normal physiological effects of either the menstrual period or pregnancy, and voice therapy is of no value in these cases. Voice clinicians must be aware, however, that such changes may be reported by patients.

A very small number of women appear to experience changes in the voice as a result of the use of birth control pills (Simkin, 1964). The quality and range of the voice may show these effects. Once again, they are usually not noted by the average speaker but may create problems for the singer. These voice changes are reversible when use of the pills is terminated.

## *Paradoxical Vocal Fold Motion or Vocal Fold Dysfunction*

This is a disability which can easily be mistaken for asthma and treated accordingly, even to the point of tracheostomy. The primary characteristic is obstruction of the airway with vocal fold closure throughout the respiratory cycle, including inspiration. A 1983 study by Christopher, Wood, Eckert, Blager, Raney, & Souhrada described five patients 14–68 years of age, of whom four were male and one female, who presented with paroxysms of wheezing and dyspnea and had initially been diagnosed as severe, uncontrollable asthmatics. However, the patients failed to respond to standard therapy for asthma and, indeed, did not test positively for the expected symptoms of asthma. All patients had a chronic history of repeated "attacks," ranging from 1 to 13 years. One patient had undergone eight tracheotomy procedures. Laryngological examination during the spasm revealed adduction of both true and ventricular folds during the full respiratory cycle and patients exhibited both inspiratory and expiratory stridor. Laryngeal function was normal during asymptomatic periods. Inhalation of a mixture of helium (80%) and oxygen (20%) was found to be effective in relieving at least the acute symptoms and frequently resulted in symptom reduction even after cessation of the treatment. All patients were found to have psychological problems, and all were referred for both speech therapy and psychological counseling. Follow-up ranged from 3 to 21 months, and no patient had had recurrence of the symptoms.

Other varieties of paradoxical vocal fold motion have been reported, in which the vocal folds seem to behave in a manner opposite to the normal, that is, adduction is observed during deep inspiration, and there is at least slight abduction on expiration (Kellman & Leopold, 1982; Rogers & Stell, 1978). One such patient had undergone tracheotomy twice for relief of symptoms that had been diagnosed as laryngospasm. Patients were reported to show significant reduction, if not elimination, of symptoms in response to various interventions, including speech therapy, intravenous injection of diazepam or of a placebo, hypnosis, and verbal support. Although voice symptoms ranging from aphonia to weak or hoarse voice may be present, restoring the airway is of primary importance. Voice therapy can be helpful in teaching these patients specific breathing techniques. Psychological treatment may also be indicated in some cases.

Although an apparently rare or under reported or misdiagnosed disability for many years, paradoxical vocal fold motion (PVFM) or vocal cord dysfunction has been reported in increasing numbers in recent years. Bless and Swift (1995) make the claim that "PVCM is a symptom with multiple determinants." Their definition of the problem is broader than has previously been reported and etiology is not limited to psychological problems, but includes (*a*) hyperreactivity of the airway; (*b*) neurogenic etiology of either central or peripheral origin; (*c*) psychological (has not been ruled out); (*d*) pharmacological; or (*e*) other unspecified medical problems. Treatment involves a combination of medical, behavioral, and psychological approaches. Gracco et al. (1995) reported instances of exercise-induced upper airway dysfunction in which the vocal folds were observed to adduct during inspiration. For further discussion see "Voice Therapy Techniques" later in this chapter.

## VOICE THERAPY TECHNIQUES: ASSOCIATED PHYSIOLOGY AND INDICATIONS FOR USE

It is important to recognize that the manner in which a therapeutic technique is used will vary from clinician to clinician. Furthermore, with experience each clinician will develop and perfect those techniques found to be most useful and effective. Clinicians bring their own personalities and approaches to the clinical process, and the techniques that fit that style and produce a level of comfort and confidence are the ones that are most likely to be adopted and well used.

It is the philosophy of this book that an understanding of laryngeal anatomy and phonatory physiology is basic to being a skilled voice clinician. Therapeutic techniques are only valid when they are used knowledgeably. The clinician must develop the knowledge base and the skill to determine what therapeutic approaches make sense for the individual patient. Indeed, a skilled clinician may make up a technique never tried before but something that makes sense for a given person.

---

### Case Study

---

J. M. was a patient whose use of ventricular phonation was felt to be of psychological origin. A variety of techniques had been tried to elicit clear voice, but to no avail. The clinician then instructed her to simply blow through her fingers while holding them in front of her mouth and to feel the stream of air. She was instructed to sustain that airstream steadily for at least 5 seconds. After a few trials of blowing, she was told to add a very slight bit of sound to the blowing while she continued to feel the airstream on her fingers. She successfully produced acceptable voice quality in doing this. Very gradually the good voice was shaped into speech, with no return of the ventricular phonation. This was a technique the clinician had never used previously.

---

There is nothing magical in the technique. For this patient, a way had been found to allow her to release laryngeal tension and produce easy voice. In this example, as in many others that might be cited, the clinician had a working hypothesis, perhaps unspoken, relating the technique to be used to the physiological effect that is desired. A patient may respond favorably to a number of approaches, all of which have the same goal. There is not a single technique that is always effective with all people. The clinician must understand what the patient is doing that is undesirable and then ask the question: "How can I get this patient to alter that specific behavior?"

Returning to the previous case study, the clinician knew from previous fiberoptic laryngoscopic studies of this patient that the ventricular phonation was produced with tight squeezing of the whole larynx, including supraglottal structures. Tension was apparent in respiratory function as well. The patient seemed to hold her breath during attempted phonation, releasing only when the effort to phonate was terminated and the vocal folds abducted fully. Perceptually, the voice sounded tight and strained, in addition to being very hoarse. It also seemed that this particular patient "froze" and became even more tense when asked to try any new activity that required phonation. Therefore, she was asked to carry out an activity, blowing, that does not require phonation and was therefore not threatening. The addition of feeling the stream of air captured J. M.'s attention and provided tangible, nonphonatory feedback. If J. M. continued to concentrate on this smooth, constant stream of air, phonation would begin softly and easily in perhaps a breathy manner. The introduction of tension and strain would surely interrupt or markedly change the airflow. For these various reasons it was hypothesized that if the patient was able to carry out the instructions, there was a good chance that she would do so with good voice.

There are few techniques that are specific to a single voice disorder because there is so much similarity in laryngeal physiology across many disorders. For example, patients who misuse their voices and those who abuse them to the point of creating mucosal changes may be engaging in the same form of vocal behavior from the physiological point of view. Thus, many of the same therapeutic techniques may be used in each instance. The specific type of misuse or abuse (i.e., talking too much versus talking too loud) will differ from patient to patient, and that issue must be addressed individually. However, the suggested means of changing those patterns may be similar across patients.

A major lack in voice research is documentation of the efficacy of therapeutic techniques and outcome data. This lack, although decried by many (Johnson, 1985; Ludlow, 1981; Moore, 1977; Perkins, 1985; Reed, 1980), is not easily corrected. Problems of terminology, of definition, of qualitative and quantitative assessment procedures, and of well-established normative standards (as discussed previously) plague the researcher who wishes to address the issue. Brewer and McCall (1974) used the fiberoptic laryngoscope to demonstrate visible changes in laryngeal physiology as patients were instructed in a therapeutic technique. Johnson (1985) reports on the efficacy of his particular program of reducing vocal abuse, which utilizes a highly structured behavior modification approach. Casper, Brewer, and Conture (1981) reported on computer-assisted measurement of specific intrasubject changes in laryngeal physiology, visible on fiberoptic images, that were felt to be the result of therapeutic intervention. The procedure, although workable, was fairly time consuming, and the results could be interpreted only relative to each individual's performance. Such research is helpful, but the approach does not lend itself to all voice problems. In the case study cited earlier, a new technique was used, and although in this case it proved to be effective, it would not necessarily be an appropriate or effective procedure with other cases of psychogenic dysphonia. If the research question to be answered is concerned not with specific techniques but rather with the question of whether the voice improved as a result of therapy, there must be some agreement on quantitative or qualitative parameters of assessment that would substantiate improved status. Such standards do not yet exist.

Thus, we are left with a variety of therapy techniques whose efficacy is acclaimed by many authors. The most often used of these will be discussed in this section, which not only will describe how they are done but also will give at least a theoretical rationale of why clinically they seem to be of value. The authors want to caution again that the techniques are only as good as the clinician who is making use of them. Clinicians should use them wisely but should continue to question their efficacy and search for ways to demonstrate it. It is not the intent of the authors to suggest that a single technique need be chosen and only that technique should be used. Quite the opposite is often the case, several techniques may be used concurrently or at different points in the therapy plan.

There is no particular meaning to be assigned to the order in which these techniques are presented. There is also no intent to make this an all-inclusive list. Indeed, most clinicians adapt procedures to fit their personal styles and develop unique ones, as do most voice coaches. The challenge is to be able to think through a problem in such a way that it is possible to devise techniques to use based on an understanding of the type of vocal behavior desired. No single technique will be equally effective with all people.

## Breathy Phonation: The Confidential Voice

We have found this technique to be widely appropriate and easy for patients to learn and to use, and it has resulted in clinical success. Producing voice is a holistic activity that is usually accomplished without conscious attention to pitch, loudness, variability, or other aspects of voice production. In light of this it seems reasonable to think that a therapy technique that can function in a holistic manner to accomplish its goals should be beneficial and easy for patients to adopt. The use of breathy phonation is such a technique (Casper, 1993). The patient has only to concentrate on making the voice very breathy and in so doing a number of other desirable goals are accomplished. These include reduction of loudness, reduction of rate, reduction of hyperfunction, and a beginning awareness of allowing the expiratory airflow to do the work of producing sound.

It is important to stress at the outset that breathy voice is being recommended here as a technique to be used for a circumscribed period of time during therapy and not as the end product of therapy. The voice is described to patients as being the softest intensity they can produce, much like the voice one would use to exchange a confidence with a friend when one does not wish others nearby to hear. It is a confidential voice. It differs from whisper in that some voicing is present. The very breathy quality of the voice is its hallmark and differentiates it from a voice just reduced in intensity.

Instruction to talk in a confidential voice and the model of that voice presented by the clinician are often all that is necessary for the patient to understand and to be able to produce the voice. However, when that is not sufficient, it is often helpful to start vocalization activities with other techniques such as the sigh and the yawn/sigh. In both of these the focus is on producing easy, unimpeded airflow and breathy voicing without stress.

There are several undesirable behaviors that may accompany a patient's use of breathy phonation that are very easily resolved if the clinician is alert. It is not enough for the voice just to be lowered in intensity; it must be breathy. The breathiness must be marked by ease of airflow without evidence of pushing or forcing air. The phonation that is produced must be "well focused" in that pitch should not be lowered nor should mouth opening be reduced. It will not and, indeed, cannot be a resonant voice at this stage.

The patient is instructed to use this voice for all speaking and is forewarned that it will be inaudible in any noisy environment. All loud talking is thus eliminated temporarily. It is also important to instruct the patient that fewer words per breath will be possible because of the increased expenditure of air. Furthermore, because one effect of the increased airflow may be a drying of the mucosa, we suggest that the patient increase fluid intake. This technique is appropriate for patients who need to eliminate vocal abuse or misuse. It is helpful as part of a vocal hygiene program whenever a period of modified voice rest or reduction of voice use is indicated.

Verdolini-Marston and her colleagues (Verdolini-Marston, Burke, Lessac, Glaze, & Caldwell, 1995) investigated the efficacy of the confidential voice therapy technique with five female patients with vocal fold nodules. The therapy was provided by two clinicians over a 2-week period. Pretreatment and post-treatment measurements of phonatory effort, auditory perceptual ratings of voice disorder severity, and visual ratings of vocal fold characteristics seen in videostroboscopic recordings were obtained. An additional five patients with nodules comprised the control group. Many patients showed improvement after the 2-week therapy period whereas there was little improvement of voice production in the control group. Most therapy patients had a decrease of phonatory effort and a decrease in the rated severity of dysphonia. Four of the five patients in the therapy group showed visible changes of the vocal folds. These data suggest that the confidential voice therapy approach can be effective in reducing vocal abuse and result in better voice production.

Another interesting finding from this study was the report that continued use of the therapeutic techniques after therapy had ended contributed to improved voice performance. Patient compliance and willingness to use the new form of voice production in routine voice usage appear to be predictive of long-term voice improvement.

***Rationale:*** *We have observed laryngeal physiology endoscopically as we have asked patients and normal speakers to use this voice and have noted the desired effect (Casper, Colton, Brewer, & Woo, 1989). The glottis remains very slightly open, thus reducing the force of contact and of medial compression of the vocal folds. The larynx seems to remain vertically at about the resting level. There is an absence of any appearance of laryngeal tightness or squeezing, and the closed phase of the glottal cycle is reduced. In some patients there may be a tendency to produce breathiness with a posterior glottal chink and Y appearance. This is not as desirable as incomplete glottal closure along the full length of the folds, and may be indicative of a greater than necessary degree of tension or strain in producing the phonation. In such cases, the use of visual biofeedback with the flexible endoscope in place can be very effective. Thus, with one maneuver the patient is provided with a type of voice production that eliminates abuse yet allows continued voice use, albeit different and reduced. It is a holistic approach that does not require that the act of speaking be broken down into its component parts, with each addressed separately and then put back together. We have also found it rather simple for patients to move gradually from the breathy, confidential voice to increased voicing without returning to abusive patterns.*

## *Sigh, Aspirate Initiation, Easy Initiation of Phonation*

These three techniques are combined under one heading because they are variations on a theme sharing a common rationale. For the sigh, the patient is instructed to produce the most relaxed, effortless, natural sigh possible. Whether or not voicing is present does not matter initially, but as this is practiced it is hoped that some voicing emerges naturally and easily. In a natural, spontaneous sigh it is not uncommon to release some air audibly before the actual voicing begins, then to produce just minimal voicing in terms of loudness and duration, and to finish the sigh with audible expiration of the rest of the breath supply. It is important that the patient not hold the breath after the inspiration. There must be a continuous flow from inhalation through exhalation, otherwise there is a tendency to close the glottis tightly as the breath is held.

From the sigh it is easy to have the patient practice aspirate initiation of voicing, using words that begin with an /h/. This should be done in a slightly exaggerated manner so that the /h/ is held and the voicing is initiated much as in the sigh and with a breathy quality. As the patient becomes adept at this maneuver, it is possible to omit the actual production of the /h/ yet continue the effortless gliding into easy initiation of phonation.

*Rationale: These techniques reduce laryngeal and vocal tract tensions, reduce the force of vocal fold contact and of medial compression, teach easy coordination of airflow and phonation, counteract abusive habits of tension and hard glottal attack, and foster resting level laryngeal posture. They may be very helpful for patients who have difficulty in learning to use a breathy voice for general conversation and appear to need more direct step-by-step work to learn to reduce tensions. In a fiberoptic and stroboscopic study of aspirate initiation of phonation, Casper et al. (1989) observed the expected physiological characteristics described above.*

## Yawn/Sigh

The patient is instructed to simulate a real yawn, or if possible, to actually trigger a real yawn. The yawn is completed with a sigh, making sure to allow air to be released in a relaxed way. This is not always easy for patients to do. We tend to be socialized into hiding and stifling public yawns. It is sometimes helpful to instruct the patient to open the mouth very wide, pull the tongue back and inhale long and deeply. Initiation of voicing should be carried out with this same oral posture, with a gradual closing of the mouth as the yawn and sigh progress. It is well to suggest that patients become aware of natural yawns and try to concentrate on how they feel when they occur spontaneously. As the patient learns the technique and can identify the tension reduction, a gradual shaping of the yawn/sigh into production of words, then phrases, and finally sentences should proceed slowly. The yawn should be gradually eliminated.

*Rationale: In a true vegetative yawn, the larynx lowers dramatically (Casper et al., 1989). This change can be observed fiberoptically. The physiology of a yawn is incompatible with the excessive laryngeal tensions that many patients exhibit. Easy, natural airflow and phonation are fostered. The intent is to eliminate abusive initiation and maintenance of phonation and to reduce laryngeal tensions. Individuals who have adopted hyperfunctional habits of voice production tend to have a high laryngeal posture. They often complain of pain in the extrinsic laryngeal muscles. The yawn/sigh maneuver, which lowers laryngeal posture serves to "stretch" those muscles, providing relief from the tightness. This is a further benefit of the technique.*

## Post BoTox Injection Therapy

Following successful injection, patients often experience a brief period of breathy voice. During that time there is a natural desire to "push" the voice so as to get the most voicing possible. The thrust of voice treatment, which should be restricted to three or four sessions, is to counteract this tendency. Easy onset of phonation is taught using techniques described earlier. The patient must be taught to concentrate on the airflow, specifically the maintenance of that flow. Pushing for increased loudness is discouraged.

## *Trill*

The trill is a sound made by the tongue tip making contact with the alveolar ridge and oscillating rapidly as sound is produced. The sound can be described as the trilled /r/ heard in many languages, including Spanish. The trill can also be made using the lips and allowing them to oscillate rapidly as voice is produced. When used as a vocal exercise the sound is sustained. It is an exercise used by many singers to "warm up" the voice. Very rapid and strong laryngeal vibrations can be felt if the fingers are placed on the larynx during production of the trill.

We have found the trill to be very useful and productive with a variety of disordered voices. We began using it with patients whose vocal folds were scarred postoperatively. The results seemed to be much better than any we had obtained with this population using other techniques. Subsequently we have used it with patients who present with a variety of disorders, particularly hypofunction and presbyphonia.

Patients are first instructed in production of the sound at a comfortable pitch and then to sustain it. Pitch variation is then introduced by sustaining the trilled sound at various pitches and then by gliding the trill through a range of pitches in both descending and ascending glides. We find it helpful as therapy progresses to extend the trilled sound into voicing without trill. This is done by instructing the patient to start the trill and go into vowel prolongation at that same pitch with no break in phonation between the two. This can be done with a variety of vowel sounds and at various pitches as well. And finally, the sound is shaped into speech. Although we extend practice beyond the trill itself, we also instruct patients to continue practice of the trill as such, and to use it as a warm-up exercise at the start of the day and prior to any extended speaking.

***Rationale:*** *The trill appears to "jump start" the vibratory behavior of the vocal folds. It is claimed that production of the trill balances resonance, fosters normal laryngeal tension by equalizing the aerodynamic and the myoelastic forces, and enhances coordination of respiration/phonation/articulation (Behlau and Pontes, 1990). McGowan (1992) described some work on modeling the tongue tip trill based on some physiological data and modeling experiments. Basically, the tongue tip acts like a springed trap door that creates pressure differences between the outside air and the cavity behind the tip constriction. These pressure differences oscillate to produce the desired effect. What happens in the cavity behind the constriction is dynamic with oscillatory changes of air pressure and air volume velocity. There appear to be oscillations on the pharyngeal walls creating small volume velocity changes of the air passing through them. These pharyngeal wall variations may be important also for vocal fold oscillation because they could create a greater pressure difference across the vocal folds producing oscillation. McGowan also suggests that the subglottal air pressures during the production of tongue trills may be greater than during normal phonation, again creating a greater force for vocal fold oscillation. There are little research data to substantiate these claims but clinical experience suggests that the technique is a very useful one which is capable of eliciting improved voice in many patients. In the patient with postoperative scarring of the vocal folds, the increased stiffness of the cover interferes with vibratory behavior. The trill appears to have the potential to reduce the effect of the stiffness probably because of the forceful but healthy vibratory behavior.*

## Pitch Extension Exercises

This technique focuses on extending the pitch range in patients who experience difficulty with restricted range. It should only be used with patients who do not have vocal fold pathology such as nodules, polyps, cysts, hemorrhage, etc. Although restricted pitch range is a characteristic sign accompanying those pathologies, the presence of the lesions acts to impede the laryngeal adjustments necessary for production of a full pitch range. When the pathology is resolved those patients generally regain a full pitch range without any therapeutic attention specifically directed to that skill. Those patients for whom the pitch extension exercises seem most appropriate and effective are those whose restricted range is due to stiffening of the vocal fold cover (as in a scar), rigidity of the entire phonatory system including vocal folds (as in some Parkinson's patients), hypofunction (as in presbyphonia), and hyperfunction or musculoskeletal tension. It is important to make certain that this activity is done in a gentle manner free of strain. The patient is instructed in producing a sustained vowel (or the syllable /la/) at a comfortable pitch level. When that is established the patient is instructed to sing one or two notes up the scale. How far this is extended depends on the patient's capabilities. Singing up and down these several notes, and perhaps extending the pitch range downward as well is used as practice material to be done several times per day. The range is extended gradually as the patient demonstrates the ability to do so.

*Rationale: The act of raising pitch, when done without strain, usually involves the elongation of the vocal folds, thereby thinning the mass and placing it under greater tension. Patients with scarred vocal folds usually have an area of stiffness of the cover that does not vibrate well. Stiffness is a characteristic of scar tissue. The intent of this exercise is to encourage active stretching of the folds, thus a stretching of the scarred area as well. This, in turn, should increase the flexibility of the scarred vocal fold and improve its vibratory behavior. In persons with Parkinson's disease, this exercise is designed to counteract the tendency toward monotonic voice production as the neurological control of the entire laryngeal mechanism becomes increasingly impaired. Patients who present with presbyphonia and those with other hypofunctional voice disorders benefit from vocal activities that increase the work of the phonatory mechanism.*

## Chewing

The act of chewing as a therapy technique was described by Froeschels in 1952. The technique requires that the patient practice the motions of chewing in an exaggerated manner and then sequentially, over time, add voicing, random sounds, words, phrases, sentences, and conversation while gradually reducing the degree of exaggeration of the mouth movements. As the technique is described, it is very important to help the patient imitate the chewing act quite exactly. This must involve constant movement of the tongue. Exaggeration of the act requires that the mouth be open while chewing. The resulting sounds produced when the activity is carried out correctly should be very variable. If the sound produced tends to be a repetitive, unchanging "yam yam," the chewing is being done with inadequate tongue movement. It has been our experience that it is often difficult for patients to learn to do this chewing. As with yawning, we have been socialized into chewing as unobtrusively as possible, and certainly with the mouth closed. If this technique is to be used, the clinician must be adept at and comfortable with modeling it for the patient. It is often helpful for the clinician to do the activity along with the patient, thereby reducing self-consciousness. The use of chewable substances can help the patient identify the components of the chewing act.

It then becomes somewhat easier to carry out that activity based on recall and imagery and without the actual substance in the mouth. (It is not a good idea for the clinician to provide chewable material. Instead, the clinician should suggest that the patient bring crackers, gum, or other chewable foods to the therapy session.) Each step of chewing as a therapy approach must be mastered before the next level is introduced. Thus, the patient must learn to chew in the most exaggerated manner while producing voicing and random sounds before being asked to practice words. It is important to realize that articulatory clarity will be reduced in the early stages of using this technique as the focus remains on the chewing motion. Use of words and phrases that begin with vowels may be the easiest to begin practice. As the patient progresses and longer utterances are introduced, the chewing motions are almost eliminated, but excess tensions associated with phonation should not be evident.

*Rationale: In adopting this technique, Froeschels sought a natural vegetative movement onto which phonation could be added without changing the totality of the act and without adding tensions or other negative behaviors the patient had habituated into the speaking act. The chewing motion has a tendency to release excess tensions in the vocal tract and laryngeal area, and when done correctly encourages mouth opening and reduction of mandibular tensions. These behaviors in turn foster easy onset of phonation without making that a specific focus of attention.*

## Chant-Talk

The name of this technique describes a manner of speaking that is a cross between speaking and singing or, from the singer's point of view, a form of singing that is a cross between singing and speaking. We tend to think of it as having limited frequency variability while retaining the flow of song. It can be used as a therapeutic technique in a number of different ways. Most simply, the patient can be asked to chant an utterance rather than speak it. If this is effective in eliciting effortless phonation of a good quality, the technique can be extended in practice with gradual reduction of the singsong quality of the chant. If a particular "voice placement" or "focus" is sought, this chanting can be one of a variety of ways of finding that focus. For example, using Cooper's "um-hum" technique (1973; see also the "um-hum" therapy technique described later), the patient may be asked to sustain that sound and chant the counting of numbers, or series of words or a sentence. It may be helpful for some patients to locate and identify the desired vocal sound through this chanting approach.

*Rationale: The chanting of an utterance encourages an easy flow of phonation, reducing the tendency toward hard glottal attack and increased force of vocal fold contact. Voicing flows continuously rather than the start/stop of speech. There may be some increased proprioceptive feedback as vibrations are felt through the nose and cheek areas, thus helping the patient to reduce focus on the larynx. It is also felt that if the voice is produced in this manner, there is usually a reduction in laryngeal and vocal tract tensions. Because chanting differs from talking and is usually a new way for patients to produce voice, it may be easier for them to alter voice production through this activity than to attempt to do so in speaking, wherein the habits are entrenched.*

## Hum and Nasal Consonants

This is another technique designed to teach easy voice production through a "natural" approach. The patient is asked to produce a hum and to be able to feel the resonance of that hum in the nose and cheeks. The pitch of the voice is generally not of direct concern, although it may seem to change as the patient searches for an easily produced, fully resonant sound. The hum is sustained, and the patient practices this until the target sound is produced without difficulty. It is often instructive to then ask the patient to lower and elevate the mandible, keeping the lips closed while sustaining the hum. This results in an almost palpable forward movement of the focus of the voice, with a tickling sensation often being reported around the lips and along the alveolar ridge of the palate. One of the authors was instructed by a voice coach to "hook" the sound in the back of the throat in order to master this kind of voice quality. The sound used for practice was the /ng/. Bear in mind that the sound being sought is not a nasal sound but rather a sound that might best be described as the "twang" that is typical of Country Western singing (Colton & Estill, 1981). Gradually the production of these sounds is shaped into speech by first using nonsense syllables and words heavily loaded with the nasal consonants. Although the early practice of this technique may result in greater nasal resonance than is desirable, that is temporary and normalizes as speech is introduced. This technique can easily be combined with the chant-talk technique.

    *Rationale: As described in the rationale for chant-talk, the act of humming is different from speaking and thus may not be encumbered with undesirable habituated behaviors. A hum encourages easy initiation of phonation and provides proprioceptive feedback of nasal and facial vibration, thus refocusing the patient's preoccupation with the laryngeal area. The continuant nasal consonant promotes ease of sustained phonation, and it can easily be coordinated with the idea of smooth airflow from inhalation through exhalation. The "twang" sound also elicits a mode of vocal fold vibration that produces a greater number of harmonics and thus a richer sound (Colton & Estill, 1981).*

## Vocal Function Exercise Program

Stemple, Glaze, and Gerdeman (1995) propose a specific program of exercises that are reported to be efficacious in the treatment of various voice disorders. Specifically, patients are instructed in four exercises and required to practice them several times a day: (*a*) sustaining the vowel /ee/ on the note F above middle C for females and below middle C for males softly and for as long as the person is capable of sustaining the voiceless /s/; (*b*) producing the word "knoll" starting on a high pitch and allowing the pitch to glide down while still holding on to the word; (*c*) the same as (b) but in reverse, starting low and gliding high; and (*d*) sustaining the vowel /o/ softly on the following notes: C, D, E, F, and G begining on middle C for females and an octave lower for males.

    *Rationale: The authors state that many etiological factors may be responsible for weakening, straining, and creating imbalance of the laryngeal mechanism. These exercises are felt to address these areas and provide a systematic exercise program to restore balance, strength, and ease of phonation.*

## Digital Manipulation, Pressure, and Massage

Aronson (1985) has described a technique that involves direct physical manipulation and massage of the laryngeal area. The clinician must identify the tips of the hyoid bone and exert light pressure in a circular motion in that area. The clinician then moves the fingers into the thyrohyoid space and carries out the circular motion massage, moving posteriorly from the thyroid notch area. The massage is then done on the posterior borders of the thyroid cartilage. With the fingers along the superior border of the thyroid cartilage, the clinician begins to gently exert pressure in a downward manner in order to move the larynx down. There should be an increase in the thyrohyoid space. During these maneuvers the patient is asked to phonate vowels.

When a positive change in the voice is noted (clearer quality and lowered pitch), the focus shifts to the production of that voice with, and then without, the manipulation. This entire activity needs to be carried out with care and with recognition that some pain might result. Patients must be reassured that the pain is temporary and is like any muscular pain associated with excessive tension and its reduction through direct manipulation and massage. According to Aronson, this technique may be effective in eliciting normal voice in a single therapy session in cases of dysphonia due to increased musculoskeletal tensions. However, when the condition has been of long standing, a longer course of treatment using this technique may be necessary.

Nelson Roy has recently described the use of this technique and reported data on its efficacy (Roy, 1994; Roy & Leeper, 1993; Roy, Tasko, & Harvey, 1995; Tasko, Roy, & Harvey, 1994). Roy confirms the finding that many patients are able to achieve normal voice in a single therapy session. The diagnoses of the patients so treated fall primarily into two categories, i.e., musculoskeletal tension and functional or psychogenic disorder. He states that 88% of the patients in his study population reported pain on palpation of the laryngeal area often radiating to the ear. His description of the technique begins with palpation of the laryngeal area to determine the degree and location of tension and pain, the mobility of the larynx in the vertical dimension, and the extent of laryngeal elevation. The technique is otherwise as described above.

**Rationale:** *This technique is based on the need to reduce "cramping" in the extrinsic and intrinsic laryngeal muscles, which is believed to be the cause of dysphonia in many patients. The massaging of muscles induces relaxation, and the technique promotes a lowered laryngeal position, permitting ease of phonation. In using this technique, it is particularly important that the clinician understand and be able to identify the specific disturbance of phonatory physiology exhibited by a patient. Many but not all voice patients who are classified as having a hyperfunctional voice disorder speak with the larynx in an elevated posture. Care must be taken not to exert undue effort in pushing the larynx lower than is comfortable for the patient.*

Boone (1983) has described a method of digital pressure that is very different in both intent and technique from that described above. Boone suggests that digital pressure be applied as a gentle inward push on the anterior aspect of the thyroid cartilage while a patient sustains a vowel. This pressure should result in lowered fundamental frequency and can be used to elicit and then habituate this lowered pitch, when that is a therapeutic goal.

**Rationale:** *Applying pressure as described tilts the thyroid cartilage posteriorly and in so doing shortens vocal fold length and increases mass. This then results in a lowered fundamental frequency of vibration, perceived as lowered pitch. Once elicited in this manner, the lowered pitch becomes the target to be practiced and produced voluntarily.*

## Easy Production of Falsetto or High Pitched Sounds

This technique is yet another one that tends to shift the patient away from habituated patterns of voice use. It is especially helpful for patients who demonstrate anteroposterior laryngeal squeezing and for some who are said to be using ventricular phonation. It may require trial and error and much suggestion on the part of the clinician to facilitate the patient's ability to produce a high pitched sound. The use of imagery can be very helpful (see "Imagery" below) as can the use of animal sounds, such as the meow of a kitten or a wolf howl. It is important to observe that there is a continuous flow from inhalation through exhalation, as the patient may have the tendency to increase tension and hold the breath prior to initiation of voicing. When the patient learns to easily produce the high pitched vowels at will, that sound can be sustained and the pitch gradually lowered in a glissando to the comfortable speaking level, without a change in voice quality. The patient is then asked to produce a sustained vowel at that targeted speaking pitch, maintaining the improved quality. As this is established, it can be shaped into speech. There is no attempt to specify a pitch level beyond that which is identified by the patient as comfortable and normal sounding.

*Rationale: Easy production of the upper frequency range is most commonly produced by a lengthening of the vocal folds, decreasing their mass. It cannot be done using ventricular phonation, for example. Therefore, if a high pitched sound is elicited from a patient who has been using ventricular phonation, the technique has successfully shifted the patient out of that phonatory mode. The same rationale may be applied to patients who tend to constrict the larynx in the anteroposterior dimension or to those whose aberrant voice production behaviors are psychologically based. Patients with psychogenic voice problems have "learned" a particular manner of phonation that produces their aberrant sound. If they are asked to produce sound in some novel way, they often must abandon their "learned" method and in so doing normal voice may be elicited. Thus, the change in laryngeal physiology from their particular behavior to that required for the production of the upper frequency range, if successful, may be sufficient to restore normal phonatory function, which can then be maintained as pitch is normalized.*

## Imagery

The use of imagery can be very helpful in describing how a particular type of sound should be produced. For example, statements of imagery such as "Make it feel as if your voice is floating effortlessly out of your throat and up into your head" can describe to the patient a way that effortless voicing might feel. Patients should be encouraged to provide their own imagery as they release tensions and change their manner of initiating phonation. The use of imagery can be combined with many of the other techniques, as it can help patients keep in mind what they are attempting to do. Imagery is often used in those techniques designated by some as "placing the voice" or finding a "focus" for the voice. It has been reported that professional singers and actors use imagery concerning their breathing, which although often in contradiction to known physiological fact, works well for them (Hixon, 1987; Watson, Hixon, & Maher, 1987).

*Rationale: The physiology of imagery is receiving increasing attention as its use grows in the training of athletes and in fighting disease (Keaton, 1983; Ungerleider, 1986). It has been used in singing pedagogy for many years, and its effectiveness is perhaps attested to by legions of superb performers. We use it in voice therapy to help a patient understand something about how to produce voice or what quality to attempt to produce, when other types of explanations are either not possible or have not been effective. Imagery, although perhaps not physiologically correct, can describe what seems to happen in a very subjective, sensory way. It is important that both the clinician and the patient recognize that the imagery being used is a means to an end, not necessarily an accurate explanation of the desired physiology.*

## Pushing, Pulling, Isometrics

These techniques are placed together because they are used interchangeably to produce the same end result. Pushing refers to any of the many ways that patients may be encouraged to push against the wall, push down on the chair, and so on, while pulling refers to the opposite maneuvers of pulling up on a very heavy desk, pulling up on the chair one is sitting in, and the like. Isometric forms of these activities include placing the palms of the hands together at chest height and pressing them together or locking the fingers of the hands together at chest height and pulling them apart. Whichever method is used, the patient is instructed to phonate at the point of maximum pull or push. The sound produced will be a forceful grunt and should be demonstrated by the clinician. All of the varieties of these techniques are designed to force effort closure of the glottis, a form of hyperfunction of the mechanism. They can often be used with surprising success in eliciting a low pitched phonation in cases of puberphonia and in eliciting voicing in patients who present with psychogenic aphonia. Once the patient has learned to carry out the push or pull, the same effect can be obtained by holding the breath, bearing down, and grunting. As the desired voicing is produced, the patient is instructed to sustain that sound as the force of the maneuver is gradually released. In a gradual stepwise fashion, the targeted sound is practiced with less and less need for the forceful push or pull activity.

Because these activities enforce a certain behavior on the larynx, patients with psychogenic problems also may have difficulty holding on to their typical mode of voice production. Thus through the use of push, pull, or isometric activities these patients may find an acceptable way to abandon their symptom and produce voice in a more typical fashion.

*Rationale: These maneuvers are designed to create effort closure of the glottis with the larynx in a lowered position. As such they are the opposite of hypofunction. Furthermore, the posture of the laryngeal mechanism is determined by the activity and dictates a particular type of vocalization. This shifts the individual from the usual manner of vocal production and introduces a behavior difficult to counteract. If tension is released prior to phonation, then the technique will be ineffective. Traditionally these types of procedures have been recommended for use in cases of unilateral vocal fold paralysis. The rationale has been that the effort closure forces a crossing of the midline of the unaffected vocal fold to approximate the paralyzed fold. Further discussion of this topic will be found later in this chapter under "Unresolved Issues and Myths." As noted earlier, we have found these techniques to be effective in eliciting a low pitched voice from patients with puberphonia. The vocal fold and laryngeal postures that naturally occur in the use of these techniques are incompatible with anything but a low pitched voice, if they are being done correctly.*

Although these techniques are potentially useful, there is a caveat. By their nature they induce hyperfunction and thus are potentially abusive. They should therefore, be used judiciously. We have found that their effectiveness will be noted fairly quickly, if indeed they are going to be effective. Thus, it is usually not necessary to prolong their use. When assigned for home practice, the amount of time involved should be clearly specified. These effort closure techniques should be used cautiously and sparingly in recognition of their potentially abusive nature.

## *Laughing, Coughing, Throat Clearing, Gargling, and Other Reflexive Acts*

In the attempt to elicit voice from the aphonic patient or to find a normal voice for the dysphonic patient when there are no positive laryngologic findings, the use of any of the above can be extremely effective. Indeed, it is important for the clinician to listen for spontaneous laughing, coughing, vocalized pauses, or throat clearing during general conversation with the patient. Patients are not aware that the mechanism used for producing the above sounds is the same as is used for producing the speaking voice. Thus, such sounds may be heard during conversation or even when the patient is asked to produce them. The skilled clinician can make use of that sound by shaping it into speech in a gradual manner. This technique may occasionally be startlingly effective. However, it may also be ineffective with some who will continue to use dysphonic voice or no voice in response to a direct request even though they may have produced such sounds spontaneously. Again, it takes the skill of the clinician to utilize all instances of good voicing to reestablish normal voice.

*Rationale: These behaviors are so automatic that the patient may perform them unaware that voice is being produced. Thus, they may be produced with a much better sound than is heard in speech. Because they are not speech behaviors, their production may be free of habituated but undesirable phonatory speech behaviors. The inability to elicit an improved voice using these behaviors also may be a meaningful finding. It may suggest that the patient is somewhat resistant to "giving up" the bad voice, or perhaps there is a problem present that has not been identified. Certainly what it means is that further exploration is necessary both for ways to elicit voice and/or for the etiology of the problem. Although throat clearing and coughing can be abusive to the laryngeal mechanism, and are thus not recommended for extensive therapeutic use, they can be used judiciously in the search for normal voicing.*

### "Um-Hum"

In this technique the patient is instructed to say "um-hum," the vocalized utterance used by a listener to indicate agreement with the speaker, in a naturally spontaneous and sincere manner. There is a deceptive simplicity to this technique and the clinician must be sure to elicit a very natural production of "um hum." This is difficult for some persons to do when it becomes a conscious and voluntary utterance. When it is captured in a natural manner, the production is then shaped by adding single words, as in "um-hum one." Gradually this is extended through the use of increasingly longer utterances until the patient is able to produce the targeted voice without needing the starting "um-hum."

*Rationale: According to Cooper (1984) this simple utterance, if said as naturally as possible, results in producing a voice at the appropriate pitch level and with the correct focus for the individual. Vibration should be perceptible along the bridge and sides of the nose and down to the lips. This technique, similar to the preceding one, capitalizes on a phonatory act that is almost reflexive in nature. The fact that a nasal component is present in the consonant /m/ adds to the appropriate focusing of the voice.*

### Whispering

Whispering is the act of moving the articulators to form words in the presence of rapid airflow but the absence of phonation. Very little instruction is usually required to elicit whispering. A quiet, unforced whisper can be used when vocal rest or minimal voice use is part of the treatment plan. It is sometimes instructive to ask patients who habitually use excessive loudness to limit themselves to a quiet whisper for part (or parts) of each day. The pronounced contrast between the whisper and the habitual loudness level may help to focus the patient's awareness and to make reducing loudness to an acceptable level easier to accomplish.

*Rationale: Despite many caveats in the literature that whispering is harmful, there is no experimental evidence to support that notion. Indeed, there is evidence that suggests otherwise. This issue is addressed more completely in the section "Unresolved Issues and Myths." An unforced whisper by definition is an absence of phonation. This suggests that the vocal folds are not fully adducting and thus collision forces are reduced. Gentle airflow is present and there should be an absence of tensions.*

### Breathing

It is sometimes helpful for direct attention to be paid to respiration. By focusing on the breathing, tensions that may be generalized throughout the chest as well as the larynx and vocal tract can be reduced. Patients should be instructed as simply as possible to sit at rest and allow their breathing to function normally. Remember that the diaphragm is a muscle of inhalation and is active during the inspiratory cycle (Fig. 9.2). But at high lung volumes it may be necessary to contract the diaphragm in order to prevent the rapid, unwanted descent of the rib cage, producing greater than needed subglottal pressures that will produce louder and uncontrolled voice production. As shown in Figure 9.2, a number of muscles are activated during a speaking event. At high lung volumes, the muscles activated will be inspiratory, but as lung volume falls, expiratory musculature will be needed to provide the proper air pressure to drive the vocal folds. Excess muscle activity in the respiratory musculature will prevent the smooth coordination of the respiratory system and the steady maintenance of subglottal air pressure and phonation.

The clinician should observe the patient's breathing pattern at rest and, assuming that it is normal, instruct the patient to gently place one hand on the area of the abdomen (diaphragm) and the other on the upper chest, while continuing to breathe quietly. The patient should be able to identify slight outward movement of the abdomen (diaphragm) area on inhalation with imperceptible movement of the upper chest. The patient's attention also needs to be directed to the continuous movement in the respiratory cycle from inspiration through expiration. If the patient exhibits a breathing pattern at rest and in general conversation that seems aberrant, additional attention needs to be addressed to pulmonary function in general. As soon as the effortless breathing has been established, the patient should be instructed to breathe in a little more deeply and to release the exhalatory cycle as a sigh without changing the manner of breathing. It should be sufficient to instruct the patient to fill the body with air. Thus, the focus on breathing leads easily into incorporation of the sigh, the yawn-sigh, aspirate initiation of phonation, and so on. As the patient learns to do these activities easily, the task can continue to be altered so that the inhalatory stage of breathing occurs more quickly, as it does normally during speech, while the exhalatory stage is lengthened. When adding the latter refinement, it is important that the patient not introduce tensions and attempts to extend exhalation beyond the available air supply. The clinician must determine whether the work on breathing has helped the patient to also reduce or eliminate laryngeal tensions. It is important that the patient be instructed in the generalization of the improved respiratory control to conversational speech. The clinician must remember that average conversational utterances on one continuous respiration tend to be very short, about 5 seconds (Boone & McFarlane, 1988), and that, therefore, nonprofessional voice users do not need to inhale as deeply as do professional voice users in singing, acting, or public speaking. The amount of therapeutic time devoted to work on breathing and, indeed, the need for any such attention, must be decided on a case-by-case basis.

Extended training in breath support and breath control is important for the professional voice user. Many activities or exercises can be designed to accomplish this, but they are beyond the scope of this book. It is important to note, however, that any such exercises must be done with an understanding of respiratory physiology and recognition of the need to build control in a gradual way, as in any activity of muscle building and training.

**Rationale:** *The respiratory system is the power source for the voice. The systems involved in phonation are closely intertwined, and tensions in one system cannot easily be isolated from the rest. Thus, reducing respiratory tensions and assuring continuous airflow from inspiration through expiration assists in reducing laryngeal tensions and avoiding closure of the glottis prior to the initiation of phonation. Most patients, with the exception of those who have chronic respiratory problems, chronic obstructive lung disease or neuromotor impairment of the control of respiration, tend to have normal respiration and adequate air supply for speech. This topic*

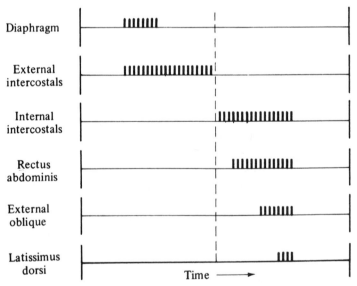

*Figure 9.2.* In the upper portion of this figure are shown the lung volume-muscle pressure relationships during the production of a sustained vowel. At high lung volumes, a large amount of inspiratory muscle pressure is needed to counteract the large lung pressures that are created. As lung volume decreases, less inspiratory effort is needed, until resting lung volume is reached (point where the curve crosses the vertical line in the middle of the graph). At still lower lung volumes, expiratory muscle effort is needed to produce the necessary subglottal pressures for speech. In the panel below, a schematic of muscle activity in the diaphragm, external intercostals, internal intercostals, rectus abdominis, external oblique, and latissimus dorsi is shown in relationship to the pressure relationships shown above.

*will be discussed later in "Unresolved Issues and Myths." Singers, actors, and other professional voice users may have demands placed on voice use that require greater control of increased volumes of air. This group of voice users will need more extended training in the management of breath support and breath control than the average speaker.*

## Relaxation

A variety of techniques are used to teach generalized relaxation. These include progressive relaxation in which the patient is instructed to concentrate on specific parts of the body one at a time and then through imagery and suggestion to release the tensions present (Jacobson, 1938). Another part of the technique involves purposefully tensing a specific body area, followed by a release of that tension. Imagery is often used in teaching relaxation and deep breathing exercises are frequently incorporated as well. The shoulders, upper back and neck are very vulnerable to muscle tightening in tense individuals (Nagler, 1987). A popular activity for relaxation of these tensions has been the head roll, in which the patient is instructed to very, very slowly allow the head to be rotated 360 degrees. However, it has been suggested that circular rotation of any part of the spine may not be helpful to the intervertebral disks, and the following exercises are recommended instead (Nagler, 1987):

1. While holding the left elbow in the right hand, pull it over to the right side, hold, then relax. Do the same with the other arm, and repeat the sequence three times for each arm.
2. Place the hands, palms in, on the upper chest, with elbows out to the sides. Circle the elbows in one direction and then reverse. Repeat three times.

**Rationale:** *The rationale for engaging in relaxation therapy as one segment of a vocal rehabilitation program is primarily to release excess tensions in systems involved with phonation. However, it must be recognized that most of our talking is done in states other than complete relaxation. Thus, it is important to use these techniques in specific ways and then to incorporate them into healthy patterns of phonation.*

## Phonating on Inhalation

The technique for creating voice in this way is just as described by the title. The patient is instructed and shown how to make sound in the reverse of the normal pattern, that is, as air is being drawn into the lungs. This is usually a fairly simple sound for most people to make. The most common use of this technique involves practice in going directly from the voice produced on inhalation into voice produced on exhalation. If this technique is successful in eliciting an improved voice quality in the exhalatory phase, then it can be continued with gradual reduction in the need to start the phonation on inhalation. This technique has been described for use with patients exhibiting ventricular fold phonation.

Another use of inspiratory speech has been described by Harrison et al. (1992) in a patient with spasmodic dysphonia. The technique of speaking on inhalation differs from that described above in that there is no attempt to transfer from the phonation produced on inhalation to similar phonation on exhalation. Rather, the focus here is on learning to use inspiratory speech to replace expiratory speech, to establish the inspiratory speech as the habitual pattern. Harrison et al. (1992) describe a patient with adductor spasmodic dysphonia who had discovered that he could produce speech during inhalation in a much more fluent and less effortful manner than his spasmodic speech. He adopted that form of speech, which was judged to be perceptually somewhat rough but intelligible and more acceptable to listeners than the strain/struggle interrupted spasmodic speech. One of the authors of the Harrison et al. paper was able to learn the inhalatory form of speech with relative ease although the authors recognize that may not be the case for all patients. Nevertheless, it is offered as an alternative to other methods of treatment for patients with spasmodic dysphonia. Use of this type of phonation for spasmodic dysphonia has been described by others through informal contacts (Freeman, Shulman, personal communication). It is a noninvasive form of treatment which, if successfully learned, may offer more consistent voice to the patient, albeit somewhat hoarse, than the improved-to-worsening cycle experienced by patients requiring periodic BoTox injection.

*Rationale: Voice produced on inhalation is said to be produced by the true vocal folds (Lehmann, 1965; Williams, Farquharson, & Anthony, 1975). Thus, in patients who are using ventricular fold phonation or those who are improperly using the vocal folds, it is theorized that this technique will stimulate more appropriate physiology. In the pattern of inspiratory speech described by Harrison et al. (1992), the vocal folds were not fully approximated and the authors believe that a posterior gap was present although not fully visible. Clearly this laryngeal posture differs from the abducted folds that we expect to see on inhalation. The authors suggest that contraction of the cricothyroid muscle, which begins along with the diaphragm, an involuntary action which is not likely to be accessible to voluntary control, may serve as a counter to the adductory forces of the laryngeal muscles, thereby reducing the force of vocal fold approximation and allowing for fluent speech. A second explanation offered by the authors has to do with the respiratory reflexes of the larynx, which may be abnormal in persons with spasmodic dysphonia.*

## Vocal Hygiene

This category will include techniques that should be incorporated into most voice therapy programs. Vocal hygiene may constitute the entire rehabilitation program, or it may be but one part of the program. In most instances of misuse and abuse of the voice, it should be a routine part of the program, and training in vocal hygiene as a preventive measure should be the final stage of voice therapy after a successful outcome has been attained (Fig. 9.3). Morrison and Rammage (1994) provide a useful listing of dos and don'ts and helpful hints about vocal hygiene.

### REDUCING THE AMOUNT OF TALKING

Patients who are excessive talkers, those who have a tendency toward vocal abuse or vocal fatigue, those who have undergone laryngeal surgery, and certainly those involved in voice therapy for conditions associated with misuse or abuse with or without tissue change, should be counseled about the need to significantly curtail their voice use, i.e., talking. This restriction may be necessary for perhaps only a specified period of time. This is sometimes referred to as modified vocal rest. Instructions should be as detailed as needed and should include all restrictions on voice use. If patients are able to eliminate all but essential talking, that is usually sufficient. Additional restrictions having to do with loudness of voice will tend to further reduce voice usage because of the limitations imposed by environmental noise levels. It may be helpful to use therapy time to work out a plan for where and when the voice will have to be used. Other behavior modification approaches, such as charting when, where, and for how long voice is used, may help accomplish this reduction in the amount of talking. The topic of complete voice rest will be discussed in greater detail in "Unresolved Issues and Myths."

*Figure 9.3.* Vocal hygiene.

## REDUCING LOUDNESS

This may involve eliminating all use of the voice when the ambient noise level requires a vocal intensity level above that permitted by a soft breathy voice. Such a restriction will not allow yelling for the dog or for children playing outside or upstairs; it will not allow talking in a car, above a television or radio, above machinery or other noise in an employment setting, at a cocktail party, or in a bar with loud music playing, and so on. Such reduction of loudness is necessary when there have been mucosal changes, whether evidenced by inflammation, edema, or vocal nodules.

There are some patients whose primary vocal abuse is the routine use of excessive loudness. This often requires different techniques and is not an easy pattern to alter. We all have a vocal image in our minds, which includes a loudness level. Patients who are excessively loud often do not believe that people will be able to hear them if they speak more softly. They must be willing to test whether this is the case by engaging in intensity reduction activities. Devices that provide visual or auditory feedback can be extremely helpful in establishing an acceptable level of loudness. A useful device known as the Voice Intensity Controller (VIC, Behavioral Controls, Inc.) is small enough to be worn by the patient and preset to beep when a specific loudness level has been exceeded. Visual feedback of loudness can also be provided with the use of the Visi-Pitch (Kay Elemetrics Corp.), the Vocal Loudness Indicator (LinguiSystems), or a number of computerized programs that permit online imaging of the voice signal.

## IDENTIFYING AND REDUCING OR ELIMINATING VOCAL ABUSE

All potentially abusive vocal use or other abusive behaviors detrimental to laryngeal health should be identified and eliminated if possible, or at least reduced to a minimum. Exploration of abuses needs to be very thorough. Abuses may include smoking of legal or illegal substances; use of certain drugs; spending large amounts of time in dry, dusty, or smoke-filled environments; exposure to airborne irritants; frequent habitual throat clearing; constant cough; excessive drinking of alcoholic beverages; as well as the abusive behaviors of excessive talking, excessive loudness, and excessive strain discussed elsewhere. All identified abuses need to be discussed, and specific plans need to be made as to how they will be reduced or eliminated. Patients should be required to monitor their performance on the agreed upon plan.

### ENVIRONMENTAL MANIPULATION

Whenever it seems appropriate, changes can be made in the environment to help patients function with reduced voice use or to make the environment itself more hospitable. For example, humidification can be increased by the use of room humidifiers, amplification can be used when there are demands on vocal loudness, whistles or bells can be adopted by teachers to obtain attention in place of typically loud voice use, the television volume can be muted when it is necessary to talk, and so on. Creativity is sometimes required in order to plan environmental changes. People may be resistant to changing their habitual modes of functioning. It is often necessary to work through this resistance and for the clinician to find ways to encourage patients to adopt the plans and give them a fair trial.

The need for adequate moisturization and humidification of the upper respiratory tract should also be discussed as part of a vocal hygiene program. Conditions that may deter and interfere with good levels of environmental humidity should be explored. These might include the use of wood stoves for home heating, a work environment that is extremely dry or dust-filled (e.g., old school buildings, theaters), extensive airplane travel, and others. When such conditions exist it becomes the individual's responsibility to take whatever remedial or compensatory actions possible, such as using room humidifiers or increasing liquid intake.

At the successful conclusion of a therapy program with voice restored to its normal state, patients should be advised about monitoring their vocal health and appropriate actions to take. Because hoarseness may accompany an upper respiratory infection or may result from an evening's overuse, patients need to understand that it need not signal a recurrence of the initial problem. However, they should be advised to immediately restrict voice use and loudness and increase liquid intake. They, of course, should follow any additional course of treatment prescribed by their physician for the condition. If such hoarseness persists for more than a week, or if it persists beyond the resolution of other symptoms of upper respiratory infection, it would be advisable to return for laryngological examination.

*Rationale: The rationale for all of the above is to help patients engage in those activities and behaviors that foster laryngeal and vocal health. Several of them serve to reduce either the force or the amount of vocal fold contact, or both. In so doing, they potentially eliminate irritation of the mucosa and change, reduce, or eliminate habitually abusive behaviors. Others have to do with maintaining the healthiest possible conditions for the mechanism to work well. Prevention of recurrence is certainly a major reason for employing these vocal hygiene procedures.*

## Energizing the Voice

This technique is a difficult one to describe because of the abstractness of the concept. It is perhaps analogous to the car engine that is chugging along on only three spark plugs rather than all six. It is akin to the desire to "set a match" under someone who is too low keyed, too subdued and laid back. It is appropriate for use with patients who are known to have normal metabolic states and a normal ear, nose, and throat examination and who are not psychiatrically depressed. It includes (*a*) the use of adequate mouth opening and movement of the articulators, (*b*) the use of more inflection or variability of pitch, (*c*) the use of adequate loudness level and increased variability of loudness as appropriate to mark meaning, and (*d*) the use of a "well-placed" and well-supported (respiration) voice. Many methods can be used to accomplish this energization of the voice. They will vary depending on the age, personality, and speaking needs of the patient. The use of scripted material from plays or other sources can be helpful, as can exercises such as practicing the role of a drill sergeant, calling out cadences, practicing in a large room, moving and using the whole body while counting, and so forth. Care must be taken so that the patient does not simply begin to shout. Whatever exercise or material is used, the patient must have specific goals that have been explained and practiced at lower levels of difficulty first. Many of these activities are often better carried out with the patient and the clinician standing some distance away from each other. Increasing mouth opening requires much work and practice. It is often helpful for the patient to practice very exaggerated movements first while receiving feedback from a mirror. The exaggeration is reduced gradually to the point where oral use is adequate. At that point, the increased mouth opening should no longer feel unusual or bizarre to the patient. Variability in pitch and loudness can be aided by the use of instruments that provide visual feedback (Visi-Pitch, computer programs, etc.) until such time as the patient has improved auditory sensitivity to and discrimination of these parameters.

*Rationale: Some patients complain about having "weak" voices that do not carry, that do not convey the desired image, and that seem to fatigue as the day goes by. In the absence of hormonal imbalance, serious psychiatric problems, laryngeal abnormality, or other organic problems, it is most likely that the problem lies in the way in which the person has learned to speak. These are behaviors that should be accessible to change. The activities described above address the types of speech patterns often seen in patients with these complaints and are designed to introduce changes in those patterns. It is clear that personality factors may be heavily involved, and the clinician must always keep this in mind.*

## Vocal Effort

The concept and technique of measuring vocal effort was described in Chapter 7. It is a simple concept that can be adapted for use as a therapy technique. It requires that the patient assign a number to represent the amount of effort being expended in habitual speech. (The only stipulation is that the numbers used increase with an increase of effort.) In order to obtain a comparative scale for that patient, have him produce phonations at a minimum effort level, a comfortable effort level, and a maximum effort level. For example, if a patient complains of feeling that it is a strain to talk and assigns the number 17 to the degree of effort involved, but phonation with minimum effort is produced at a number 5, suggest that he talk with a degree of effort corresponding to a number 8 or 10. Patients can learn to internally monitor their effort levels and modify their behavior accordingly, thereby achieving an increased measure of control over phonation. They are able to experiment with how they produce sound in order to achieve a more efficient and vocally less tiring, and probably less abusive, mode of phonation. Yet another benefit of this technique is the ease with which progress can be tracked. After a period of use of either reduced or increased effort (whichever was the goal), patients can again be asked to assign a number to their habitual phonations. This can be compared to the previous judgment.

*Rationale: Because it has been determined that patients are able to estimate vocal effort and that their estimates are manifested acoustically by variation in sound pressure level and fundamental frequency (Colton & Brown, 1973; Wright & Colton, 1972a, 1972b), using that ability in a therapeutic manner is quite appropriate. This approach accomplishes its desired goals in a holistic manner without fragmenting the various components of producing voice. It is also a technique that is easy for patients to understand and to retain in memory, thereby increasing the likelihood that they will be able to put it to use. It does not require extensive practice and provides almost immediate reinforcement both through a sense of accomplishment and control and awareness of the reduction in strain.*

## The Resonant Voice

Resonant voice therapy is based on techniques used to improve voice production in actors and singers (Cooper, 1973; Lessac, 1987). It is a form of sound production that is based on "sensations on the alveolar ridge and other facial plates during phonation." It appears to result from a tuning of F1 to individual components of the glottal tone (Raphael & Scherer, 1987) or it may be a change in the source spectrum. It is produced with a slightly abducted vocal fold posture; thus, it should not be abusive. There are a variety of exercises that can be used to teach the technique although some patients may require a period of time to learn the desired sound.

Tone placement seems to be the main goal of the resonant therapy program (Lessac, 1987). Patients with dysphonic voices often report feeling the voice vibrating in the throat. In the resonant therapy program, the patient is taught to produce a more forward placement so that the sensations of voice production can be felt in the palate, tongue, and lips. The technique produces a sound that is louder and more easily heard in a noisy environment. Its disadvantages include the time to master the technique and a hesitancy on the part of patients to use what is to them such an unusual sound.

Verdolini-Marston, Burke, Lessac, Glaze, and Caldwell (1995) compared the resonant therapy technique to the confidential voice therapy technique described earlier in this chapter. Measures of phonatory effort, auditory-perceptual ratings of severity of dysphonia, and visual impressions of the appearance of the vocal folds were obtained from 13 patients with vocal fold nodules. Three patients comprised the resonant therapy group whereas 5 patients were part of the confidential therapy group. In addition, 5 patients received no therapy (control group). The results showed that both therapy programs improved the voice. Phonatory effort was reduced in both groups with little change in the control group. Two of the 5 patients in the confidential therapy group showed improvement on ratings of the severity of dysphonia whereas all 3 patients showed improvement in the resonant therapy group. Four of the 5 patients in the confidential therapy group showed visual changes in appearance of the nodule as viewed stroboscopically whereas 2 of the 3 patients in the resonant therapy groups showed similar changes. There were few changes on any of the measures studied for patients in the control group.

The authors of this study also reported that patient compliance was predictive of voice improvement, more so than the type of therapy program. Although preliminary, these results suggest that the resonant voice therapy approach is viable for the treatment of vocal fold nodules and perhaps similar lesions.

***Rationale:*** *It has been reported (Verdolini & Titze, 1995; Verdolini-Marston et al., 1995) that this type of phonation results in limited vocal fold adduction as compared to "pressed voice." It is theorized, therefore, that the impact forces of the vocal folds as they adduct are also reduced. Such an effect is desirable when attempting to change hyperfunctional voice behaviors. Despite the reduced adductory forces the voice remains strong.*

## Voice Therapy for Patients with Parkinson's Disease

Traditional speech therapy has been provided for patients with Parkinson's disease for many years and with less than resounding success. That therapy focused on rate of speech and on the dysarthric components as they affect articulation. However, several authors have reported therapeutic success by targeting phonation (Johnson & Pring, 1990; Ramig, Mead, Scherer, Horii, Larson & Kohler, 1988; Robertson & Thompson, 1984; Scott & Caird, 1983). Building on these beginnings, Ramig and her colleagues have developed and shown the efficacy of a very specific therapy protocol (Ramig, 1995; Ramig et al., 1994; Ramig & Scherer, 1992; Smith et al., 1994) called the Lee Silverman Voice Treatment program. While this program focuses entirely on phonation, improvement in clarity of articulation, rate, and overall intelligibility has been documented. Countryman, Ramig, and Pawlas (1994) studied the efficacy of this program with three patients diagnosed with Parkinson's plus syndromes. Patients so diagnosed often have more severely debilitating symptomatology and more rapidly progressive decline of function than those with idiopathic parkinsonism. Nevertheless, all three patients demonstrated improvement in overall speech intelligibility, functional communication and voice deficits. All three patients maintained some carryover above pretreatment levels at 6 months post-treatment.

The Lee Silverman Voice Treatment program is based on an intensive program of 4 individual sessions per week for 1 month during which loudness, maximum phonatory effort, high therapeutic effort, and voice awareness are targeted. The methods used include some of the techniques already described in this chapter as well as others as follows: maximum duration sustained loud phonation; maximum frequency range (sustained highest and lowest pitches); posture; and maximal loudness. Patient's receive immediate reinforcement from their productions. The method is simple, making it possible for patients to practice at home and to remember to incorporate the new learning into all speech events. Patients are advised to "think loud, think shout."

**Rationale:** *Vocal fold bowing and incomplete glottal closure are characteristic of the phonatory behavior of parkinsonian patients as is reduction in respiratory support. Some of the exercises are designed to increase vocal fold adduction. The high effort and stress on "maximum" performance are necessary to override the rigidity and hypokinesia of Parkinson's disease. The intensity of the therapy maintains consistency of the high effort over the course of a month. It is reinforcing for the patient as progress is seen thereby motivating him to continue to put forth the effort maximizing habituation and carry over.*

## Voice Therapy for Patients with Paradoxical Vocal Fold Motion (PVFM)

Treatment described by Florence Blager (Martin, Blager, Gay, & Wood, 1987) has been found to be effective with many patients who display PVFM. The therapy consists of

1. inhalation through the nose with lips closed
2. relaxed tongue posture
3. prolonged audible exhalation through pursed lips or production of /s/
4. diaphragmatic breathing with emphasis on exhalation

*Rationale: These activities focus the patient's attention on a breathing technique, thus reducing the tendency to panic and increase tension. Nasal rather than oral inhalation increases full glottal abduction and attention to exhalation helps relax the system.*

## Voice Therapy for the Patient with Presbyphonia

These are treatment approaches for those often described as the well elderly, people usually over 65 years of age who are in generally good health (in that they are not suffering from any progressive neurological problems), do not have severe emphysema or significant hearing loss, and can participate in general physical conditioning activities and have no laryngeal pathology.

The approaches to treatment with these patients can be similar to the therapy program described for parkinsonian patients but adapted to the needs of this population. Therapy need not be intensive, although patient practice and involvement in the treatment requires full effort. The concept of vocal effort can be incorporated into the therapy as can other techniques that "push" the system and are effective for hypofunctional voice disorders. Posture is an important consideration and respiratory support may need some attention. It has also been our experience that encouraging these individuals to become involved in a program of fitness conditioning or regular exercise, including some aerobic activities, is beneficial to the voice.

*Rationale: Biological aging is different from chronological aging. Some individuals who are age 65 or older are healthy, active, and seem younger than their years, while others of the same age may show very obvious signs of aging. These differences are also revealed in the voice (Ramig & Ringel, 1983). The voice described as presbyphonic is usually lacking in stability, as evidenced by increased aperiodicity and pitch breaks, reduced intensity, and a "muffled" quality lacking in resonance. The laryngeal or stroboscopic findings usually reveal glottic incompetence, reduced amplitude of excursion, and reduced mucosal wave. All of the activities described above should potentially "push" the system to greater performance, thereby increasing glottal competence and improving all other functions.*

## CRITERIA FOR TERMINATION OF THERAPY

When undertaking any treatment plan it is necessary to consider possible outcomes and how they are to be handled. In the current climate of accountability and stress on outcomes of treatment, documentation of the therapy process, beginning with the evaluation and all test data, is essential in helping to determine and to support the decision to continue or to terminate therapy. If comparison of the data reveals positive changes that can logically be attributed to the therapy although the desired endpoint has not been reached, it is possible to make a good case for continuation of the treatment plan. Furthermore, awareness of such progress can be effectively used to motivate the patient and inspire an added measure of confidence—confidence the patient has in the clinician and self-confidence the patient gains based on the progress made. If the data are negative, revealing essentially no change, the door is opened for discussion of possible reasons, and support is lent to the need for additional testing, examination, or in some instances, termination of therapy. The following sections will set forth some criteria for the termination of therapy.

## Elimination or Reduction of Vocally Asymptomatic Tissue Changes

For some patients, a significant reduction in the size, extent, or severity of mucosal pathology may lead to essentially normal voice. We have known of patients who, although totally asymptomatic for voice problems, were found (during routine ear, nose, and throat examination) to have vocal fold nodules. These patients were not only vocally asymptomatic at the time of the examination but denied experiencing any change in voice in the past. It appears that certain small lesions may be so situated as to have minimal effect on glottal closure or on mucosal vibratory behavior, leaving the voice perceptually unchanged. This then may also be the case with a patient who has reached a stage in therapy where the voice is normal-sounding and a complete vocal range has been restored despite the continued presence of some mucosal pathology. In the first example voice therapy may take the form of a single session in which vocal hygiene concepts are taught. In the second example vocal hygiene should be taught prior to termination of treatment in order to prevent a recurrence or worsening of the laryngeal condition. The patient who experiences full resolution and elimination of signs of pathology and return of good voice is obviously also a candidate for termination of voice therapy.

### Improved Voice of a Quality Acceptable to Patient

In clinical practice, a patient may experience a degree of improvement that is looked upon by the clinician as only a point along the road to the "best" voice but that is accepted by the patient as being totally adequate. This may be a form of resistance to therapy, or it may be related to the expense incurred in continuation of the therapy, or it may reflect the patient's view and expectation quite precisely. At some point it is important for the clinician to raise the self-directed question, "Whose needs am I interested in fulfilling, mine or this patient's?"

There are also many situations in which restoration of normal voice is not a realistic goal. For those patients, the attainment of an acceptable voice should signal the consideration of termination of therapy.

### Elimination of Physical Symptoms of Pain, Discomfort, and Fatigue

Patients sometimes complain of pain, discomfort, and fatigue associated with voice production more vigorously than they do of voice symptoms such as hoarseness and pitch breaks. Indeed, the voice symptoms may be fairly minimal perceptually. Thus, for such patients, the relief of pain, discomfort, and fatigue associated with phonation is the goal, and attainment of that goal may be the proper time to terminate therapy. Incidentally, when these symptoms are relieved, patients have usually changed phonatory behavior in ways that are also reflected in improved voice production.

### Habituation of Changed Vocal Behaviors with No Return of Symptoms

When a patient has fully adopted the desired vocal behaviors and no longer complains of any of the initial phonatory problems that brought him or her to treatment, therapy should be terminated.

### Lack of Improvement after an Appropriate Therapy Trial

Voice therapy is generally not a long term process. Some improvement should be perceptually discernible with most voice patients within a month of therapy, assuming at least one session per week and a patient who complies with the therapeutic protocol.

If that is not the case, the clinician should review the case thoroughly. Every attempt should be made to resist adopting the facile excuse that the patient is resistant to therapy and is not practicing. Indeed, that may sometimes be the case, but it is incumbent upon the clinician to fully explore all other possibilities as well. These may include an erroneous initial diagnosis, an inappropriate therapeutic approach, the presence of psychological factors that do not allow the patient to abandon a symptom, environmental or medical factors helping to maintain a problem that have not been identified or dealt with, or the presence of a condition that is not responsive to a voice therapy approach. Possible actions to be taken would include consultation with the referring physician, referral to a voice laboratory for additional testing, reassessment and alteration of the therapy approach, and referral for additional consultations (neurological, psychiatric, etc.). It may well be that after all of the appropriate steps have been taken, a decision to terminate therapy may be the correct one.

## UNRESOLVED ISSUES AND MYTHS

### Clavicular Breathing: The Cause of Voice Problems?

After many years of experience in examining and working with voice-disordered patients, we are struck by the absence of clavicular breathing as a symptom or a sign. This is especially so in view of the frequent mention of this breathing pattern in many texts. Moreover, despite the claims, there is an absence of data to support this notion.

Clavicular breathing may be present in patients whose respiratory function is compromised as a result of chronic obstructive airway disease or neurological impairment. It may also be apparent in persons who are anxious and extremely tense. It is difficult to understand what the nature of the pathophysiology would be for an otherwise healthy individual to develop true clavicular breathing.

It is often the case, indeed it happens almost universally, that when people are asked to take a deep breath during examination, they will lift the shoulders and give a good example of clavicular breathing. However, if the patient's breathing pattern is carefully observed (without comment) during general conversation and at rest, we would submit that clavicular breathing will rarely be seen. That is not to say that a patient's manner of voice production does not affect respiratory function or is not affected by it. It is difficult to isolate excess tension only to the larynx and supraglottal vocal tract. Increased generalized thoracic tensions, thus, might be a part of the total voice production behavior, disrupting effective respiratory support for phonation. This should not be interpreted, however, as a basic respiratory problem or abnormality.

### Talking from the Diaphragm

"Talking from the diaphragm" seems to have become a phrase known to all whether or not any understanding of its meaning is attached to its utterance. It no doubt stems from singing pedagogy and early elocution training. If taken literally, it is physiologically impossible. However, it seems to be understood to mean that exhalation may be controlled in some way by the diaphragm. Physiologically, we know that the diaphragm is the primary muscle of inspiration, acting to enlarge the thoracic cavity in the vertical dimension. It is not an active muscle of expiration. When it is important to fully enlarge the thoracic cavity in order to be able to fill the lungs, then it would seem to be of value to spend time working on "diaphragmatic breathing." In addition, it has been shown that the diaphragm is active during the initial expiratory phase of respiration when phonation is begun on high lung volumes (Hixon, 1987). There is no doubt that professional voice users should be well trained in respiratory control. However, the average speaker is rarely called upon to have that degree of control. The normal speaker adjusts inspiration (speed and amount) and expiration (rate) to the demands of the utterance (Bless & Miller, 1972). Daniloff, Schuckers, and Feth (1980) state that speakers tend to breathe deeper when the utterance ahead is a long one, and less deeply when the anticipated utterance is short. In soft speech, the average duration of expiratory airflow is reported to be 2.4–3.5 seconds, as compared with the well-trained singer's ability to phonate loudly for more than 15–20 seconds (Daniloff et al., 1980). It is at high (or low) lung volumes that greater muscular control of respiration needs to be exercised. However, for normal speech activity, great diaphragmatic breaths are not required.

It is our impression that a great deal more emphasis has been placed on "teaching" or "correcting" breathing than is usually necessary in working with the voice-disordered patient who is not a professional voice user. Occasionally, attention to easy and relaxed breathing can be helpful in reducing tensions and diverting focus from the larynx. We would suggest that more attention should be paid to the ways in which the speaker uses the air supply.

For example, does the person release a lot of the available air supply before initiating phonation? Or does he keep talking after the easily available air supply has been exhausted, and in so doing increase tension? Or does she tend to stop in mid-sentence without releasing the air supply or replenishing it before starting up again? Is there a tendency to hold the breath before starting to talk? Direct work on such behaviorswill help to indirectly change respiratory behavior and improve smooth respiratory/phonatory coordination.

## Ventricular Phonation: Diagnosis or Description?

The term "dysphonia plica ventricularis," or dysphonia resulting from ventricular fold phonation, has typically been used as a diagnosis. We suggest that it is really a description based on visual observation, through indirect, flexible fiberoptic or stroboscopic laryngoscopy, of greater than expected approximation of the ventricular folds during phonation. The descriptive term does not reveal the underlying etiology of the behavior. The name given to this problem, "ventricular phonation," implies that the ventricular folds are the actual source of sound, which would suggest that the true vocal folds are not fully adducting. However, we have observed full true vocal fold adduction in the presence of compression of the ventricular folds, suggesting perhaps that the ventricular folds, rather than being the source of sound, may produce a damping effect on the sound emitted at the true vocal fold level or a restraining effect on the vibratory behavior of the true vocal folds. We have also observed ventricular fold vibratory behavior in some instances. Often the medialization of the ventricular folds obscures visualization of the true vocal folds, making it difficult to determine their movement characteristics. When it can be seen that the true vocal folds are not adducting, it appears that the ventricular fold activity is a compensatory behavior and may actually result in the best voice a person is capable of producing. It is important, however, to attempt to determine the reason for the impairment of true vocal fold adduction.

Caution should be exercised in diagnosing ventricular phonation based on indirect mirror examination alone. The positioning of the oropharyngeal structures required for indirect laryngoscopy, with the tongue held firmly in a fully protruded posture, may result in laryngeal adjustments that may not be typical for that person during conversational speech. Flexible fiberoptic laryngoscopic examination allows for habitual phonatory physiology to be observed.

Much is yet to be learned about the physiology, acoustics, and etiology of ventricular phonation. When the observation of excessive ventricular fold activity is made, it is necessary to continue the process of differential diagnosis in an attempt to uncover its etiology.

## *Unilateral Vocal Fold Paralysis: Does It Cross the Midline?*

It has been stated for many years that the compensatory behavior involved in the restoration of good voice in the presence of unilateral vocal fold paralysis is a crossing beyond the midline of the uninvolved fold to make contact with the paralyzed fold. As a result, the goal of therapeutic procedures that have been espoused for use with this population has been a strengthening of the normal vocal fold through activities of forceful effort closure of the glottis. There have been scant data to support the crossover effect in the presence of unilateral vocal fold paralysis. The question must also be raised as to whether return of voice has been in some instances inappropriately credited to the therapy program when the patient has, in fact, experienced spontaneous return of function (as is often the case with an idiopathic paralysis). Or perhaps the therapy hastened or assisted the return of function. Answers to these speculations are unavailable. And, indeed, there are those patients who, despite continued paralysis, have experienced return of good voice. How? What makes the difference between those who experience return of voice in the presence of paralysis and those whose voices continue to be aberrant?

Although the notion of the crossover effect is an appealing one, we have been impressed by the lack of its occurrence in many patients we have examined using flexible fiberoptic endoscopy (Casper, Colton, & Brewer, 1985), whether or not they exhibited return of voice. We explored whether the crossover could be elicited through various voice therapy maneuvers and failed to observe its occurrence in the few patients we studied. Schematic representations based on information obtained from high speed films of the behavior of the vocal folds in the presence of unilateral paralysis have shown that the glottis remains open, with the normal vocal fold approaching the midline but not crossing it, while the affected fold has a motion described as being like a "flag flapping in the wind" (Hirano, Kakita, Kawasaki, & Matsushita, 1977). More recently, using the rigid stroboscope, which permits an enlarged image, we have become aware of instances that appeared to show a crossover effect of the intact vocal fold. Further investigation of this effect is needed to determine whether in fact the vocal fold crosses the midline, whether there is a shifting of the entire larynx, how this is accomplished and learned by some individuals but apparently unavailable to others, and many other questions.

Paralysis of the vocal fold not only results in its inability to be moved by contraction of the affected muscle(s) but also changes its level and shape. These parameters—the level, tension, thickness, and eventual position relative to midline—of a paralyzed vocal fold will be determined by a variety of factors, including muscle fibrosis and contractures (Ballenger, 1985). These effects must be better understood in order to be factored into an understanding of the variability of vocal performance in the presence of paralysis.

Some authors (Yamaguchi, Yotsukura, Sata, Watanabe, Hirose, & Kobayashi, 1993) report good success with pushing exercises to achieve greater glottal closure. In our own experience, we have not been impressed by the results obtained in voice therapy using effort closure techniques. Indeed, many patients have reported such exercises to be fatiguing to the voice and seeming to result in poorer vocal performance for a period of time during and after their execution. In view of these many concerns, we feel constrained not to recommend the routine use of such exercises in these cases. Other techniques have been incidentally reported to be effective in producing clearer and less breathy voice. Among these is the use of a high pitch. When the superior branch of the recurrent laryngeal nerve is intact and functional, stretching and thinning of the affected vocal fold will still occur due to the action of the cricothyroid muscle. This action has a component of adduction and results in greater approximation of the folds and increased tension in the lax paralyzed fold. The problem with this technique is that the effect and the improved voice quality that it allows is not transferrable to a modal register phonation at an acceptable frequency level for general communication.

Often patients with unilateral paralysis attempt to compensate for the loss of the ability to increase loudness level by increasing subglottic pressure and phonatory effort. The effect that this particular compensatory behavior has is to worsen the voice and make the patient fatigued with the effort of talking. In such instances, therapy designed to reduce effort and increase tension and pressures can result in improved phonation. Methods of treating unilateral vocal fold paralysis through the use of phonosurgical techniques were described in Chapter 8.

## *The Myth of Optimum Pitch*

The concept of an optimum pitch dates back to at least 1940, when it was described by Fairbanks (1940). It has been defined variously as (*a*) that pitch at which the voice has good quality and maximum intensity with the least effort, (*b*) that pitch at which there is a "vocal swell," and (*c*) a biologically determined ideal pitch for an individual, determined by the anatomical and physiological characteristics of individual larynges. The methods for its determination have also varied somewhat, and include

1.  Listening for that pitch at which the quality of the voice is best and intensity is the greatest;
2.  Counting the number of musical notes in a person's full range (optimum pitch will be that which is 25% of the way up from the bottom of the range);
3.  Using the same technique as in (2) above and going up one-third of the way from the bottom of the range;
4.  Having the patient say "um-hum" naturally, with the lips closed and a rising inflection, while feeling the oronasopharyngeal surfaces for the most resonant frequency;
5.  Finding the pitch at which the sustained phonation of the vowel /ah/ is the longest and loudest;
6.  Finding the lowest pitch a person can produce and counting at least four notes up the scale;
7.  Listening for the pitch of the sigh of a yawn/sigh maneuver, which is said to represent a person's optimal pitch.

Experimental attempts have been made to explore the claims made about optimum pitch. In 1958 Thurman measured intensity at the various frequencies as subjects hummed a scale. Only 11% of the highest intensity levels occurred within the range of frequencies that might be considered to be appropriate for an adult's optimum pitch. A number of other investigators have examined frequency-intensity relationships (Coleman, Mabis, & Hinson, 1977; Damste, 1970; Komiyama, Watanabe, & Ryu, 1984), and have reported maximum intensity occurring about 70% up from the subject's lowest sustainable frequency (not the 25–30% claimed for optimum pitch). Vocal efficiency, another tenet of optimum pitch, can be measured as the ratio of the total output (acoustic) power over the total input (aerodynamic) power at the glottis. Van den Berg (1956), using a catheter between the vocal folds to obtain a direct measure of subglottal pressure and an esophageal catheter for an indirect measure, found a positive relationship between subglottal pressure and sound pressure level (SPL). He converted the SPL into speech power in watts to measure laryngeal efficiency at various frequencies and intensities. If optimum pitch exists, the expectation would be that an increased output power would be obtained for the same level of input power at a given frequency. This did not occur. Using slightly different methodology, Isshiki (1964) reported results similar to van den Berg's. House (1959) demonstrated an important contribution of the vocal tract when he reported that a perceptible change in overall intensity occurred when a vocal harmonic coincided with the center of a vocal tract resonance. The so-called "vocal swell" thus does not appear to be related to the concept of laryngeal efficiency. Another line of questioning was pursued by Stone (1983) when he questioned the perceptibility of the intensity change that was claimed to mark the optimum pitch. He found that the intensity changes between 100 and 200 Hz, the range in which optimum pitch would be expected to fall for adult males, were very minimal and thus imperceptible. Similar to previous reports, Stone also found greatest intensity for half of his subjects to occur at frequencies well above the level at which optimum pitch would be anticipated. And still further, using the Fairbanks method for measuring optimum pitch, Stone reported that in 23 of 30 trials (N = 10 × 3 trials each), the "optimal pitch" fell above the speaker's modal pitch. Minifie (1984) reported that the efficiency of the power conversion increased with intensity rather than with frequency. This author could find no evidence to support the concept of an optimal pitch as being most efficient. All of the studies cited thus far used normal-speaking subjects. However, Ludlow, Connor, and Coulter (1984) explored the viability of the optimum pitch concept in patients with laryngeal pathology. Their results suggest that vocal function is best at the frequencies in the upper 50% of the speaking range for normal speakers, but not for those with laryngeal pathology. They interpret their findings to mean that a set of lawful relationships exists between several measures of phonatory function and frequency in normal speakers, which are disturbed in the presence of pathology. Pathology compromises phonatory function, limiting it to a particular range in frequencies. Thus, in pathological states it is the disturbance of the lawful relationships that is meaningful rather than the existence of a particular fundamental frequency range at which phonation can be expected with least effort.

These data all seem to substantially reject the notion of an optimum pitch, at least as currently defined. Finally, it is important to be wary of subjective perceptions of pitch level. Murry (1978) demonstrated that judgments of pitch in dysphonic voices may be confounded by other voice signal parameters, such as loudness, effort, and voice quality. He found a reduction in phonational range in patients with laryngeal paralysis but did not find speaking fundamental frequency in dysphonic patients to be significantly lower than in the normal-speaking population. In Chapter 5 it was reported that a prominent perceptual characteristic of voice in Huntington's chorea was low pitch. However, actual measurements of fundamental frequency in this population showed it to be within the normal range. Wilson, Wellen, and Kimbarow (1983) demonstrated that trained listeners were not better than untrained listeners in judgments of perceived fundamental frequency (pitch) of children's voices and that neither group could identify differences of less than 20 Hz at better than chance level. It is also important to recognize that raising pitch level may appear to reduce breathiness or hoarseness, but that this happens at the expense of, not for the benefit of, the larynx. The extra effort put forth by the patient may serve to override some of the vocal symptoms. Reduction of loudness is physiologically a much sounder approach. It seems quite logical that even an optimum pitch, if there were one, could be used in improper, abusive ways.

It is the philosophical approach of this book that if phonatory physiology is normalized, the voice that emerges will be at an appropriate pitch level for that individual. Therefore, approaching the rehabilitation of disordered voice by attempting to impose an arbitrary pitch level seems inappropriate, perhaps incorrect, and often unproductive.

## *Whispering: Is It Harmful?*

Some authors believe that whispering should be avoided during periods of voice rest or as a therapeutic technique because they claim that it results in vocal fold adduction that is undesirable, or that extreme glottal friction characterizes the whisper, and that is undesirable. Are there available experimental data to support these contentions? There have been a number of investigations of laryngeal configurations during whisper (Hamlet, 1972; Monoson & Zemlin, 1984; Pressman, 1942; Pressman & Kelemen, 1955; Solomon, McCall, Trosset, & Gray, 1989; Zemlin, 1988), describing a variety of configurations including (*a*) lack of complete adduction along the full length of the glottis, (*b*) an inverted V shape, (*c*) a bowed appearance, (*d*) a Y shape with a posterior chink, (*e*) a bimodal (anterior and posterior) chink, (*f*) a parallel configuration with some adduction, and (*g*) toeing in of the vocal processes. Various reasons have been suggested for these differences in glottal configuration. Some have suggested that the glottal shape is a function of the effort involved in the whisper, others suggest it has to do with the type of whisper (quiet versus forceful whisper), while yet others claim a relationship to the phonetic context.

Monoson and Zemlin (1984) compared laryngeal appearance (high speed films), electromyograms, acoustic, and airflow data for four conditions: quiet whisper, forced whisper, breathy phonation, and conversational phonation. Glottal configurations varied to some extent among the conditions and were believed to be at least partially determined by the effort level involved. Vibratory behavior was absent in both whisper conditions and present in both breathy and conversational phonation. Airflow was greatest in forced whispering, which was felt to be due in part to an increase in activity of the expiratory muscles in that condition. The data do not support the thesis that whispering is an abusive behavior. However, the increases in expiratory muscle activity and in airflow attributed to the forced whisper suggest an increase in effort and perhaps in tension.

Solomon et al. (1989) report on a study of laryngeal configurations for two types of whispering (high effort and low effort) in 10 speakers using consonant-vowel units and running speech. The laryngeal configurations were visualized via a fiberoptic bronchoscope and videotaped for analysis. Significant individual variability was reported. Intrasubject inconsistency was also noted, although most subjects exhibited a preferred configuration. A medium-sized glottal opening was described for most subjects, with a large glottal size occurring more frequently in the high effort whisper than in the low effort whisper. Although some constriction of supraglottal structures was reported, it apparently occurred less than half of the time, even in high effort whispering. The glottal configurations described by these authors were primarily of two types: a straight edge, parallel configuration or a toeing in of the vocal processes. It is still not clear how such approximation of the vocal folds occurs during whisper, although these authors report observation of more contact during running speech than in the production of consonant-vowel units. Four of the 10 subjects displayed the straight margin configuration of the glottis, and these same subjects did not approximate the vocal folds. These authors suggest that the determination regarding the use of whisper as a therapeutic technique or during periods of vocal rest should be made on an individual basis, depending on the type of glottal configuration assumed for whisper by that patient. The efficacy of whispering as a therapeutic approach was not addressed in this study. Hufnagle and Hufnagle (1988) reported that patients demonstrated improved voice quality following a period of whispering, suggesting therefore that the behavior is not harmful and, indeed, may be helpful.

There is not yet sufficient evidence available to state unequivocally that whispering is not harmful. However, our clinical intuition suggests that it may be helpful for some patients, with a few caveats. Because the high effort forced whisper tends to suggest increased tension and effort somewhere in the system, and because tension and force are precisely the behaviors that most patients need to reduce or eliminate, it seems to us that the use of the forced whisper could be counterproductive. It is also important that the patient recognize that whispering may have a drying effect on the mucosa of the vocal folds, which should be counteracted by an increase of fluid intake.

The available evidence about the whisper is not nearly as frightening as some of the strongly stated admonitions against its use. However, much remains to be learned about the mechanism of whispering. The amount of force in medial compression of the folds when they appear to make contact during whispering has not been addressed and remains an open question, as does the degree of expiratory muscle effort involved.

## PREVENTION OF VOICE PROBLEMS

We can discuss the prevention of voice problems by addressing both primary prevention—preventing the occurrence of the problem in the first place—or secondary prevention—preventing the recurrence of a problem. In the category of primary prevention, an understanding of the deleterious effects of cigarette smoking has been effective in convincing many people to change their habits and eliminate smoking. Throughout American society, steps have been taken to minimize the spread of the effects of inhaling environmental cigarette smoke by establishing prohibitions against smoking in theaters, planes, certain sections of restaurants, and other places of public gathering. Much more needs to be done, however, as it appears that in absolute numbers, the population of smokers has not decreased significantly. The evidence linking smoking with laryngeal cancer is impressive.

Greater strides need to be made in recognizing the aversive effects of certain noxious gases. However, in the absence of widespread information, it behooves professionals to suggest safeguards that individuals may take when knowingly exposed to a variety of potentially harmful agents. Such safeguards include wearing appropriate protective masks, avoidance of unnecessary exposure, introducing air purifying systems or improved ventilation.

Education is the primary need in decreasing vocal abuse and misuse. We know that cheerleading constitutes a very stressful, abusive use of the voice that often results in mucosal damage. However, this knowledge seems not to have penetrated the cheerleading world so that training in voice use and voice conservation might be provided. There are other abusive activities that could be similarly identified. Some, such as rock singing in the presence of highly amplified sound, may not be amenable to change. Despite, or perhaps due to, laryngeal pathology such as nodules or polyps, some rock singers have a "sound" uniquely theirs that would not be possible without abuse.

Another group of people who would benefit from increased education about the voice are choir singers. Many have untrained voices and abuse them with regularity but without awareness. Choir directors frequently have limited backgrounds in vocal pedagogy and are thus ill-equipped to train their choirs in healthy habits of singing and voice use. This becomes increasingly critical when the choir is composed of or includes prepubertal children.

Primary prevention through education needs to be increased in the public schools so that children learn to recognize beginning signs of vocal abuse and are trained in voice conservation. In addition to education of the children, all school personnel should have a greater understanding of vocal abuse, its harmful effects, and ways to avoid or eliminate it. Such education not only would be helpful to them in managing their own voice production but also would make them more capable of identifying the problem in children. Such a program, which had impressive results, is described by Nilson and Schneiderman (1983). Their program was directed at 2nd and 3rd grade students and their teachers and included discussion of the vocal mechanism and voice production, voice qualities both normal and abnormal, and learning to identify vocal abuse. Both the children and the teachers were found to have gained and retained significant knowledge about the voice, and when the children who had been part of the program were retested for voice, no new cases of dysphonia were identified. A primary prevention plan has been proposed by Flynn (1983), and Marge (1984) has addressed prevention of voice disorders as one area under the broader topic of prevention of communication disorders.

Secondary prevention, for those who have experienced even a single episode of vocal disturbance that required treatment, is essential. It is incumbent upon laryngologists who successfully treat a patient with a preventable problem that they either take the time to clearly instruct the patient in a program of vocal hygiene or refer that patient to a speech-language pathologist for such education and counseling. Indeed, failure to do so might leave the door open for medical-legal problems.

## MALPRACTICE

In the current litigious climate, it is important that all those who treat patients with voice problems, including speech-language pathologists, recognize how they may be vulnerable to malpractice actions and take appropriate steps to safeguard themselves. Instances of persons with voice problems bringing suit against otolaryngologists or speech-language pathologists and of speech-language pathologists being called upon to testify as "expert witnesses" in suits brought against others have already occurred. During the years 1980–1985, there was a 10% increase in claims against speech-language pathologists (Kooper & Sullivan, 1986).

Prime candidates to bring such suits are persons who claim that the treatment provided, surgical or otherwise, created or resulted in a permanent condition no better or worse than the original problem, and that they had not been advised of the possibility of that outcome. Others might claim damages for a missed diagnosis that resulted in unnecessary treatment and/or delayed initiation of appropriate treatment. The extent of liability for a disabling condition appears to be directly related to the severity of the injury as measured by its duration (Kooper & Sullivan, 1986). Thus, if a voice disorder is present and is not expected to abate or change over the person's lifespan, its severity will be judged to be greater if the patient is 25 years old than if she is 85. The extent of liability will be related to the perception of the degree of severity of the problem.

It is of utmost importance that very complete, dated records be maintained on each patient. Such records should contain the results of all testing and examination, case history material, statements of diagnosis or a listing of the differential diagnosis if full exploration has not been completed, a treatment plan, statements of prognosis specific to planned treatment modalities, and a record of all contacts with the patient or about the patient. Furthermore, whenever surgical intervention is planned, a recorded sample of the patient's voice should be a part of the record. A second recording should be made postoperatively, with additional recordings made periodically as changes in voice occur. The speech-language pathologist should make audio recordings of the patient's voice at the time of the initial visit and periodically after that.

Those who work with voice-disordered patients, when called upon to testify in court as an expert witness, must establish their expertise. They must be knowledgeable and articulate about phonatory physiology, as well as about testing and treatment procedures, the nature of voice disorders, and the emotional ramifications of disturbed communication skills or loss of the source of a livelihood. The primary question to which they will be expected to respond deals with the acceptability of the treatment that was provided in the case. This does not require that the witness agree with the course of treatment, as long as it is an accepted form of treatment for the problem.

## SUMMARY

Vocal rehabilitation in its broadest sense is discussed in this chapter. Concepts, principles, and guidelines basic to vocal rehabilitation receive attention, then specific therapeutic techniques are presented. The role of voice therapy in the treatment of voice disorders, the appropriate goals of such treatment, and the nature of the therapeutic process is proposed for the various categories of voice disorders, such as those associated with mucosal changes, those involving misuse and abuse, and those with neurological involvement. A section is devoted to discussion of some special voice problems that do not fit into these categories. The discussion of specific therapeutic techniques includes a description of how they are done, with suggestions and cautions gained from clinical practice. A rationale is presented for each technique that relates its physiological implications to the disturbed physiology typical of the voice disorders to which it is applicable. The considerations that must be taken into account in developing a prognostic statement are discussed, and some criteria for termination of therapy are suggested. The authors raise some issues in vocal rehabilitation that are based on unresolved questions and for which no substantiating data are available and question the continued use of optimum pitch as a viable concept. Discussions of the prevention of voice disorders and of malpractice concerns complete the chapter.

# Chapter 10

---

# Anatomy of the Vocal Fold Mechanism

## INTRODUCTION

In the human body, structure determines function. That is, the shape and form of a structure determine the manner in which the structure will operate. Thus, it is important to understand the anatomy of a structure in order to understand how it works. Such is the case for understanding the larynx and voice production.

A brief review of the anatomy of the larynx will be presented in this chapter. The focus will be on functional anatomy, that is, the determination of how a structure functions based on its anatomy. It is not the intent of this chapter to present full anatomical details of structures, their articulation with other structures, and their blood and nerve supply. Such details may be found in many complete anatomy texts (Dickson & Dickson, 1982; Zemlin, 1988). Rather, it is our purpose to present those details needed to understand the structure and how it functions in voice production. This information is presented so that clinicians can rapidly review a segment of anatomy and use that information to better understand a given voice problem. It is hoped that this section will be actively used during the process of differential diagnosis and in the management plan. Anatomy need not be memorized if it is understood and if reference materials are consulted in a meaningful manner.

We will begin our discussion of laryngeal anatomy from the outside and proceed to the inside; that is, we will first consider the extrinsic muscles of the larynx, then move inward to the cartilages of the larynx and the intrinsic muscles. A brief overview of the internal structures and cavities of the larynx will follow and, finally, we will consider the body cover model of vocal fold structure and laryngeal anatomy as viewed through a flexible fiberoptic laryngoscope.

## EXTRINSIC MUSCLES OF THE LARYNX

The extrinsic muscles of the larynx are those muscles that have one attachment to a structure within the larynx and one attachment to a structure outside the larynx. It is necessary to understand that the hyoid bone, which is a rather distinct structure, is considered to be part of the larynx. Some of its features are shown in the upper panel of Figure 10.1. All extrinsic muscles have their laryngeal attachments on the hyoid bone. The attachments outside of the larynx include many different structures, such as the mandible, the mastoid, and structures in the thorax. Recall that in

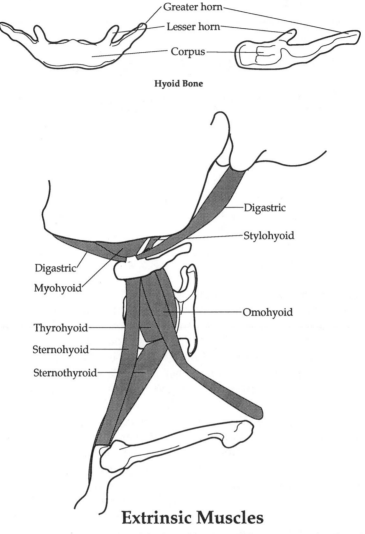

**Hyoid Bone**

## Extrinsic Muscles

*Figure 10.1*. Schematic representation of the hyoid bone and the extrinsic muscles of the larynx. Part of the extrinsic muscle group forms a sling to support the hyoid bone and larynx from above. These muscles can move the hyoid and larynx upward, forward, or backward. The other group of extrinsic muscles can pull the hyoid and larynx down.

anatomy the origin of a muscle refers to its least moveable attachment, whereas the insertion refers to its more moveable attachment.

There are eight extrinsic muscles, four that lie below the hyoid bone and four that lie above it. For those reasons, they are divided into the suprahyoid and infrahyoid groups. The muscles that comprise these two groups are listed in Table 10.1 and shown in Figure 10.1.

### Suprahyoid Group

In Figure 10.1, note how the suprahyoid group forms a sling supporting the hyoid bone and, secondarily, the larynx. The anterior part of the sling is formed by portions of the digastric (anterior belly), the geniohyoid, and the mylohyoid muscles. When

*Table 10.1.* Extrinsic Muscles of the Larynx

---

*Suprahyoid Muscles*

| | |
|---|---|
| **Digastric** | A two-part muscle consisting of a posterior belly and an anterior belly. |
| Origin | Anterior belly: originates on the lower border of the mandible near the mandibular symphysis. |
| | Posterior belly: originates on the mastoid process. |
| Insertion | Anterior belly: intermediate tendon. |
| | Posterior belly: intermediate tendon connecting to the hyoid bone. |
| Function | Anterior belly: pulls hyoid bone anteriorly and slightly upward. |
| | Posterior belly: pulls hyoid bone posteriorly and upward. |
| | |
| **Mylohyoid** | A thin muscle forming the floor of the mouth. |
| Origin | Along the mylohyoid line on the inner surface of the mandible. |
| Insertion | Most fibers meet with fibers of the opposite side at the midline raphe. |
| Function | Pulls hyoid bone anteriorly and slightly upward, depending on position of jaw. |
| | |
| **Geniohyoid** | A cylindrical muscle located above the mylohyoid muscle. |
| Origin | On the mental spine at the mental symphysis of the mandible. |
| Insertion | Anterior surface of the corpus of the hyoid bone. |
| Function | Pulls hyoid bone anteriorly and slightly upward. |
| | |
| **Stylohyoid** | A long slender muscle located superficially to the posterior belly of the digastric. |
| Origin | On the styloid process of the temporal bone. |
| Insertion | On the body of the hyoid bone. |
| Function | Pulls hyoid bone posteriorly and upward. |

*Infrahyoid Muscles*

| | |
|---|---|
| **Thyrohyoid** | A thin muscle that lies deep to the omohyoid. |
| Origin | From the oblique line on the thyroid lamina. |
| Insertion | On the lower border of the greater horn of the hyoid bone. |
| Function | Decreases distance between thyroid and hyoid, especially anteriorly. |
| | |
| **Sternothyroid** | A long, thin muscle on the anterior side of the neck. |
| Origin | Posterior surface of the manubrium of the sternum and the first costal cartilage. |
| Insertion | On the oblique line of the thyroid. |
| Function | Pulls down on the thyroid cartilage. |
| | |
| **Sternohyoid** | A thin muscle lying on anterior side of the neck. |
| Origin | On the posterior surface of the manubrium of the sternum and end of the clavicle. |
| Insertion | On the lower border of the body of the hyoid bone. |
| Function | Pulls down on the hyoid bone. |
| | |
| **Omohyoid** | A long, narrow, two-part muscle on the anterior and lateral surfaces of the neck. |
| Origin | Inferior belly: along the upper surface of the scapula. |
| | Superior belly: intermediate tendon. |
| Insertion | Inferior belly: intermediate tendon. |
| | Superior belly: the border of the great horn of the hyoid bone. |
| Function | Both divisions pull down on the hyoid, although the superior belly has a more pronounced effect in this direction than the inferior belly. |

contracted, this group of muscles pulls the hyoid bone (and thus the larynx) forward. These muscles are active during the production of a front vowel or a consonant that requires a high front tongue position. The posterior belly of the digastric and the stylohyoid form the rear part of the sling. Their contraction pulls the hyoid posteriorly. Note that the angle of pull is steep for this muscle group, whereas the angle of pull of the anterior muscle group is shallow. Thus, the action of the posterior group is to pull up on the larynx, while the anterior muscle group exerts a pull on the hyoid bone that is more forward than upward. In fact, if the jaw is lowered, it is possible that the anterior group could lower the larynx slightly.

## Infrahyoid Group

This group is made up of four muscles: the thyrohyoid, sternohyoid, omohyoid, and sternothyroid. With the exception of the thyrohyoid, the other muscles in this group have attachments from the hyoid to structures below the larynx. As a result, their contraction has the effect of pulling the larynx downward. The lowered laryngeal position results in a lengthening of the vocal tract, which has a primary effect on vocal resonance characteristics affecting the formant frequencies. A more direct effect on the voice may result from the restriction of thyroid cartilage movement that is caused by contraction of this muscle group. This restriction of movement has directly to do with vocal fold length, mass, and tension, and thereby affects vocal pitch regulation. Other muscles are also involved in pitch regulation, and they will be discussed later.

The thyrohyoid muscle connects to the larynx, and its action contributes to determining the angle of the thyroid with respect to the cricoid cartilage. If the thyroid cartilage is fixed (by other muscles) so that it cannot move, then contraction of the thyrohyoid would contribute to pulling the hyoid bone down. If, however, the hyoid bone is fixed (by contraction of muscles above it), then contraction of the thyrohyoid would pull upward on the thyroid, increasing the distance between it and the cricoid cartilage (especially anteriorly). Thus, most of the effect of the thyrohyoid muscle is to rock the thyroid cartilage upward and in so doing to potentially alter length, mass, and tension of the vocal folds, thereby affecting the pitch of the voice.

Positioning of the larynx in the vertical dimension during speaking is primarily related to vowel or consonant production. There is some variation of position in singing, and good singers may vary the vertical position of the larynx considerably, depending on their style of singing and the music (Shipp, 1975; Shipp & Izdebski, 1975). Speakers with voice problems may have a tendency to maintain higher than normal laryngeal position. This may be indicative of excessive muscle tension (Aronson, 1985; Morrison, Rammage, Belisle, Pullan, & Nichol, 1983) in the extrinsic muscles of the larynx.

## Cartilages of the Larynx

The framework of the larynx is composed of hyaline cartilage. Cartilage is softer and more flexible than bone. Hyaline refers to the type of cells that make up the cartilage. (See Chapter 3 for more details.)

The cartilages of the larynx are presented in Figure 10.2. The major cartilages are the thyroid, cricoid, and arytenoid. The other cartilages are much smaller and form parts of other structures. For example, the corniculates are small cartilages attached to the arytenoid at their apices. The cuneiforms are small cartilages embedded in the muscle tissue that connects the arytenoids to the epiglottis.

Thyroid

Cricoid

Arytenoid

*Figure 10.2.* Schematic of the cartilages of the larynx.

## THYROID CARTILAGE

The thyroid cartilage is the largest cartilage of the larynx. The most anterior angle of this cartilage, commonly referred to as the Adam's apple, is a very prominent feature in some men. It is shaped like a shield and can be thought of as shielding the structures inside. The thyroid is actually composed of two plates of cartilage, called lamina, joined at the midline to form an angle of about 80 degrees in men and about 90 degrees in women (Zemlin, 1988). The more acute angle of the thyroid together with laryngeal size accounts for the more pronounced outline of the larynx in the male neck.

Posteriorly, the thyroid cartilage has two horns or cornua. The superior horn connects the thyroid to the hyoid bone, and the inferior horn connects it to the cricoid cartilage below. Along the lateral surface of the thyroid lamina is a ridge identified as the oblique line. It is here that the thyrohyoid and sternothyroid muscles attach.

## CRICOID CARTILAGE

The second largest laryngeal cartilage is the cricoid, which completely surrounds the trachea. Sometimes it is referred to as the uppermost tracheal ring, but it is quite different in configuration from the other tracheal rings. It is larger and higher posteriorly, while anteriorly it tapers to the cricoid arch. The thyroid cartilage articulates with the cricoid on its posterolateral surface. Two kinds of movements of the thyroid on the cricoid cartilage are permitted, as illustrated in Figure 10.3. The arytenoids articulate with the cricoid on its posterosuperior surface. The details of this articulation are important and will be discussed further in the next section.

## ARYTENOID CARTILAGES

There are two arytenoid cartilages, each positioned on either side of the midline on the supraposterior surface of the cricoid cartilage. The arytenoids are roughly pyramidal in shape and have four surfaces, three angles at the base, and, of course, a single point at the apex. The basal surface is important to consider because essential musculature attaches at two of its angles.

The most anterior angle of the base of the arytenoid is referred to as the vocal process. It is here that the true vocal folds attach. The more lateral angle, referred to as the muscle process, is the point of attachment for the posterior cricoarytenoid and the lateral cricoarytenoid muscles.

The surface of the arytenoid that articulates with the cricoid cartilage is concave in appearance. The surface of the cricoid that meets the arytenoid is convex. These surfaces help to determine how the arytenoid will move on the surface of the cricoid. Because of the shape of these surfaces, a rotating motion is not permitted, but a rocking motion can occur (Broad, 1973; von Leden & Moore, 1961). Broad has described the permitted motions by comparing them to the movement of two matching cylinders, as shown in Figure 10.4. Two kinds of motion are permitted, a gliding motion along an anteroposterior plane and a rocking motion in a mediolateral direction. When these two motions occur together, there is the appearance of a rocking motion either medially and anteriorly directed (if the arytenoids are moving in) or posteriorly (if the arytenoids are moving out). Depending on speed of medial movement relative to anterior

*Figure 10.3.* Movements permitted by the articulation of the thyroid and cricoid cartilages. A rocking motion of the thyroid on the cricoid is the major movement permitted (left panel). In addition, a slight anteroposterior movement is possible (right panel).

movement of the arytenoids, it is possible for the vocal processes to be the first point of contact during adduction of the vocal folds.

### EPIGLOTTIS

The epiglottis is a leaf-shaped cartilage attached on the mesial surface of the thyroid cartilage at the juncture of the two thyroid plates. The anterior surface of the epiglottis attaches to the hyoid bone via a ligament.

The epiglottis assists in directing food and liquids into the esophagus during swallowing. During phonation, it is usually out of the way of the egressive airstream. However, it moves considerably during the production of different vowels and consonants. In some cases, it will obscure the view of the vocal folds. However, tongue position in the production of vowels like /ee/ and /oo/ usually results in forward movement of the epiglottis, thereby allowing a good view of the vocal folds. There is no evidence to support the contention that the shape of the epiglottis will alter the voice. Certainly, pulling the epiglottis over the laryngeal opening will affect sound transmission and intensity level.

The epiglottis can vary considerably in shape and curvature. Usually it is slightly concave when viewed via a laryngeal mirror or fiberscope. Sometimes it may have a very pronounced omega shape. The so-called omega-shaped epiglottis appears to be found most often in immature larynges or children's larynges. However, it may also be simply a variation of normal human laryngeal anatomy.

### OTHER CARTILAGES

The remaining cartilages are the corniculate and the cuneiform cartilages. The corniculates are small cone-shaped cartilages that form the apex of the arytenoid. The cuneiforms are small rod-shaped cartilages found within the aryepiglottic fold, a fold of tissue and muscle coursing from the arytenoids to the epiglottis.

## Intrinsic Muscles of the Larynx

Muscles that have both of their attachments to structures within the larynx are called intrinsic laryngeal muscles. The five muscles, along with their origins and insertions, are shown in Table 10.2. In this review they will be discussed roughly in order of their activation when a person produces voice.

*Figure 10.4.* Type of movements permitted by the cricoarytenoid joint.

*Table 10.2.* Intrinsic Muscles of the Larynx

| | |
|---|---|
| **Arytenoideus** | An unpaired muscle consisting of fibers oriented in two directions, oblique and transverse. |
| Origin | Oblique fibers originate at the base of one arytenoid and course to the apex of the other arytenoid. Transverse fibers originate along the lateral margin of one arytenoid and course to the lateral margin of the other arytenoid. |
| Insertion | Arytenoid of opposite side. |
| Function | Adducts arytenoids, thus closing the cartilaginous glottis. |
| **Lateral Cricoarytenoid** | A fan-shaped muscle lying along the upper surface of the cricoid cartilage. |
| Origin | On the upper border of the cricoid. |
| Insertion | Anterior surface of the muscular process of the arytenoid. |
| Function | Adducts the vocal processes of the arytenoids, thus closing the membranous glottis. |
| **Posterior Cricoarytenoid** | A fan-shaped muscle located on the posterior surface of the cricoid. |
| Origin | On the posterior lamina of the cricoid. |
| Insertion | Posterior surface of the muscular process of the arytenoid. |
| Function | Abducts the arytenoids, thus opening the glottis. |
| **Cricothyroid** | A fan-shaped muscle located between the cricoid and thyroid cartilages, consisting of two divisions, pars oblique and pars recta. These divisions refer to the different orientation of the fibers. |
| Origin | Arch of the cricoid. |
| Insertion | Inner inferior margin of the thyroid. |
| Function | Decreases the space between the thyroid and cricoid, thus increasing the distance between the thyroid and arytenoid cartilages; increasing the length of the vocal folds, decreasing their mass, and increasing their tension; and increasing vocal pitch. |
| **Thyroarytenoid** | A bundle of muscle fibers making up the true vocal folds. |
| Origin | Anteriorly, from the posterior surface of the thyroid at its angle. |
| Insertion | Along the lateral base of an arytenoid from the vocal process to the muscle process. |
| Function | Decreases the distance between the thyroid and arytenoid cartilages, shortening the vocal folds, increasing their mass, decreasing their tension, and decreasing vocal pitch. |

## ARYTENOIDEUS

The arytenoideus or interarytenoid muscle is a two-part muscle lying between the two arytenoid cartilages. One part consists of muscle fibers that course in a horizontal direction. The effect of these fibers is to pull the bases of the two arytenoids toward each other, thus adducting them. The other part consists of fibers that course from the base of one arytenoid to the apex of the other arytenoid. The effect of these fibers is to pull the tips of the arytenoids together. Together, the two parts adduct the arytenoids and close off the extreme posterior airway. Although the time when these muscles are activated depends on the speech task, in general, activity in the arytenoideus occurs anywhere from 0.5–0.3 seconds before sound is produced.

## LATERAL CRICOARYTENOID

The lateral cricoarytenoid muscle is a paired muscle coursing from the sides and upper surface of the cricoid cartilage to the muscle process of the arytenoid. The effect of this muscle is to pull the muscle process anteriorly, rocking the arytenoid medially and adducting the vocal folds themselves. Time of activation may be about 0.1 second after activity in the arytenoideus.

These two muscles (arytenoideus and lateral cricoarytenoid) function together to adduct the vocal folds. It is not necessary to completely adduct the folds for phonation to commence. Rather, there need only be sufficient adduction to impose an obstruction to the flow of air coming from the lungs, for phonation to begin.

## POSTERIOR CRICOARYTENOID

This is the only intrinsic muscle that abducts the vocal folds. From its origin on the posterior lamina of the cricoid, the muscle fibers converge to insert on the muscle process. Contraction of the muscle will pull the muscle process posteriorly, thus opening the vocal folds.

The posterior cricoarytenoid is active at the end of phonation in order to open the folds. However, it is also active during speech since there are many speech sounds that require an absence of vocal fold vibration (e.g., the stop consonants /p/, /t/, and /k/; the fricative consonants /s/ and /sh/, etc.). Thus, a short burst of activity in the posterior cricoarytenoid quickly abducts the vocal folds enough to stop their vibration.

## CRICOTHYROID

The origin of the cricothyroid muscle is along the upper surface of the sides of the cricoid cartilage. Its insertion is along the lower border of the thyroid cartilage. It is considered to be the main muscle for pitch control and its major function is to raise vocal pitch. It does so by rocking the cricoid cartilage upward or the thyroid cartilage downward, thereby increasing the distance between the thyroid cartilage and the vocal processes of the arytenoids, which are situated on the rear surface of the cricoid. The vocal folds, which are attached anteriorly on the inner surface of the thyroid cartilage and posteriorly on the vocal processes of the arytenoids, are stretched and elongated by either of these actions. Stretching the vocal folds decreases their cross-sectional area and subjects the folds to greater longitudinal tension. The decrease of area and increase of tension permit the vocal folds to vibrate at higher frequencies and thus produce the perception of higher pitch.

Decreasing the level of activity in the cricothyroid will result in a decrease of tension, resulting in a slower vibratory rate and a decrease of fundamental frequency. However, the rate of decay of muscle activity in the cricothyroid may be too slow for speech purposes. That is, it may be necessary, for linguistic purposes, to lower pitch more rapidly than would be possible by waiting for the decay of cricothyroid activity. Thus, other physiological mechanisms of frequency change may be operating to actively lower vocal pitch during speech.

## THYROARYTENOID

The thyroarytenoid muscle comprises the bulk of the vocal folds. Its contraction decreases the length of the vocal folds, increases their cross-sectional area, and decreases longitudinal tension. The action of this muscle represents one way to actively lower vocal pitch. Of course, contraction of this muscle also changes the configuration of the vocal folds themselves, thereby affecting how they will move within the vibratory cycle.

The thyroarytenoid may be divided into two muscle groups. The medial portion of the muscle is called the thyrovocalis muscle, and the more lateral portion is referred to as the thyromuscularis muscle. There is some controversy about whether or not the two parts are anatomically distinct (Dickson & Dickson, 1982). From a functional point of view, the medial portion of the thyroarytenoid (or thyrovocalis) is most active during the vibratory activity of the vocal folds and therefore may have a significant effect on phonation. The lateral (or thyromuscularis) portion may exhibit little movement during vibration, and thus its action may have minimal effect on the vibratory characteristics of the vocal folds.

## DETAILED ANATOMY OF THE VOCAL FOLDS: THE BODY COVER MODEL

Hirano (1974, 1981a) has proposed a model of the vocal folds that has considerable merit in explaining the variation of human voice production. Simply stated, the vocal folds consist of three layers: (*a*) the outer cover, consisting of epithelium; (*b*) a middle layer, the lamina propria; and (*c*) the body. A schematic diagram of the three layers is shown in Figure 10.5.

The cover of the vocal folds is composed of squamous cell epithelium. Mechanically, epithelium is very stiff, making this layer much stiffer than its neighbor, the lamina propria (Kakita, Hirano, & Okmaru, 1976). It is this difference of stiffness that determines the manner in which the layers will respond to deformation during vibration. In some modes of vibration, the degree of coupling between the epithelium and the lamina propria is very small (as in low frequency speech activities). In other modes of vibration, the degree of coupling between the cover, the lamina propria, and the body may be very great (as may be the case in falsetto voice). Thus, the combination of the mechanical characteristics of the three layers will ultimately determine the mode of vocal fold vibration.(See Fujimura, 1981, for a good discussion of the relationships between biomechanical characteristics of the vocal folds and sound production.)

The lamina propria is actually a three-layered area lying between the cover and the body. Its superficial layer is very pliable, consisting of loose fibrous components. The intermediate layer consists primarily of elastic fibers. The deepest layer consists of collagenous fibers. Mechanically, each layer will exhibit different characteristics, and variation in the composition of each of the three layers of the lamina propria will alter the manner of vocal fold vibration.

The body of the vocal fold is the vocalis muscle. Although muscle cells are the primary components of muscle, blood cells, collagen cells, and inorganic material are also present. Muscle fibers themselves exhibit different mechanical characteristics when they are in the process of contracting than when they are contracted or at rest (Colton, 1988). Thus, there can be considerable variation in the mechanical characteristics of the body, depending on the amount of muscle activation, the amount of collagenous or elastic fibers present, the amount of heat generated (Cooper & Titze, 1985; Hill, 1938; Titze, 1981), and other variations due to blood flow, oxygen consumption, and the like.

## FOLDS AND CAVITIES OF THE LARYNX

### *Folds*

The folds and cavities of the larynx are shown in Figure 10.6, sagittal and coronal cross-sections of the larynx. The major folds of interest are the true vocal folds. Superior and lateral to the true vocal folds are the false or ventricular folds. The false vocal

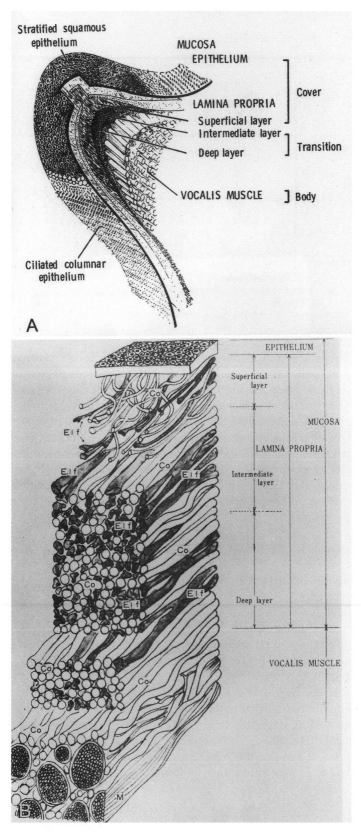

*Figure 10.5.* Schematic representation of the vocal folds as a body and cover. **A,** Cross-sectional representation. **B,** The kinds of fibers present in each layer.

*Figure 10.6.* Cross-sectional representation of the larynx.

folds do not usually vibrate in normal voice production, except perhaps at very low fundamental frequencies (50 Hz or below). They have few muscle fibers, and it is very difficult to regulate their tension, mass, and length. Occasionally they are seen to adduct partially or almost completely and obscure the true vocal folds. Only infrequently is vibration of the ventricular folds observed.

The aryepiglottic folds comprise a ring of muscle and connective tissue extending from the tips of the arytenoids to the epiglottis. In effect, they form a sphincter enclosing the entrance to the larynx. During swallowing and protective acts, the aryepiglottic folds contract to reduce the diameter of the laryngeal entrance and thus protect the airway. We have occasionally observed sphincteric movement of these folds during phonation.

### Cavities

The major cavities of the larynx are (*a*) the supraglottal cavity, (*b*) the subglottal cavity, and (*c*) the ventricles.

The supraglottal cavity lies above the glottis or the opening between the vocal folds. Its superior boundary is the aryepiglottic sphincter. This cavity could potentially act as a resonator of the sound produced by the vibrating vocal folds, although it is usually considered to be part of the entire vocal tract acoustically.

The subglottal cavity lies beneath the true vocal folds. Its lower boundary is the first tracheal ring. It is in this cavity that pressure increases beneath the closed vocal folds until it becomes sufficient to force the vocal folds open and begin phonation.

The ventricles, often referred to as the ventricles of Morgagni, are paired cavities lying above and slightly lateral to the true vocal folds. The opening of these cavities is usually very small, and thus they seem to have little effect on the sound produced at the vocal folds. However, in some conditions encountered in singing, the opening may be sufficient to permit meaningful resonance and thus add to the glottal tone. Sundberg (1974) has shown that under certain conditions, it could resonate frequencies in the vicinity of 2800 Hz. In most speech conditions, however, its resonant effect on sound is minimal.

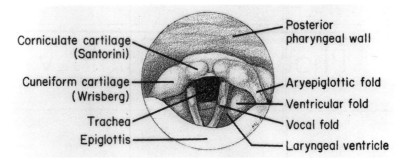

Corniculate cartilage (Santorini)
Cuneiform cartilage (Wrisberg)
Trachea
Epiglottis
Posterior pharyngeal wall
Aryepiglottic fold
Ventricular fold
Vocal fold
Laryngeal ventricle

*Figure 10.7.* Laryngoscopic view of the larynx. This is a view typically seen during indirect mirror, fiberoptic, or stroboscopic examination of the larynx.

## LARYNGOSCOPIC VIEW OF THE LARYNX

Figure 10.7 presents a view of the larynx typically seen when observing the larynx either through a laryngeal mirror or a laryngeal endoscope (flexible or rigid). It is a common view to most otolaryngologists and should be to speech-langugage pathologists and voice scientists. The various structures that can be viewed are identified in this figure. It is essential to know these landmarks to properly interpret images of the larynx. A good knowledge of normal anatomy and its variations is needed in order to correctly identify laryngeal pathology. It is important to recognize that there is much variability in normal anatomic structures. Examples of this variability as seen fiberscopically were discussed by Casper, Brewer, and Colton (1987a). The most marked structural variability occurred in the configuration of the "arytenoid complex" (arytenoids, cuneiforms, corniculates). There were obvious movement differences among the subjects in this area. Some subjects exhibited symmetrical movement whereas in others the movements were asymmetrical. There was also asymmetry in the apparent length of the true vocal folds. Notably, the marked anteroposterior movement and twisting of the larynx, often seen in patients with voice disorders, were not observed in normal speakers. Normal can span a broad range of differences in both structure and function. Asymmetry is not necessarily a sign of an abnormal larynx.

## SUMMARY

A brief review of the anatomy of the larynx and the vocal folds is presented. The extrinsic muscles of the larynx help to support and adjust the position of the larynx. The intrinsic muscles of the larynx attach to the various cartilages of the larynx (thyroid, cricoid, arytenoid) and serve to adjust the length, tension, and mass of the vocal folds, as well as to adduct them. A brief discussion of the cavities and folds of the larynx is presented, concluding with a presentation of the laryngoscopic view of laryngeal anatomy.

# Chapter 11

# Phonatory Physiology

The vibrating vocal folds are the major source of periodic sound for speech. There are other periodic sound sources (e.g., flapping lips), but these are minor compared to the sound produced from the vocal folds. In addition, there are aperiodic sound sources such as those used for the production of voiceless consonants. The vocal folds may be also involved in the production of aperiodic sound, as, for example, in the consonant /h/.

In this chapter, we will review the basic concepts of phonatory physiology. First, the conditions that must exist before sound can be produced will be presented, followed by discussion of the mechanisms necessary for initiating and sustaining sound. The third and fourth sections will be brief outlines of the physiological mechanisms for control of vocal pitch and intensity control by the vocal folds, respectively. Finally, a review of some of the mechanisms for control of voice quality will be presented. The reader interested in further information on these topics is referred to the excellent text by Titze (1994).

GLOTTAL TONE INITIATION Before sound can be produced from the vocal folds, several conditions must be established. First, the vocal folds must be approximated or almost approximated in the phonatory position. This position, in comparison to the inspiratory position of the vocal folds (Fig. 11.1A), is shown in Figure 11.1B. Phonation may also be initiated after completely closing the vocal folds.

It is also necessary to properly tense and elongate the vocal folds prior to actually producing sound. Length and tension are important determinants of the fundamental vibrating rate of the vocal folds, in ways that will be discussed later under "Mechanisms of Vocal Frequency Change."

Finally, there must be airflow from the lungs. In order to be able to produce the required flow of air from the lungs, there must be a sufficient quantity of air in the lungs. Typically we inhale before we begin producing sound for an utterance.

Once these initial conditions have been established, phonation can start. When the vocal folds are in the phonatory position, it is necessary to close them in order to start vibration. If one starts with the vocal folds fully closed, it is necessary to open them in order to start vibration. Whatever the starting point, the process thereafter is similar and is simply described as a series of alternate openings and closings of the vocal folds. The opening and closing is regulated by the degree of tension in the vocal folds and

**A**

**B**

*Figure 11.1.* Schematic representation of the stages of vocal fold adduction. **A,** During inspiration. **B,** At start of phonation.

two aerodynamic events.

The aerodynamic event important for closing the vocal folds is called the Bernoulli effect, named after a famous 18th-century Swiss physicist. Bernoulli was most interested in fluid flows, but his principles hold for gas flows as well. Simply stated, Bernoulli's second law of fluid mechanics states that the sum of the static pressures and the kinetic pressures in a gas is always equal to a constant. The constant may vary according to the temperature, pressure, or molecular structure of the gas. But within these conditions, when motion of the molecules changes, there is a change in the static pressure exerted by the molecules. Stating the principle another way, when there is increased motion of gas molecules, there will be decreased pressure.

The Bernoulli effect is often evoked to explain how airplanes rise in the air. The undersurface of the wing of an airplane is rather flat, whereas the upper surface is markedly convex in shape. This curvature on the upper wing surface means that the air molecules passing over the top of the wing have a greater distance to travel to pass over the wing than those molecules that pass under the wing. The velocity of the molecules traveling along the surface of the upper wing must increase in order to travel the distance in the same time as the molecules traveling under the wing. In short, their kinetic "pressure" has been increased. According to Bernoulli's principle, when the kinetic pressure increases, the static pressure must decrease. Thus, there is less pressure along the upper surface of the wing. By the same token, there is greater pressure below the wing, and this greater pressure will lift the wing (and the airplane) into the sky.

The same principle holds for the vocal folds. The vocal folds impose a partial obstruction to the flow of air. The molecules traveling along the sides of the trachea, when meeting the vocal folds, must travel a greater distance around the fold to meet the molecules traveling up the center of the trachea. The molecules along the surface of the vocal folds must increase their velocity and kinetic pressure. Again, static pressure on the surface of the vocal folds will be decreased. The vocal folds, being pliable and movable, will begin to move toward the center of the trachea because of this pressure differential. Eventually, the two vocal folds will meet at the midline, and airflow will cease.

The trick that needs to be performed to produce vibration is to create the Bernoulli effect when you wish to close the vocal folds and a positive pressure when you wish to open them (Titze, 1994). When the vocal folds close, there is a sudden decrease of air-flow. When the vocal folds open, there is a momentary delay in the start of the airflow due to this inertia. This explains the characteristic shape of the airflow pulse through the glottis where the rising airflow phase is slower than the opening of the vocal folds (Fig. 11.2A and B). Air particle velocities through the glottis also shows asymmetry (Fig. 11.2C). Generally, these velocities increase as the vocal folds open and change direction when the airflow pulse shuts off at closure. Intraglottal air pressure is solely dependent on air particle velocity (Titze, 1994). The classic Bernoulli equation states that as kinetic energy increases, static "energy" must decrease as both sum to a con-stant. Thus, as air particle velocity increases, intraglottal pressure decreases. Air parti-cle directional change results in an abrupt negative change of intraglottal pressure (Fig. 11.2C and D) just when we need it to produce vocal fold closure. Positive pres-

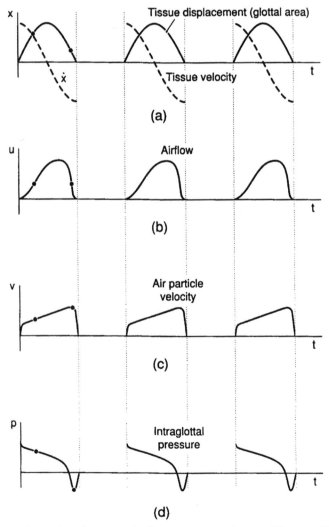

*Figure 11.2.* Relationships between displacement and velocity of the vocal folds, airflow, air particle velocity, and intraglottal air pressures.

sure below the vocal folds forces them open.

The tension and mass of the vocal folds create a resistance to vibration. Consequently, there is a minimum pressure required to force the folds into vibration. Titze (1992b) calls this pressure phonation threshold pressure (PTP). PTP is dependent on the frequency of phonation and may be slightly different for males and females (and probably for children as well). PTP is also dependent on hydration levels of vocal fold tissues (Verdolini-Marston, Titze, & Druker, 1990). Intensity control is also related to PTP.

## MECHANISMS OF VOCAL FREQUENCY CHANGE

The human vocal mechanism is capable of producing a wide range of frequencies, sometimes in excess of three octaves. In this section, we will review some of the physiological mechanisms that determine the fundamental vibrating rate of the vocal folds.

Early in the study of phonation, individuals compared the vocal folds to vibrating strings. After all, both the vocal folds and strings had a length and a mass and were under tension. Furthermore, much was known about the determinants of frequency in strings, and the analogy appeared to be a good one.

As research on voice physiology progressed, evidence accumulated that prompted a reevaluation of the analogy between the mechanism of frequency variation by the vocal folds and by a string. Recent evidence has confirmed that the physical properties that determine the frequency of a vibrating string also determine the vibrating frequency of the vocal folds. The vibratory frequency of a string and of the vocal folds is determined by its length, tension, and mass. Actually, in the case of the vocal folds, it is not their total mass that is significant but rather the mass that is set into vibration. The amount of mass set into vibration will depend on fundamental frequency, intensity, and mode of vibration. Furthermore, the amount of mass varies as a function of the length of the string of the vocal fold. The relationship of vocal fold thickness to length is similar to that observed in a rubber band. As the band is stretched, the thickness of the band decreases.

### *Vocal Fold Length and Fundamental Frequency*

A convenient way of understanding the relationships between length, mass, and tension in a string and in the vocal folds is by graphing the parameters as a function of frequency. A plot of fundamental frequency as a function of vocal fold length is shown in Figure 11.3. In the modal register, as vocal fold length increases, frequency increases. This relationship is clearly opposite to that predicted by the classic equation for determining the frequency of a vibrating string. However, when phonation is produced in the falsetto or upper register, fundamental frequency appears to decrease as vocal fold length is increased. Subsequent research has shown that the length of the vibrating portion of the vocal folds decreases as frequency is increased (Rubin & Hirt, 1960). These opposite effects, at least for modal register phonation, is why the string analogy was thought by some to be inappropriate for the control of fundamental frequency by the vocal folds. But length is not the sole mechanism for control of fundamental frequency either in strings or the vocal folds.

### *Vocal Fold Mass and Fundamental Frequency*

The mass of the vocal folds may also play a role in frequency control. Figure 11.4

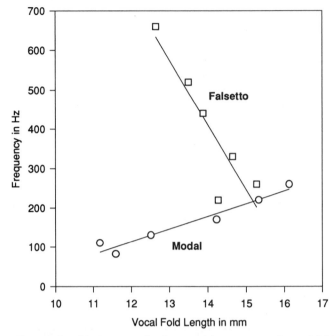

*Figure 11.3.* The relationship between fundamental frequency and vocal fold length.

shows the relationship between thickness of the vocal folds and frequency. Note that for the vocal folds, vocal frequency decreases as mass increases, a relationship similar to that for a vibrating string.

## Vocal Fold Tension and Fundamental Frequency

Tension affects the vibrating frequency of a string and the vocal folds. The relationship between tension and frequency of the vocal folds is shown in Figure 11.5. As tension increases, so too does frequency. In general, the effect of tension on the vocal folds produces changes of frequency much like in a string.

It is very difficult to measure tension directly in the living human vocal fold. Indirect evidence must be obtained from recordings of muscle activity or measurements made on dog or excised human larynges (Perlman & Titze, 1988; Perlman, Titze, & Cooper, 1984). Moreover, the variations of tension produced by muscle contraction must also be considered (Colton, 1988) when trying to understand how tension determines the fundamental frequency of phonation.

Tension becomes more important in the determination of fundamental frequency at certain areas of an individual's total phonational range. Van den Berg and Tan (1959) have shown that the largest variation of tension occurs at upper frequencies, most often produced in the falsetto register. A small amount of tension variation occurs at frequencies typically heard in speech. Thus, although tension is an important determinant of fundamental frequency variation, it is not the only determinant. As has been shown, the mass of the vocal folds (or more accurately, their mass per unit length) has a pronounced influence on the fundamental frequency of the vibration.

It is clear that there may be several mechanisms determining fundamental frequency in the human voice. At some frequencies (usually in the modal register), overall mass may be the most important determinant (Allen & Hollien, 1973), whereas at

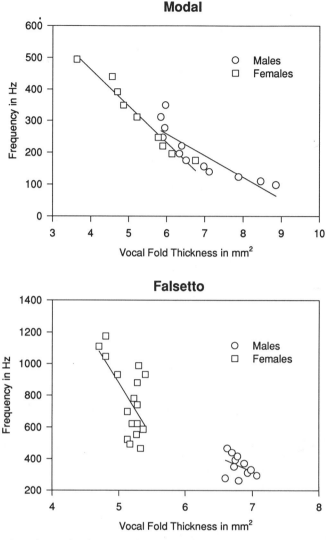

*Figure 11.4.* The relationship between fundamental frequency and vocal fold thickness.

other frequencies (usually in the falsetto register), tension may be the dominant factor. It is the combination of these factors that ultimately determines the fundamental frequency of vocal fold vibration.

The data from van den Berg and Tan also show that the relationship between tension and fundamental frequency differs as airflow rates differ (Fig. 11.5). Thus, airflow appears to be another contributing factor in the physiological mechanisms of vocal frequency control. In some cases, airflow may be the major determinant of frequency, much as it is for aeolian tones. You may have walked through an open field in which telephone or electrical wires passed overhead and heard the sound the wind makes when striking the wires. This is an example of an aeolian tone whose frequency is determined by the speed of the airflow rushing across the wire. In many patients with phonatory disorders, there is excessive airflow. Although the speed of the airflow may not directly affect the fundamental frequency of the vocal folds as in an aeolian tone, it may be a sign of an inefficient mechanism being used for the variation of vocal pitch. Or it may be that the patient is using a combination of tension, mass,

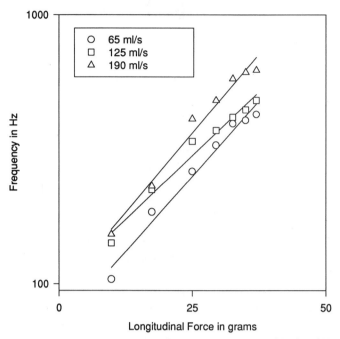

*Figure 11.5.* The relationship between fundamental frequency and vocal fold tension.

and airflow that causes or contributes to the voice problem. These possibilities point to the need for information about all of these parameters with voice patients. The availability of such information may help in understanding the bases for the patient's vocal problem.

As in a string, the fundamental frequency of the vocal folds is determined by a complex interaction between length, mass, and tension. There may be various combinations of these parameters that produce the same fundamental frequency. However, not all combinations of length, mass, and tension may be efficient for the production of voice.

## MECHANISMS OF LOUDNESS CHANGE

The human voice is capable of producing a wide range of vocal intensities, sometimes exceeding 60 dB. Additional changes of intensity result from variation in the size and shape of the vocal tract, which acts as a resonator of sound. The mechanisms for the control of vocal intensity, much as those of pitch control, involve muscular activity in combination with airflows and pressures.

Vocal intensity is usually reported in decibels of sound pressure level. Since sound is basically a pressure disturbance, we would expect that increased pressures beneath the vocal folds, when released by the folds, would produce a greater intensity, and indeed, experimental evidence supports this expectation (Ladefoged & McKinney, 1963). As shown in Figure 11.6, when the subglottal air pressure increases, intensity increases, although the exact relationship will vary for different vowels and voice qualities.

However, the controlling mechanism of vocal intensity is not subglottal air pressure. Rather, the controlling mechanism is the degree and time of closure of the vocal folds themselves. That is, by maintaining closure of the vocal folds, there is more time to build up pressure beneath them. More intense sound results when the subglottal

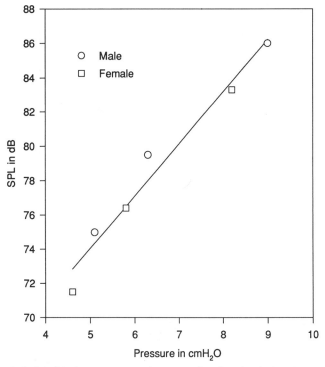

*Figure 11.6.* Relationship between sound pressure level and subglottal air pressure.

air pressure is sufficient to overcome the resistance of the vocal folds. Resistance is the important factor in intensity control. The more vocal fold resistance there is to opening, the greater the pressure disturbance when the resistance is overcome and the folds are forced to open. Thus, intensity is most often controlled by the vocal folds through variations of glottal resistance. Glottal resistance is defined as the ratio of the pressure divided by the flow. Measuring these two quantities will allow the calculation of resistance.

Isshiki (1964, 1965) has shown that glottal resistance is a major controlling mechanism of vocal intensities for low fundamental frequencies, that is, fundamental frequencies produced in the lower part of an individual's phonational range or in the modal register. At higher frequencies, especially frequencies produced in falsetto, glottal resistance is no longer the major factor. Rather, it appears that airflow becomes the dominant variable in intensity variation at these high fundamental frequencies. Furthermore, the range of intensities an individual can produce in the falsetto register is much smaller than can be produced in the modal register (Colton, 1973). This finding would suggest, or at least be in consonance with, the existence of a different controlling mechanism for intensity control in falsetto.

Another mechanism of intensity control has been described (Sundberg, Titze, & Scherer, 1993; Titze, 1994). The vocal folds produce sound when they close. The intensity (and spectra) of the sound is dependent on the velocity of closure of the vocal folds. Glottal power is directly related to the rate of change of the airflow pulse at the moment of closure (Titze & Sundberg, 1992). This rate of change of airflow at closure is often referred to as maximum declination rate or simply airflow closing slope. The relationship between the airflow closing slope of the airflow pulse and intensity is shown in Figure 11.7. Therefore, intensity control by the vocal folds may be dependent on at least two factors, glottal resistance and the rate of airflow change at the mo-

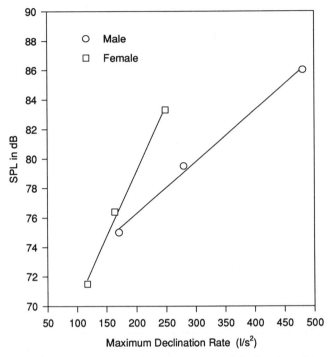

*Figure 11.7.* Sound pressure levels and maximum rate of declination of the airflow pulse (or the slope of the closing portion of the airflow pulse) as derived from inverse filtering.

ment of closure.

For a variety of reasons, some patients have difficulty in completely closing their vocal folds. In an attempt to speak at a normal vocal intensity, these patients increase air pressure by increasing the expiratory force from the thorax-abdomen system. The patient may also attempt to increase glottal closure in an effort to increase glottal resistance and to maintain an adequate level of tension in the vocal folds. As a result of this effortful vocal behavior, greater than normal subglottal pressures are developed, and there is increased tension in the vocal folds. Because greater than normal muscle activity is involved, these conditions may create vocal fatigue as well as excessive air rushing across the vocal folds. The latter creates greater noise levels in the voice. A vicious cycle ensues, as the vocal fatigue may result in even poorer vocal fold adduction and the need for even greater effort on the patient's part, leading cyclically to poorer voice.

There is another factor that will affect the sound pressure level (SPL) of phonation. That factor is the spectral characteristics of the tone produced by the vocal folds. It is well known that variation of the frequency composition of a tone will vary its intensity. Adding frequencies or varying the amplitude of the components of the tone will affect the intensity of the complex tone. Similarly, the spectrum of the vocal folds can be varied within limits and thus alter the overall intensity of the vocal fold tone. Consequently, the vocal folds can affect the intensity of the tone by variation of the frequency components in the tone. Speed of closure of the vocal folds will affect the spectral features of the glottal tone (Löfqvist, 1993).

In some patients with phonatory disorders, the spectral characteristics of the tone produced are markedly different from normal. Usually, but not always, the number of frequency components in the pathological voice is much smaller than in the normal voice. When that is the case, then lower intensities would be expected. In order to

*Figure 11.8.* Inverse filtered airflow waveform of the vocal folds (top panel) and its corresponding frequency spectrum (bottom panel) from a phonation produced by a male subject.

compensate for the different spectral characteristics and their effect on intensity, a patient may try to increase subglottal pressures or adductory forces, resulting in increased strain and subsequent abuse of the vocal folds.

Loudness is the perceptual correlate of intensity, but intensity is not the only physical factor that affects loudness. The pitch of the voice and its spectral composition may also affect its perceived loudness. Of course, factors such as the distance from the speaker, room acoustics, diffraction, and interference may also affect the loudness of a voice as perceived by a listener.

## MECHANISMS OF QUALITY VARIATION

Voice quality is an important attribute of normal and abnormal voices. Voice quality identifies the individual and sets him or her apart from another. A change of voice quality may signal the presence of a benign problem or one that could be life threatening. But defining voice quality can be difficult and imprecise.

Many adjectives are used to describe voice quality: pleasant and unpleasant, normal and pathological. Singers, actors, professional speakers, and those who work with the voice use jargon to describe the variation of normal voice quality. Quantification of these terms either acoustically or physiologically has proven to be very difficult.

Acoustically, the important parameter concerned with voice quality is spectrum. Spectrum refers to the number and amplitude of the frequencies present in a complex tone, such as the vocal fold tone. Figure 11.8 presents the spectrum of a typical vocal fold tone produced during speech. However, the vocal folds can produce many different voice qualities, each with its own spectral characteristics (Fig. 11.9).

Other factors may be important in describing a voice quality acoustically. Although pitch would be expected to be one such factor, it is interesting to note that it apparently is not used in distinguishing one voice quality from another (Colton, 1987). This finding is similar to the influence of pitch in the perception of nonphonatory sounds like complex sounds (Plomp, 1976) and noise bands (Chipman & Carey, 1975). Varying the pitch level may alter some of the details of a voice, but not its basic voice quality.

Voice quality is not solely determined by the vibratory characteristics of the vocal folds. The shape and configuration of the vocal tract are also determinants of voice

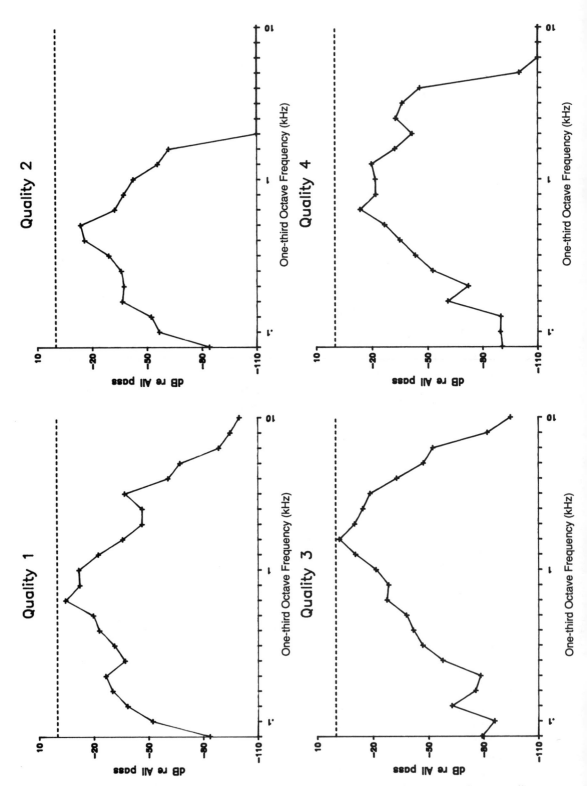

*Figure 11.9.* Some spectra of different voice qualities. Mode 1 refers to a quality typically heard during speech, mode 2 to a quality of a sound heard during sobbing or during the singing of a lullaby, mode 3 to a quality typically heard in Country Western singing, and mode 4 to a quality heard in operatic singing.

quality. For example, females have slightly different vocal tract configurations than males, and as a result, female voices can still be recognized as female even when the obvious pitch difference is removed (Coleman, 1971, 1973, 1976). The overall characteristics of an individual's vocal tract, such as the length, cross-sectional area, ratio of oral to pharyngeal cavity size, and so on, would also determine that individual's voice quality.

Physiological change in laryngeal and vocal tract configurations and characteristics have been observed in individuals as they produced various voice qualities (Colton & Estill, 1981; Painter, 1986, 1991). For example, in some voice qualities, the size of the pharyngeal cavity is much larger than in other voice qualities. Many of these differences appear to occur in the larynx itself, as well as in the pharynx. We have little information about the vocal tract characteristics of patients with voice disorders.

## SUMMARY

In this chapter, a brief review of the mechanisms for voice production, frequency control, intensity variation, and the generation of voice quality have been reviewed. The tone produced by the vocal folds results from the complex interaction of airflow, air pressure, and muscular activity, which regulate the length, mass, and tension of the vocal folds. Variation in these parameters will affect the fundamental frequency of the voice, as well as its intensity and voice quality. Measurement of these acoustic parameters of the voice will assist in the quantification of the vocal behavior and help to determine the nature of the problem. Accurate measurement of acoustic, perceptual, or physiological parameters can play a part in understanding disorders and planning treatment.

# Chapter 12

# Neuroanatomy of the Vocal Mechanism

Volitional control of the muscles of the larynx resides in the brain. However, there are many connecting points or stations within the brain, including the cortex, subcortical areas, midbrain, and medulla, that play an important role in the ultimate control of phonation. Thus, saying that phonation is controlled by the brain is much too simplistic and underemphasizes the roles various structures play in integrating information and coordinating the activity of the muscles active in phonation. In this chapter, a brief review of the neuroanatomy and neurophysiology of phonation will be presented. A further and more detailed review of brain mechanisms controlling vocalization may be found in Larson (1988).

## CORTICAL MECHANISMS OF PHONATORY CONTROL

The cerebral cortex is that portion of the brain responsible for the conceptualization, planning, and execution of the speech act, including phonation. Some areas of the cortex may be responsible for creating the act, others for its linguistic characteristics, and still others for the emotionality of the act. Penfield and Roberts (1959) have identified three major areas of the cortex directly responsible for vocalization. These are, in decreasing order of importance, (a) the precentral and postcentral gyrus (Rolandic area), (b) the anterior (or Broca's) area, and (c) the supplementary motor area. These areas are shown in Figure 12.1. Experiments have demonstrated that vocalization occurs when certain spots within these areas are stimulated in both the dominant and nondominant hemispheres (Fig. 12.2). Within these areas, depending on the specific areas stimulated, it has been shown that vocalization can be initiated or stopped and speech can be slurred or distorted. These behaviors occur as the result of stimulation in either the dominant or the nondominant hemisphere. Speech and phonation are complex motor acts involving simultaneous activation and control of many muscles. Although the control of these motor acts occurs primarily in the cortex, control of individual muscles seems to occur at a much lower level in the brain. There is no evidence to suggest that cortical stimulation produces a response in a single solitary muscle. Higher brain function is concerned with idealization of the event, integration of sensory information, feedback control, and coordination of various muscles required for the motor act.

*Figure 12.1.* Diagram of the cortical areas involved in speech movement control. Area 4 (primary motor cortex), areas 3, 1, and 2 (somatosensory cortex), area 44 (Broca's area), and area 6 (premotor cortex and supplementary motor area).

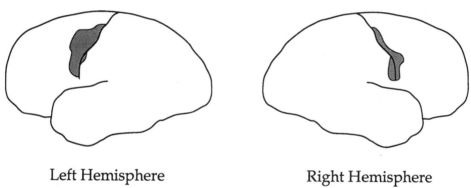

## Left Hemisphere                         Right Hemisphere

*Figure 12.2.* Areas on the left and right hemispheres that produce vocalization when stimulated.

## SUBCORTICAL MECHANISMS

The motor cortex has numerous connections to the thalamus, a major portion of the diencephalon or interbrain. Other parts of the diencephalon include the hypothalamus, metathalamus, epithalamus, and subthalamus (Riklan & Levita, 1969). The third ventricle is also part of the diencephalon (Gardner, 1963). The thalamus has major pathways to the motor cortex and Broca's area (Penfield & Roberts, 1959). In addition, the thalamus has numerous connections to the cerebellum, midbrain, and other structures in the diencephalon (Fig. 12.3). There are various nuclei in the thalamus that project to parts of the cerebral cortex. These are shown in Figure 12.4. Note that the motor area (precentral gyrus) located anterior to the central sulcus receives much of its projection from the ventral lateral nucleus of the thalamus. Botez and Barbeau (1971) concluded that the ventrolateral nucleus was responsible for the initiation of speech movements as well as control of loudness, pitch, rate, and articulation. Broca's area

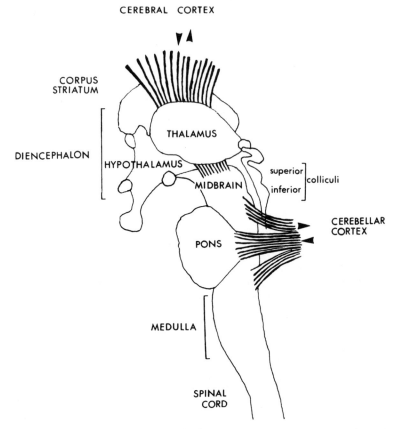

*Figure 12.3.* Diagrammatic representation of the brainstem.

receives connections from the dorsal median and centromedian nuclei of the thalamus. (The centromedian nuclei help form the massa intermedia shown in Figure 12.4.)

The thalamus is a most fascinating structure in the diencephalon since it appears to act both as a relay for impulses occurring in lower areas of the brain and as an integrator of information (Riklan & Levita, 1969). Furthermore, the thalamus is involved in the maintenance of consciousness, alertness, and attention and may also integrate emotion into a complex motor act. Some of the thalamic nuclei are nonspecific and project to many areas on the cortex (Fig. 12.5). Thus, insofar as speech and voice are concerned, the thalamus plays a major role in integrating incoming sensory information, coordinating outgoing information from the cortex and other areas of the brain, and, perhaps, adding emotionality to speech and voice.

## MIDBRAIN STRUCTURES

The midbrain or mesencephalon lies beneath the thalamus (House & Pansky, 1967). On the anterior surface of the midbrain are the cerebral peduncles that connect the cerebrum with the brainstem and spinal cord. On its posterior surface, there are four rounded areas called the colliculi. The superior colliculi are concerned with visual function, whereas the inferior colliculi are concerned with audition. Within the midbrain there is a cavity called the cerebral aqueduct of Sylvius, which is surrounded by a thick zone of gray matter. An important area of this gray matter, dorsal to the aqueduct, is called the periaqueductal gray.

*Figure 12.4.* Diagram of the major thalamic nuclei and their projections.

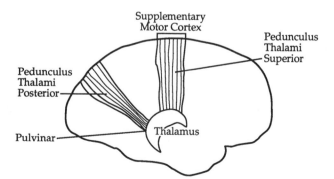

*Figure 12.5.* Drawing showing the connections between the pulvinar nuclei of the thalamus and the posterior speech area of the cortex. Diagram also shows the pathway between the thalamus and the superior speech cortex (supplementary motor area).

Several investigators have shown that stimulation of the dorsal and ventrolateral areas of the periaqueductal gray produces activity in some laryngeal muscles (Larson, 1985; Larson & Kistler, 1986; Ortega, DeRosier, Park, & Larson, 1988). Larson (1985) has reported that some cells in the ventrolateral area stimulate muscle activity, whereas other cells suppress activity. He suggested that the periaqueductal gray may be an intermediate area between the recognition of a stimulus or event and the subsequent production of the motor act. Other areas, such as the hypothalamus, amygdala, and anterior cingulate gyrus, are responsible for vocalizations but of a kind that Larson (1985) notes are species specific. Botez and Barbeau (1971) also implicated the periaqueductal gray in disorders involving mutism.

Lesions in the PAG and adjacent areas have produced mutism (Adametz & O'Leary, 1959; Randall, 1964). Moreover, electrical stimulation of the PAG has produced natural sounding vocalizations in a variety of species (Jürgens & Pratt, 1979; Kelly, Beaton, & Magoun, 1946; Yajima, Hayashi, & Yoshii, 1982). Chemical stimulation of the PAG has elicited two kinds of vocalizations in cats (Zhang, Davis, Bandler, & Carrive, 1994). One vocalization type (Type A) consisted of meows, howls, and growls remarkably similar to normal feline vocalizations. The other vocalization type (Type B) was described as a hiss, also found in normal feline repertoire. Type A vocalizations were all voiced with a fundamental frequency and strong harmonics. It involved activity in the cricothyroid, genioglossus, and internal oblique muscles. Type B has no voicing and no activity in the cricothyroid muscles but normal activity in the genioglossus and internal oblique muscles. Zhang and his colleagues point out that these vocalization types are very similar to voiced and unvoiced sounds produced by humans.

Zhang et al. (1994) found strong evidence for the PAG to be involved in the control of patterns of muscle activity involving muscles of respiration, vocalization and in the orofacial area. They specifically pointed out that no PAG sites were found that activated individual muscles. They concluded that the PAG contains neurons involved in the control of at least two kinds of vocalization.

## BRAINSTEM

The major bilateral structures in the brainstem implicated in the neural control of phonation include the nucleus ambiguus, nucleus tractus solitarii, and nucleus parabrachialis. Yoshida, Mitsumasu, Hirano, Morimoto, and Kanaseki (1987) performed an elegant study in which they traced the connections among these structures. When they injected a tracer chemical into one nucleus ambiguus, they found evidence of the tracer throughout the contralateral nuclei, in the nuclei tractus solitarii bilaterally, in the nuclei parabrachialis, and bilaterally in the lateral and ventrolateral parts of the periaqueductal gray area, with a predominance ipsilaterally. Injection of a tracer into the nucleus tractus solitarii resulted in labeled cells throughout the nucleus itself, as well as in the dorsal motor nucleus of the vagus, part of the hypoglossal nucleus, the medial portion of the nucleus gracilis, and the dorsal part of the reticular formation. Clearly, there are many interconnections bilaterally among the nucleus ambiguus, nucleus tractus solitarii, reticular formation around the nucleus ambiguus, motor roots of the vagus, and periaqueductal gray area.

Zhang, Davis, Carrive, and Bandler (1992) have also implicated the nucleus retroambigualis in the control of vocalization. This "structure" is actually the caudal 1/3 of the ventral respiratory group located in the ventrolateral medulla. Neurons in this area have been long implicated in the control of respiration (von Euler, 1986) but it has been shown that they also have an important role in the control of laryngeal muscles and vocalization.

## CEREBELLUM

The cerebellum, a structure lying immediately posterior to the midbrain area, is strongly implicated in the control of movement. Its location is shown in Figure 12.6A. Figure 12.6B shows the cerebellum from a dorsal view after the cerebrum has been removed. The three main portions of the cerebellum are seen in this diagram: the vermis (V), the pars intermedia (PI), and the hemispheres (H). The cerebellum consists of many transverse folia, shown in Figure 12.6C, whose complex infolding vastly increases the surface area of the cerebellum in much the same way as is seen in the cerebrum. The fissura prima (FP) is a deep fissure separating the anterior and posterior lobes.

Two major areas of the cerebellum are instrumental in the control of movement (von Euler, 1986). The first, the pars intermedia, has many direct connections via midbrain nuclei with the cerebrum (Fig. 12.7A). Impulses from the motor cortex are quickly relayed from the pyramidal tracts (PT) to the pars intermedia via the nuclei pontis, lateral reticular nucleus, and inferior olive. The pars intermedia analyzes the movement patterns and quickly returns the results of its analysis to the cerebral cortex via connections through the interpositus nucleus, the ventral lateral nuclei of the thalamus, and the red nucleus. As such, the pars intermedia acts like a computer controlling a missile. It may not have given the original command to fire, but it constantly monitors the missile, taking small corrective actions whenever the missile deviates from its intended flight plan (Eccles, 1977).

The role of the cerebellar hemispheres in movement control seems to be one of planning the stages of a movement pattern. As shown in Fig. 12.7B, there are few direct connections to tracts that lead to lower motoneurons, as was the case for the connections between the cerebrum and pars intermedia of the cerebellum. Rather, the connections from the motor cortex pass through the nuclei pontis and inferior olive directly to cells within the cerebellar hemispheres, and impulses from the cerebellar hemispheres pass through the nucleus dentatus to the ventral lateral nuclei of the thalamus and red nucleus back to the cerebral hemispheres, where movement is initiated. It appears that the command center, after drafting a movement plan, sends it on to the cerebellar hemispheres for revision and refinement before adopting it. According to

*Figure 12.6.* **A,** Human cerebrum and cerebellum. **B,** The cerebellum from its dorsal aspect. **C,** Midline view after sagittal section. *Legend:* H, hemispheres; V, vermis; PI, the pars intermedia; FP, fissura prima.

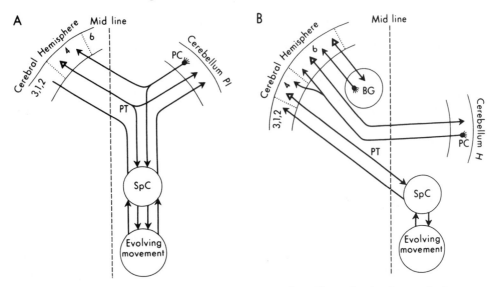

Figure 12.7. Cerebrocerebellar circuits in motor control. **A,** The main circuit starts in the motor cortex (4) and travels down the pyramidal tract (PT) to the spinal cord, with side branches via the pars intermedia (PI) to the cerebellum. Impulses from Purkinje cells (PC) in the cerebellum communicate with the motor cortex and down to the spinal cord. **B,** Circuits from area 6 in the cerebrum to the cerebellar hemispheres (H). A return circuit from the Purkinje cells (PC) back to areas 4 and 6 is shown. Also shown is a circuit from area 6 to the basal ganglia (BG) and its return to the cerebrum. Spinal centers (SpC) are indicated. Evolving movement refers to the desired movement pattern of a structure.

Eccles (1977), the cerebellar hemispheres are concerned with anticipatory planning based on learning, experience, and sensory information they receive from other brain centers.

The importance of the cerebellum in the control of speech movement cannot be emphasized enough. Kornhuber (1977) believes that without it (and other midbrain areas) the cerebral cortex could not function and would be ineffective in the generation of movements. The cerebellum acts to regulate motor movement continuously and quickly, requiring some degree of preprogramming and adjustment by learning. Certainly, coordination of muscles within the larynx is necessary for phonation, as is coordination with other systems involved in speech production.

## PERIPHERAL CONNECTIONS: THE VAGUS NERVE

The vagus nerve is the major nerve that supplies the larynx (and other parts of the body as well). The vagus provides sensory fibers within the larynx, as well as fibers that control all the muscles of the larynx. The cell bodies of the vagus are located in the nucleus ambiguus. Laryngeal muscles are controlled by cells in the more caudal portions of the nucleus. The vagus emerges from the surface of the medulla between the cerebellar peduncle and the inferior olives in the midbrain. It exits the skull through the jugular foramen.

After exiting the skull, the vagus divides into many branches that serve the head, neck, thorax, and abdomen. These are shown schematically in Figure 12.8. Shortly after exiting the jugular foramen, a small filament (the meningeal filament) exits the nerve to serve the dura mater on the posterior fossa of the base of the skull. The auricular branch provides sensory fibers to the skin behind the pinna and to the posterior

## FUNCTIONAL COMPONENTS OF PERIPHERAL NERVES

*Figure 12.8.* The vagus nerve.

part of the external auditory meatus. The pharyngeal branch provides motor fibers to the muscles of the pharynx and soft palate.

The major portions of the vagus serving the larynx are the superior laryngeal and the recurrent laryngeal nerves. The superior laryngeal is the primary sensory nerve for the larynx. It arises from the inferior ganglion of the vagus and descends along the side of the pharynx behind the internal carotid artery, where it sends off two branches. The external branch descends along the side of the larynx to serve the cricothyroid muscle. The internal branch descends to an opening in the thyrohyoid membrane and enters the larynx to serve the mucous membrane of the larynx down to the true vocal folds. The recurrent laryngeal nerve follows a different course on either side of the body. On the right side, the recurrent descends in the neck to loop

*Table 12.1.* Branches of the Vagus (10th Cranial Nerve)

| | |
|---|---|
| *In the jugular fossa* | |
| Meningeal | Serves dura mater in posterior fossa at the base of the skull. |
| Auricular | Serves skin on back of outer ear (auricle) and posterior part of the external acoustic meatus. |
| Pharyngeal | Joins with glossopharyngeal, sympathetic, and external laryngeal nerves to form pharyngeal plexus, which serves the muscles and membranes of the pharynx and muscles of the soft palate, with the exception of the tensor. |
| *In the neck* | |
| Superior laryngeal | |
| External | Supplies cricothyroid. |
| Internal | Pierces the hyothyroid membrane to supply the mucous membrane of the larynx down to the true vocal folds. |
| Recurrent | |
| Right side | Arises in front of the subclavian artery to travel upward along the trachea. |
| Left side | Arises on the left side of the arch of the aorta. |
| Both | Enter the larynx behind the articulation of the inferior cornu of the thyroid with the cricoid. |
| | Serve all intrinsic muscles with the exception of the cricothyroid. |
| Superior cardiac | Serves cardiac plexus. |
| Inferior cardiac | Serves cardiac plexus. |
| *In the thorax* | |
| Anterior bronchial | Sensory to the lung. |
| Posterior bronchial | Sensory to the lung. |
| Esophageal | Sensory to the esophagus. |
| *In the abdomen* | |
| Gastric | Sensory to the stomach. |
| Celiac | Sensory to the pancreas, spleen, kidneys, suprarenal bodies, and intestine. |
| Hepatic | Sensory to the liver. |

around the subclavian artery (just below the clavicle) and then ascends alongside the trachea to serve the remaining intrinsic muscles of the larynx. On the left side, the recurrent laryngeal nerve takes a much more circuitous route, descending into the thorax, looping around the aorta, and then ascending alongside the trachea until it reaches the larynx. It also provides motor fibers to the remaining intrinsic laryngeal muscles.

There are other branches of the vagus nerve in the neck, thorax, and abdomen that provide sensory innervation to various structures within these areas. These branches of the vagus are shown in Table 12.1.

The extrinsic laryngeal muscles are innervated by several nerves. The anterior belly of the digastric muscle receives its innervation from the mylohyoid branch of the inferior alveolar nerve, whereas the posterior belly is innervated by the 7th cranial nerve (the facial). The mylohyoid muscle is innervated by the mylohyoid branch of the inferior alveolar nerve, and the geniohyoid, sternohyoid, sternothyroid, and omohyoid muscles by the ansa cervicalis (C1). The thyrohyoid is innervated by ansa cervicalis (C1) via the hypoglossal nerve.

There are numerous protective mechanisms within the respiratory tract, but the most vigorous exist in the larynx. Some are mechanical and act to close off the airway; others are expulsive and serve to force foreign substances from the airway. All are reflexive and operate under involuntary control.

There are many sensory endings within the larynx that collect information about the state of the larynx and respiratory tract and transmit this information via several reflex arcs as well as directly to the central nervous system. Wyke (1967, 1969) has written extensively about these reflex control mechanisms. The complexity of these control systems and their interactions with the respiratory and other body systems make this a fascinating area of study. For example, sensory endings exist in the mucosa or lining of the larynx that respond to mechanical forces or air pressure changes within the tract. These nerve endings are capable of sending information to the central nervous system about the mechanical state of the lining of the respiratory tract. Furthermore, reflex endings exist within the joints of the various cartilages of the larynx that discharge when these joints are moved. These discharges have been shown to affect the ongoing electrical activity of some intrinsic laryngeal muscles (Wyke, 1967). Finally, the intrinsic laryngeal muscles contain specialized stretch receptors that discharge when the muscle is stretched or contracted (Wyke, 1969). The various levels of reflex mechanisms within the larynx suggest that elaborate precautions are in place to protect the airway and maintain life. From our perspective in voice pathology and its treatment, they are important to consider when trying to understand the physiology of normal and aberrant human phonation and laryngeal behavior. Wyke (1969) hypothesizes that some types of stuttering may be related to disorders of the various reflex mechanisms within the larynx.

## SUMMARY

Proper control of the muscles of the larynx is critical in the production of voice. The levels of control within the central nervous system are multiple and complex. Lesions in some parts of the system, especially in the cortex and thalamus (and related structures) would be expected to have profound effects on speech and voice production. However, the fact that cortical and some subcortical controls are present bilaterally provides some measure of safety when lesions are unilateral. Indeed, cases have been reported wherein portions of the cerebral cortex were surgically removed with little lasting effect on speech and phonation. Lesions farther down in the brain might be expected to have a more singular effect on a specific muscle or set of muscles. However, innervation is still bilateral and redundant in some lower level brain areas, thus affording considerable protection of the systems involved in speech production. Once the nerves exit the skull, lesions of a nerve will have more specific effects involving, perhaps, a single muscle or small number of muscles bilaterally or unilaterally.

# Chapter 13

# Some Normative Data on the Voice

In this chapter some normative data on the voice are presented. Our purpose is not to present all the available data, much of which is incomplete and confusing, but rather to provide the most meaningful data against which patient data may be compared clinically. The data reported here were gathered from a variety of sources, all of which are referenced for those seeking further information. An invaluable source for more complete data is Baken (1987). The sources of the data in several of this chapter's tables are indicated by numbers in the body of the table, keyed to references below the table. The full citation for these sources appears in the reference list at the end of the book. Other reference information can be found in the "Figure and Table Credits" at the end of the book. Additional information about these measures and how they are obtained can be found in Chapter 7.

## FUNDAMENTAL FREQUENCY

The measure of fundamental frequency, reflecting the vibratory rate of the vocal folds, is useful for comparing intra- and intersubject pitch levels. Fundamental frequency can be measured during production of sustained vowels or during a reading passage. It is important to note, however, that fundamental frequency will vary depending on the type of speech material used. There are considerable data on fundamental frequency, covering ages from birth to death. At many ages, however, fundamental frequency plateaus and may not change for many years. The data in Table 13.1 represent a summary of fundamental frequencies. There have been several studies reported of fundamental frequency at certain ages or within certain age ranges. The data in Table 13.1 represent the average of these studies. Table 13.2 presents summary data for untrained and trained speakers.

### Fundamental Frequency Variation

The standard deviations of fundamental frequency, often referred to as the variability of fundamental frequency or pitch sigma, are also shown in Table 13.1. Variability is much smaller for sustained vowels than for reading passages. Fundamental frequency variability or lack thereof may be a physical measure that relates to the perception of voice monotone, a perceptual sign noted in some voice disorders.

*Table 13.1.* Fundamental Frequencies

| Age Range | Mean $F_0$ | Standard Deviation[a] | Range | Reference[b] |
|-----------|-----------|-----------|-------|-----------|
| | | *Males Reading* | | |
| 7 | 294 | 2.2 | | 1 |
| 8 | 297 | 2.0 | | 1 |
| 10 | 270 | 2.4 | | 1 |
| 11 | 227 | 1.5 | 192–268 | 2 |
| 14 | 242 | 3.4 | | 1 |
| 19 | 117 | 2.1 | 85–155 | 3 |
| Adult | 132 | 3.3 | | 4 |
| 20–29 | 120 | | | 5 |
| 30–39 | 112 | | | 5 |
| 40–49 | 107 | | | 5 |
| 50–59 | 118 | | | 5 |
| 60–69 | 112 | | | 5 |
| 70–79 | 132 | | | 5 |
| 80–89 | 146 | | | 5 |
| | | *Females Reading* | | |
| 7 | 281 | 2.0 | | 6 |
| 8 | 288 | 2.8 | | 6 |
| 11 | 238 | 1.51 | 98–271 | 2 |
| 19 | 217 | 1.71 | 65–255 | 3 |
| 20–29 | 224 | 3.8 | 192–275 | 7 |
| 30–40 | 196 | 2.5 | 171–222 | 8 |
| 40–50 | 189 | 2.8 | 168–208 | 8 |
| 60–69 | 200 | 4.3 | 143–235 | 7 |
| 70+ | 202 | 4.7 | 170–249 | 7 |
| 80–94 | 200 | 2.7 | 183–225 | 9 |

[a]*Standard deviation (SD) is expressed in semitones.*
[b]*Reference key:*
1. *Fairbanks, Wiley, and Lassman, 1949.*
2. *Horii, 1983.*
3. *Fitch and Holbrook, 1970.*
4. *Snidecor, 1943.*
5. *Hollien and Shipp, 1972; Shipp and Hollien, 1969.*
6. *Fairbanks, Herbert, and Hammond, 1949.*
7. *Stoicheff, 1981.*
8. *Saxman and Burk, 1967.*
9. *McGlone and Hollien, 1963.*

## Frequency Perturbation

Frequency perturbation or jitter refers to the variation of fundamental frequency present in all speakers to some degree and detected when the subject is attempting to produce a steady, sustained vowel. The frequency variations are the result of instability of the vocal folds during vibration. As such, perturbation reflects the biomechanical characteristics of the vocal folds, as well as variations of neuromuscular control. Normal speakers have a small amount of frequency perturbation, which may vary according to age, physical condition, and in, some cases, sex. These variables are included in Table 13.3, obtained from data reported by Casper (1983).

## *Maximum Phonational Range*

Maximum phonational range refers to the range of frequencies, from lowest to highest, that an individual can produce. The intensity of the tone is usually not controlled, and the person may be asked to sustain the tone for about 1 second. Placing further demands on the production of the sound (i.e., production at a specific intensity or for a longer duration) may be expected to alter the magnitude of the range obtained. The data reported in Table 13.4 were obtained from many sources and represent the means of several studies. Note that there are no data for children.

## VOCAL INTENSITY

The intensity of phonation observed during speech is dependent on several factors. These include the intensity produced at the glottis, the shape of the vocal tract, the

*Table 13.2.* Mean Speaking Fundamental Frequencies for Various Age Groups

| Age Groups | | 20–35 | | 40–55 | | 65–85 | |
|---|---|---|---|---|---|---|---|
| | | Mean | SD | Mean | SD | Mean | SD |
| Females | | | | | | | |
| | Naive | 192.00 | 2.00 | 195.00 | 3.40 | 175.00 | 2.40 |
| | Trained | 217.00 | 3.60 | 205.00 | 4.10 | 201.00 | 5.20 |
| Males | | | | | | | |
| | Naive | 118.00 | 2.60 | 100.00 | 2.60 | 127.00 | 3.10 |
| | Trained | 131.00 | 3.10 | 126.00 | 3.90 | 125.00 | 4.00 |

*Table 13.3.* Frequency Perturbation Data

| Age Range | Measure | Jitter Factor | | Directional Perturbation Factor | | Pitch Perturbation Quotient | |
|---|---|---|---|---|---|---|---|
| | | /ee/ | /oo/ | /ee/ | /oo/ | /ee/ | /oo/ |
| *Males* | | | | | | | |
| 20–29 | Mean | 0.78 | 0.72 | 70.73 | 6,948 | 0.65 | 0.57 |
| | SD | 0.4 | 0.36 | 11.25 | 14.87 | 0.3 | 0.26 |
| 40–49 | Mean | 0.99 | 0.87 | 74.37 | 72.49 | 0.77 | 0.7 |
| | SD | 0.61 | 0.51 | 10.86 | 14.84 | 0.38 | 0.32 |
| 60–69 | Mean | 0.91 | 0.87 | 67.77 | 69.43 | 0.77 | 0.74 |
| | SD | 0.63 | 0.56 | 15.46 | 14.55 | 0.5 | 0.43 |
| *Females* | | | | | | | |
| 20–29 | Mean | 0.55 | 0.56 | 46.3 | 47.83 | 0.56 | 0.57 |
| | SD | 0.41 | 0.41 | 19.67 | 19.68 | 0.39 | 0.37 |
| 40–49 | Mean | 0.63 | 0.61 | 53.06 | 51.67 | 0.65 | 0.61 |
| | SD | 0.4 | 0.42 | 16.57 | 19.76 | 0.41 | 0.4 |
| 60–69 | Mean | 0.66 | 0.7 | 49.91 | 48.88 | 0.65 | 0.69 |
| | SD | 0.52 | 0.59 | 19.1 | 18.64 | 0.49 | 0.56 |

amount of lip opening and the distance of the microphone from the lips of the speaker. Physical and emotional characteristics of the speaker may also affect vocal intensity. Thus, the data presented in Table 13.5 should be used with caution. It may be useful as an indicator of approximate intensity levels expected but be sure to check the specific vowel or syllable used and the lip-microphone distance.

## Amplitude Perturbation

During sustained vibration, the vocal folds will exhibit slight variation of amplitude from one cycle to the next. This is called amplitude perturbation or shimmer. Normal speakers will present a small amount of shimmer, which depends both on the vowel used and the sex of the person. Some typical shimmer values are shown in Table 13.6.

## Maximum Intensity Level

Patients may vary considerably in their ability to produce loud tones. This may be a helpful diagnostic sign or a measure of change following treatment. Thus, it may be useful to measure maximum intensity output. Normal speakers can usually produce maximum outputs in excess of 110 dB; this is somewhat dependent upon sex, age, the frequency at which the phonation is produced, and the measurement procedure. Table 13.7 presents a summary of maximum intensity levels for different ages and both sexes.

## S/z Ratio

The s/z ratio is a simple measure designed to examine the effect of pathology on phonation. Although there is some variation among normal speakers, generally ratios greater than 1.4 are considered abnormal. Ratios around 1 are normal and expected

*Table 13.4.* Maximum Phonational Range

| Age Range | Low Frequency | High Frequency | Range | Reference[a] |
|---|---|---|---|---|
| | | *Males* | | |
| 17–26 | 80 | 764 | 39.06 | 1 |
| 18–36 | 80 | 675 | 36.92 | 2 |
| 35–75 | 80 | 260 | 20.4 | 3 |
| 40–65 | 83 | 443 | 28.99 | 5 |
| 68–89 | 85 | 394 | 26.55 | 4 |
| | | *Females* | | |
| 18–38 | 140 | 1,122 | 36.03 | 2 |
| 66–93 | 134 | 571 | 25.09 | 4 |
| 35–70 | 136 | 803 | 30.75 | 5 |

[a]Reference key:
1. Hollien and Jackson, 1973.
2. Hollien, Dew, and Phillips, 1971.
3. Canter, 1965.
4. Ptacek, Sander, Maloney, and Jackson, 1966.
5. Colton and Hollien, 1972.

for both children and adults of different ages (Table 13.8). The clinician is cautioned to use this measure as one of a battery of measures rather than as a single definitive measure. Numerous authors (Case, 1991; Hufnagle & Hufnagle, 1988; Mueller, Larson, & Summers, 1993; Sorensen & Parker, 1993) have raised concerns about the validity of the measure.

## Maximum Phonation Duration

Maximum phonation duration is the maximum time a person can sustain a tone on one continuous expiratory breath. It supposedly is a measure of phonatory control and respiratory "support." As Kent, Kent, and Rosenbek (1987) have pointed out, maximum phonation duration can be influenced by variables that have little to do with phonatory control. Important variables include age, sex, and, of course, the physical characteristics of the respiratory system. Table 13.9 presents a summary of the data reported on maximum phonation duration from many studies. This measure should be used with care because of uncertainty about its validity and stability on repeat trials (Kent et al., 1987).

*Table 13.5.* Vocal Intensity in Monosyllables and Reading Passage

| Utterance Type | Loudness Level | N | Age | Mean dB | SD (dB) | Reference[a] |
|---|---|---|---|---|---|---|
| | | Females | | | | |
| /pa/ | | | | | | |
| | Soft | 10 | 20–30 | 65.35 | 1.84 | 1 |
| | Comfortable | 10 | 20–30 | 70.44 | 1.88 | 1 |
| | Loud | 10 | 20–30 | 76.75 | 3.38 | 1 |
| /pœ/ | | | | | | |
| | Soft | 20 | 18–36 | 83.30[b] | 3.20 | 2 |
| | Comfortable | 20 | 18–36 | 76.40 | 4.00 | 2 |
| | Loud | 20 | 18–36 | 71.50 | 4.90 | 2 |
| Rainbow Passage | | | 20–30 | 68.15 | | 3 |
| | | Males | | | | |
| /pa/ | | | | | | |
| | Soft | 10 | 20–30 | 70.42 | 3.19 | 1 |
| | Comfortable | 10 | 20–30 | 74.69 | 3.08 | 1 |
| | Loud | 10 | 20–30 | 80.72 | 3.51 | 1 |
| /pœ/ | | | | | | |
| | Soft | 25 | 17–30 | 75.00 | 2.50 | 2 |
| | Comfortable | 25 | 17–30 | 79.50 | 3.30 | 2 |
| | Loud | 25 | 17–30 | 86.00 | 4.30 | 2 |
| Rainbow Passage | | | 20–30 | 70.42 | | 3 |

[a]*Reference key:*
1. *Stathopoulos and Sapienza, 1993. SPL was measured from a pressure transducer placed in a circumferentially exhausted face mask. Therefore, distance of the microphone to the lips of the speaker is estimated to be about 1 inch.*
2. *Holmberg, Hillman, and Perkell, 1988.*
3. *Ryan and Gelfer, 1993.*
[b]*Averaged over 15 syllable repetitions.*

Table 13.6. Amplitude Perturbation Data

| Vowel | Mean | SD |
|---|---|---|
| | *Males* | |
| /ah/ | 0.47 | 0.34 |
| /ee/ | 0.37 | 0.28 |
| /oo/ | 0.33 | 0.31 |
| Mean | 0.33 | 0.31 |
| | *Females* | |
| /ah/ | 0.33 | 0.22 |
| /ee/ | 0.23 | 0.08 |
| /oo/ | 0.19 | 0.04 |
| Mean | 0.25 | 0.11 |

Table 13.7. Maximum Intensity Levels

| Age | Mean | SD | Range | Reference[a] |
|---|---|---|---|---|
| | | *Males* | | |
| 18–39 | 106 | 5.1 | 92–116 | 1 |
| 45–65 | 110 | 7.1 | 99–129 | 2 |
| 68–89 | 101 | 5.9 | 88–110 | 1 |
| | | *Females* | | |
| 18–38 | 106 | 3 | 99–112 | 1 |
| 40–70 | 101 | 18.2 | 93–115 | 2 |
| 66–93 | 99 | 4.5 | 90–104 | 1 |

[a]Reference key:
1. Ptacek, Sander, Maloney, and Jackson, 1966.
2. Colton, Reed, Sagerman, and Chung, 1982.

Table 13.8. S/Z Ratios

| Age | Mean | Range | Reference[a] |
|---|---|---|---|
| | | *Males* | |
| 5 | 0.92 | 0.82–1.08 | 1 |
| 7 | 0.7 | 0.52–0.97 | 1 |
| 9 | 0.92 | 0.66–1.5 | 1 |
| | | *Females* | |
| 5 | 0.83 | 0.50–1.14 | 1 |
| 7 | 0.78 | 0.51–1.10 | 1 |
| 9 | 0.91 | 0.75–1.26 | 1 |
| Adults | 0.99 | 0.41–2.67 | 2 |
| Aged | 0.76 | | 3 |
| | 0.82 | | 3 |

[a]Reference key:
1. Tait, Michel, and Carpenter, 1980.
2. Eckel and Boone, 1981.
3. Young, Bless, McNeil, and Braun, 1983.

## AIRFLOW

### *Average Airflow Rates*

Measurements of physiological parameters such as airflow and air pressure have some face validity in that vocal pathology will affect their magnitude. Both airflow and air pressure are dependent on a number of factors, however, including respiratory drive, vocal fold valving, frequency, and intensity. Thus, the conditions under which these measurements are obtained must be understood and controlled in order to be properly interpreted.

Average airflow measures are shown in Table 13.10. Average airflow may be reported in cubic centimeters per second or as is the case in this table milliliters per sec-

*Table 13.9.* Maximum Phonation Duration

| Group | Ages | Mean (sec) | SD |
|---|---|---|---|
| *Males* | | | |
| Young children | 3–4 | 8.95 | 2.16 |
| Children | 5–12 | 17.74 | 4.14 |
| Adults | 13–65 | 25.89 | 7.41 |
| Aged | 65+ | 14.68 | 6.25 |
| *Females* | | | |
| Young children | 3–4 | 7.5 | 1.8 |
| Children | 5–12 | 14.97 | 3.87 |
| Adults | 13–65 | 21.34 | 5.66 |
| Aged | 65+ | 13.55 | 5.7 |

*Table 13.10.* Average Flow Rates (ml/sec)

| Age | Task | Mean | Range | N | Reference[a] |
|---|---|---|---|---|---|
| *Males* | | | | | |
| 7 | /ah/ | 96 | 51–128 | 10 | 3 |
| Adult | /ah/ | 119 | 96–141 | 5–36 | 1 |
| | /ee/ | 144 | 89–136 | 30 | 4 |
| | Reading | 177 | 141–218 | 4 | 2 |
| Adult | /pah/ | | | | |
| | Soft | 130 | | 10 | 5 |
| | Comfortable | 120 | | 10 | 5 |
| | Loud | 140 | | 10 | 5 |
| *Females* | | | | | |
| 7 | /ah/ | 72 | 45–115 | 10 | 3 |
| Adult | /ah/ | 112 | 89–136 | 5–36 | 1 |
| | /ee/ | 177 | | 30 | 4 |
| | Reading | 191 | 152–170 | 4 | 2 |

[a]Reference key:
1. Based on data presented in Table 3.1 of Hirano, 1981a.
2. Horii and Cooke, 1978.
3. Beckett, Thoelke, and Cowan, 1971.
4. Woo, Colton, and Shangold, 1987.
5. Stahopoulos & Sapienza, 1993.

ond. Many researchers and clinicians have reported data on airflow for both normal speakers and those with vocal pathology. Some of the data for normal-speaking subjects are reported in Table 13.10. There is some variation depending on the task the subject performs, and there is some suggestion that children have much smaller flows than adults. Females tend to have slightly lower flows than males.

### Vibratory Airflow

Vibratory airflow refers to the variations of airflow during a cycle of vibration. Two major aspects of vibratory flow have been measured and are reported in Table 13.11. The first, AC flow, refers to the peak airflow during vibration. The second, minimum or DC flow, refers to any airflow that occurs when the vocal folds are supposedly closed. Both appear to be correlated with breathiness in the voice. AC flow varies both as a function of sex and of the intensity level at which the phonation is produced. Females have much lower AC flows than males, and there is a tendency for minimum or DC flow to be lower for female speakers also. As intensity levels increase, so too does airflow.

### Air Pressure

The amount of air pressure used in producing phonation will, in large measure, determine the intensity of the voice. In normal speakers, air pressure ranges between 4 and 5 cm/$H_2O$ for normal conversational or moderate level phonations (Table 13.12). Air pressure will also affect the magnitude of airflow; thus, it is important to know at what pressures airflow measures have been collected. These data were derived

*Table 13.11.* Vibratory Airflows Based on Inverse Filtering of Oral Airflow Data (ml/sec)

| Age Range | N | Condition[a] | AC Flow | DC Flow | Reference[b] |
|---|---|---|---|---|---|
| | | | *Males* | | |
| 17–30 | 25 | Normal | 260 | 120 | 1 |
| | 25 | Soft | 220 | 180 | 1 |
| | 25 | Loud | 490 | 110 | 1 |
| 21–30 | 8 | Normal | 303 | 68 | 2 |
| 20–31 | 10 | Comfortable | 250 | | 3 |
| 69+ | 10 | Comfortable | 330 | | 3 |
| | | | *Females* | | |
| 17–30 | 20 | Normal | 140 | 90 | 1 |
| | 20 | Soft | 110 | 120 | 1 |
| | 20 | Loud | 180 | 90 | 1 |
| 21–30 | 8 | Normal | 189 | 75 | 2 |
| 20–31 | 10 | Comfortable | 140 | | 3 |
| 69+ | 10 | Comfortable | 150 | | 3 |

[a]*Normal, soft, and loud refer to the loudness level at which the speakers were asked to produce the phonation.*
[b]*Reference key:*
*1. Holmberg, Hillman, and Perkell, 1988; tables AI–AVI.*
*2. Brodie, Colton, and Swisher, 1988.*
*3. Higgins and Saxman, 1993; phonation was a series of /bœp/s.*

*Table 13.12.* Air Pressure Measurements Based on Intraoral
Pressure Estimates (cm/H$_2$O)

| Age Range | N | Condition[a] | Pressure[b] | SD | Reference[c] |
|---|---|---|---|---|---|
| | | *Males* | | | |
| 17–30 | 25 | Normal | 5.91 | | 1 |
| | 25 | Soft | 4.79 | | 1 |
| | 25 | Loud | 8.39 | | 1 |
| 21–30 | 8 | Normal | 4.12 | 1 | 2 |
| 20–31 | 10 | Comfortable | 5.81 | 1.4 | 3 |
| 69+ | 10 | Comfortable | 7.99 | 2.73 | 3 |
| | | *Females* | | | |
| 17–32 | 25 | Normal | 6.09 | | 1 |
| | 25 | Soft | 4.79 | | 1 |
| | 25 | Loud | 8.46 | | 1 |
| 21–30 | 8 | Normal | 4.28 | 0.88 | 2 |
| 20–31 | 10 | Comfortable | 6.51 | 0.8 | 3 |
| 69+ | 10 | Comfortable | 6.35 | 1.71 | 3 |

[a]*Loudness level at which the phonation was produced. All used the indirect intraoral air pressure method for estimating lung pressure (Smitheran and Hixon, 1981).*
[b]*To convert cmH$_2$O to kPa, multiply cmH$_2$O by 10.197.*
[c]*Reference key:*
*1. Holmberg, Hillman, and Perkell, 1988.*
*2. Brodie, Colton, and Swisher, 1988.*
*3. Higgins and Saxman, 1993.*

from measurement of intraoral air pressure according to techniques described by Rothenberg (1968, 1982) and Smitheran and Hixon (1981). In some current literature, pressure is reported in kiloPascals (kPa). To convert pressure in cm/H$_2$O to kPa, multiply by 10.197.

## *Maximum Flow Declination Rate (Closing Slope)*

Maximum Flow Declination Rate (MFDR) or the closing slope of the inverse-filtered airflow waveform reflects the closing rate of the vocal folds. The faster the closing rate, the greater the amplitude in the higher frequencies. Thus, MFDR is related to vocal intensity production by the vocal folds and their spectrum. Table 13.13 presents some data from normal speakers at three intensity levels.

*Table 13.13.* Maximum Flow Declination Rates (or Closing Slope of the Inverse Filtered Airflow Waveform Pulse) for Normal Speakers

| Syllable | N | Age | Mean | SD | Reference[a] |
|---|---|---|---|---|---|
| Males | | | | | |
| /pœ/ | | | | | |
| Soft | 25 | 17–30 | 171.1 | 71.30 | 1 |
| Comfortable | 25 | | 279.6 | 90.40 | 1 |
| Loud | 25 | | 481.1 | 162.60 | 1 |
| /pa/ | | | | | |
| Soft | 10 | 20–30 | 218.43 | 100.03 | 2 |
| Comfortable | 10 | | 367.78 | 130.20 | 2 |
| Loud | 10 | | 573.16 | 186.22 | 2 |
| Females | | | | | |
| /pœ/ | | | | | |
| Soft | 20 | 18–36 | 117.2 | 57.80 | 1 |
| Comfortable | 20 | | 164.00 | 57.50 | 1 |
| Loud | 20 | | 248.90 | 84.00 | 1 |
| /pa/ | | | | | |
| Soft | 10 | 10–20 | 148.05 | 70.62 | 2 |
| Comfortable | 10 | | 248.42 | 87.20 | 2 |
| Loud | 10 | | 397.21 | 168.56 | 2 |

[a]*Reference key:*
*1. Holmberg, Hillman, and Perkell, 1988.*
*2. Stathopoulos and Sapienza, 1993.*

*Appendix*

---

# Forms Used in
# Voice Evaluation Clinic
# and Laboratory

**VOICE EVALUATION LABORATORY**
**Department of Otolaryngology and Communication Sciences**
**SUNY Health Science Center at Syracuse**
**Syracuse, New York 13210**
**(315) 464-5573 or 464-4678**

### TELEPHONE CONTACT SHEET

Name _____ Age_____

Telephone _____

Address _____

Referred by _____

        M.D. _____    Speech Path. _____    Voice Coach _____    Other (who?) _____

Referring Complaint:
        Hoarseness _____        Pain in Throat _____
        Loss of Voice _____        Difficulty Singing _____
        Other _____

Services Desired (check appropriate items)

        _____ Complete Evaluation & Diagnosis*        _____ Pre-op Documentation
        _____ Second Opinion/Consult                        _____ Post-op Documentation
        _____ Diagnosis and Treatment                       _____ Voice Recording Only

* (Complete evaluation includes: ENT examination, fiberoptic study, speech pathology consult,
air flow studies, EGG, and voice recording)

If medical referral: pertinent history, treatment and physical findings:




If not medical referral:  Name of doctor: _____

Are records available?_____

— — — — — — — — — — — — — — — — — — — — — — — — — — — — — — — — —

Appt. Date _____        History form mailed _____
                                                                                                                        (date)

Appt. Time _____        Appointment card mailed_____
                                                                                                                        (date)

**VOICE EVALUATION LABORATORY**
**Department of Otolaryngology and Communication Sciences**
**SUNY Health Science Center at Syracuse**
**Syracuse, New York 13210**
**(315) 464-5573 or 464-4678**

## <u>REFERRAL FORM</u>

Patient's Name_____ Age _____ Date of Referral_____

Address _____ Tel. (___) _____

Chief Complaint: _____

SERVICES DESIRED (check appropriate items)

_____ COMPLETE EVAL & DIAGNOSIS*          _____ Pre-op Documentation
_____ Second Opinion                       _____ Post-op Documentation
_____ Dx and Treatment                     _____ Voice Recording Only

*Complete evaluation includes: ENT Examination, Videotaped Fiberoptic Study, Speech Pathology Consult, Air Flow Studies, Electroglottography, Voice Recording.

PERTINENT HISTORY (physical findings, previous treatment, surgery, etc.)

_____

_____

_____

_____

(Please submit copies of pertinent reports, operative notes, etc.)

Report sent to: ___ You;  ___ School; ____ Other: _____

If other examinations are indicated, (e.g., Neurological, Psychiatric) should patient be informed?
___Yes ___No

Do you wish to discuss our findings and recommendations with the patient?
_____Yes _____No

___Patient will call for appointment.
___Please contact patient for appointment.

FOR APPOINTMENT CALL: (315) 464-5573

_____
referral source-print

_____
address

_____
telephone number

**VOICE EVALUATION LABORATORY**
**Department of Otolaryngology and Communication Sciences**
**SUNY Health Science Center at Syracuse**
**Syracuse, New York 13210**
**(315) 464-5573 or 464-4678**

## VOICE HISTORY

Name _____ Date of Birth _____ Age _____ Date _____

Complaint (please state the main concern in your own words)

_____

_____

When did you first notice a problem with your voice?_____

Please describe the course of the problem, the treatment you have had, where, and who treated you.

_____

_____

Please describe any feelings you have in your throat (such as tickle, lump, pain, difficulty swallowing, strain, fatigue, etc.) _____

_____

Does your voice get better, worse, stay the same?_____

      When is it better? _____

      When is it worse? _____

Do you have any of the following?

      _____ Allergies       _____ Neurological Problems

      _____ Respiratory Problems       _____ Endocrine/Hormone Problems

Have you had any of the following?

      _____ Surgery on your larynx? When _____

      _____ Heart Surgery? When_____

      _____ Chest Surgery? When_____

      _____ Thyroid Surgery? When_____

      _____ Stroke? When _____

      _____ Injury to the Neck? When _____

      _____ Chemical or Inhalation Exposure? When _____

Do You:

      _____ Smoke? (Tobacco or other substances)

      How much?_____

      _____ Drink? (Beer, wine, other alcoholic substances)

      How much?_____

      _____ Take any medication regularly? (Include aspirin)

      What?_____

      _____ Talk above noise? What noise?_____

      How much? _____

      _____ Talk loud, scream, yell? How much?_____

      _____ Sing: _____Choir, _____ Solo, _____with musical group

Are you employed? _____ Yes _____ No

What kind of work do you do?_____

Is talking required for your job? _____ Yes _____ No

Please add any other information which you think may be pertinent.

Department of Otolaryngology & Communication Sciences
SUNY Health Science Center
Syracuse, NY 13210                    **Voice Evaluation Clinic**

### Stroboscopic Examination

Name of Patient: _____    Date: _____

History: _____

_____

_____

Type of Exam: ☐: Rigid  ☐: Flexible  Comments on Exam: _____

| **Voice Measurements** | Modal | High | Low | Loud |
|---|---|---|---|---|
| Fundamental Frequency | ____ | ____ | ____ | ____ |
| SPL | ____ | ____ | ____ | ____ |

**Severity of Dysphonia**: ☐: Normal  ☐: Mild  ☐: Moderate  ☐: Severe  ☐: Aphonic

**Vocal Fold Edge**    Right: ☐: Smooth  ☐: Slightly rough  ☐: Moderately rough ☐: Ext Rough
                            Left: ☐: Smooth  ☐: Slightly rough  ☐: Moderately rough ☐: Ext Rough

**Glottal Closure Pattern**:    ☐: Complete ☐: Incomplete ☐: Hourglass ☐: Irregular ☐: Bowed
                            ☐: Anterior Chink        ☐: Posterior Chink

**Phase Closure:** ☐: Normal   ☐: Predom Open  ☐: Predom Closed  Frame Count: _____

| **Mucosal Wave** | | **Amplitude of Vibration** | | **Vibratory Behavior** | |
|---|---|---|---|---|---|
| Right Fold | Left Fold | Right Fold | Left Fold | | |
| ☐: Normal | ☐:Normal | ☐: Normal | ☐:Normal | Right Fold | Left Fold |
| ☐: Absent | ☐: Absent | ☐: Absent | ☐: Absent | ☐: Always Present | ☐: Always Present |
| ☐: Slightly | ☐: Slightly | ☐: Slightly | ☐: Slightly | ☐: Partial Absence | ☐: Partial Absence |
| ☐: Moderately | ☐: Moderately | ☐: Moderately | ☐: Moderately | ☐: Complete Ab | ☐: Complete Ab |
| ☐: Severely | ☐: Severely | ☐: Severely | ☐: Severely | | |
| and | | and | | | |
| ☐: Increased | ☐: Increased | ☐: Increased | ☐: Increased | | |
| ☐: Decreased | ☐: Decreased | ☐: Decreased | ☐: Decreased | | |

**Periodicity:** ☐: Regular  ☐: Sometimes Irregular  ☐: Mostly Irregular
☐: Always Irregular

**Phase Symmetry**
☐: Regular        ☐: Stm Irr
☐: Most Irr        ☐: Al irreg

Observations and Impressions: _____

_____

_____

Diagnosis: _____

Recommendations: _____

_____

**VOICE EVALUATION LABORATORY**
**Department of Otolaryngology and Communication Sciences**
**SUNY Health Science Center at Syracuse**
**Syracuse, New York 13210**
**(315) 464-5573**

Patient Number_____     Recorded on _____

Last Name _____     First Name _____

Address _____

City_____ State_____ Zip_____

Phone (___)_____ Occupation _____

Date of Birth _____ Sex _____ SS# _____

Hospital Number_____ Smoker_____ Drinker_____

Video Tape Number_____ Counter_____ Additional Videos?_____

Problem_____
_____
_____
_____

Major Category_____ Minor Category_____

Referred by_____ Examined by _____

ENT Exam_____
_____
_____
_____

Acoustic Data?_____ Strobe Data_____ Air Flow Data _____

Comments:

**COMMUNICATION DISORDER UNIT**
**SUNY Health Science Center**
**Syracuse, New York**

## VOICE HISTORY AND EVALUATION

Patient's name:_____ DOB:_____ Age:_____ Date of Eval:_____

Referred by:_____ Medical Dx _____

Complaint as stated by patient:_____

HISTORY OF PROBLEM:  [onset, duration, prior episodes, treatment, effect]

I. VOICE SYMPTOM HISTORY:
   A. Variability/Consistency [use related, situational, physical well-being, time of day]:

   B. Associated Symptoms and Sensations [pain, dryness, tickle, lump, strain, fatigue, dysphagia, weight loss, heartburns slurred speech]:

- - - - - - - - - - - - - - - - - - - - - - - - - - - - - - - - - - -

   CLINICAL OBSERVATIONS AND PHYSIOLOGICAL IMPLICATIONS:
     1. Perceptual Observations:          Physiological Correlates:

     2. Behavioral Observations:          Physiological Correlates:

- - - - - - - - - - - - - - - - - - - - - - - - - - - - - - - - - - -

II. VOICE USE HISTORY:
   A. Talking [how much, where, how, to whom]

   B. Other voice use [singing, acting, sound effects, throat clear]

III. HEALTH HISTORY:
   A. Present health [neurological, respiratory, allergy, psychiatric, gastrointestinal, endocrine/hormonal, chronic conditions]:

   B. Past health [relevant to present problems]:

   C. Surgery [laryngeal, thyroid, cardiac, thoracic, intubation]:

   D. Trauma/Substance or Environmental Exposure [accident, assault, chemical ingestion, smoke, noxious gasses, burn, inhalation, noise]:

E. Substance Use [tobacco, alcohol, medications, illicit drugs]:

— — — — — — — — — — — — — — — — — — — — — — — — — —

CLINICAL OBSERVATIONS:
    IMPRESSIONS OF GENERAL HEALTH              PHYSIOLOGICAL IMPLICATIONS

— — — — — — — — — — — — — — — — — — — — — — — — — —

IV. SOCIAL, OCCUPATION, RECREATION HISTORY [family constellation, living arrangements, life style, job
    description, exercise programs, hobbies]

V. VOCAL FUNCTION TESTING:
    A. Phonational Range: low: _____ Hz        high: _____ Hz
    B. Speaking Fundamental Frequency: _____ Hz
    C. Dynamic Range:    low: _____ dB       high _____ dB
    D. S/Z Ratio  [3x each]

        s _____ sec.        z _____ sec.        Mean s = _____ sec.
        s _____ sec.        z _____ sec.        Mean z = _____ sec.
        s _____ sec.        z _____ sec.        S/Z ratio = _____ sec.

    E. Sustained /a/ [3x]

        1. _____ sec   2. _____ sec   3. _____ sec   Mean = _____ sec
        steady _____      interrupted _____      tremor _____

    F. Frequency Perturbation [jitter]:
    G. Amplitude Perturbation [shimmer]:
    H. Lab Studies:
        1. Airflow data

        2. EGG

        3. Spectrography

        4. Fiberoptic, Stroboscopic etc.

VI. AUDIOLOGICAL EVALUATION [attach report or summarize]

VII. PERCEPTUAL CHARACTERISTICS:
    A. Quality:

    B. Pitch:

    C. Inflection:

    D. Rate:

VIII. ABILITY TO MODIFY VOCAL BEHAVIOR [pitch and loudness variability, easy onset, reflexive acts, etc.]

IX. DIAGNOSTIC IMPRESSIONS:

X. RECOMMENDATIONS:

XI. PROGNOSTIC CONSIDERATIONS

REPORTS TO:

_____
SPEECH PATHOLOGIST

**SUNY HEALTH SCIENCE CENTER**
**Dept. Of Otolaryngology and**
**Communication Sciences**
**Voice Evaluation Clinic**

**STANDARD PROTOCOL - FIBEROPTIC ASSESSMENT**

1.  Observe larynx at rest.
    Instructions to patient.        Just sit quietly for a moment.

2.  Observe deep inspiration.
    Instruction to patient:         I want you to take a deep breath, and release it. Then do it
                                    two more times.

3.  Observe sustained vowel phonation at comfortable (modal) pitch (3x) repetitions.
    Instruction to patient:         I'd like you to say /ee/ at a pitch that is comforable for you
                                    and hold on to it for a few seconds. (Can be modelled).
                                    May be repeated using /oo/).

4.  Observe sustained vowel phonation at elevated (modal) pitch (3x) repetitions.
    Instruction to patient:         Now I'd like you to do the same thing, hold on to that /ee/ but at
                                    a high pitch. (Can be modelled) (may be repeated using /oo/.)
    Alternate instruction:          If patient does not elevate pitch, request the sound of a
                                    baby kitten, the squeal of a mouse, etc. It may be helpful to
                                    model these sounds.

5.  Observe dynamics of pitch change.
    Instruction to patient:         I want you to start with that high sound and let your voice glide
                                    down to a deep sound, like this: model a downward glissando.
                                    (3x) repetitions. Now let's start at the bottom low note and let your
                                    voice glide upward, like this: model an upward glide (3x)
                                    repetitions.
    Alternate instruction:          If patient has difficulty with this task, request a wolf howl sound
                                    that starts on a low /ah/ and glides up on an /oo/. It is helpful to
                                    model.

6.  Observe speech.
    Instruction to patient:         Please repeat each of these sentences twice.
                                    a.  See the busy bees.
                                    b.  We eat green beans.
                                    c.  Do queens eat honey?
                                    d.  Who hoots at the moon?
                                    e.  Do you chew your food?

7.  Observe non-phonatory laryngeal behavior.
    Instruction to patient:         I'd like you to whistle for me like this: (model a few short
                                    interrupted bursts of whistle).Now I'd like you to whistle a little bit of
                                    Happy Birthday.If patient cannot whistle, a "pretend" whistle is
                                    acceptable.

8.  Period of diagnostic therapy. The instructions to the patient will depend on the vocal maneuvers
    you wish to elicit. It is appropriate at this time to follow-up on any of the above activities if
    behaviors of interest were noted, or if you wish to make another attempt to teach a task. If a
    particular type of voice usage is of concern, for example, the high notes in singing or during
    lecturing, it is helpful to obtain a sample of that behavior.

# References

Adametz, J., & O'Leary, J. L. (1959). Experimental mutism resulting from periaqueductal lesions in cats. *Neurology, 9,* 636–642.

Adran, G. M., Demp, F. H., & Marland, P. M. (1954). Laryngeal palsy. *British Journal of Radiology, 27,* 201–209.

Alberti, P. W. (1978). The diagnostic role of laryngeal stroboscopy. *Otolaryngology Clinics of North America, 11,* 347–354.

Allen, E. L., & Hollien, H. (1973). A laminagraphic study of pulse (vocal fry) register phonation. *Folia Phoniatrica, 25,* 241–250.

American Joint Committee for Cancer Staging and End Results Reporting. (1983). Philadelphia: JB Lippincott.

American Speech-Language-Hearing Association. (1992). Vocal tract visualization and imaging. *ASHA, 34*(3, Suppl. 7), 37–40.

Aminoff, M. J., Dedo, H. H., & Izdebski, K. (1978). Clinical aspects of spasmodic dysphonia. *Journal of Neurosurgery and Psychiatry, 41,* 361–365.

Ardran, G., Kinsbourne, M., & Rushworth, G. (1966). Dysphonia due to tremor. *Journal of Neurology, Neurosurgery and Psychiatry, 29,* 219–223.

Aring, C. D. (1965). Supranuclear (pseudobulbar) palsy. *Archives of Internal Medicine, 115,* 198–199.

Arnold, G. E. (1959). Spastic dysphonia I: changing interpretation of a persistent affliction. *Logos, 2,* 3–14.

Arnold, G. E. (1962). Vocal nodules and polyps: laryngeal tissue reaction to habitual hyperkinetic dysphonia. *Journal of Speech and Hearing Disorders, 27,* 205–217.

Arnold, G. E. (1980). Disorders of laryngeal function. In M. M. Paparella & D. Shumrick (Eds.), *Otolaryngology* (pp. 631–648). Philadelphia: WB Saunders.

Arnold, J. (1894). Myelocyste, Transposition von Gewebskeimen und Sympodie. *Beitr Pathol Anat Allg Pathol, 51,* 259–275.

Arnold, K. S., & Emanuel, F. W. (1979). Spectral noise levels and roughness severity ratings for vowels produced by male children. *Journal of Speech and Hearing Research, 22,* 613–626.

Aronson, A. E. (1973). *Psychogenic voice disorders.* Philadelphia: WB Saunders.

Aronson, A. E. (1985). *Clinical voice disorders: an interdisciplinary approach.* New York: BC Decker.

Aronson, A. E. (1990). *Clinical voice disorders: an interdisciplinary approach* (3rd ed.). New York: Thieme.

Aronson, A. E., Brown, J. R., Litin, E. M., & Pearson, J. S. (1968a). Spastic dysphonia. I. Voice, neurologic, and psychiatric aspects. *Journal of Speech and Hearing Disorders, 33,* 203–218.

Aronson, A. E., Brown, J. R., Litin, E. M., & Pearson, J. S. (1968b). Spastic dysphonia II. Comparison with essential (voice) tremor and other neurologic and psychogenic dysphonias. *Journal of Speech and Hearing Disorders, 33,* 219–231.

Aronson, A. E., & DeSanto, L. W. (1981). Adductor spastic dysphonia: 1½ years after recurrent laryngeal nerve resection. *Annals of Otology, Rhinology and Laryngology, 90,* 1–6.

Aronson, A. E., & DeSanto, L. W. (1983). Adductor spastic dysphonia: three years after recurrent laryngeal nerve resection. *Laryngoscope, 93,* 1–8.

Aronson, A. E., & Hartman, D. E. (1981). Adductor spastic dysphonia as a sign of essential (voice) tremor. *Journal of Speech and Hearing Disorders, 46,* 52–58.

Aronson, A. E., Peterson, H. W., & Litin, E. M. (1966). Psychiatric symptomatology in functional dysphonia and aphonia. *Journal of Speech and Hearing Disorders, 31,* 115–127.

Baer, T. (1979). Vocal jitter: a neuromuscular explanation. In V. Lawrence (Ed.), *Transcripts of the 8th symposium: care of the professional voice* (pp. 19–22). New York: Voice Foundation.

Baer, T., Gore, J. C., Boyce, S., & Nye, P. W. (1987). Application of MRI to the analysis of speech production. *Magnetic Resonance Imaging, 5,* 1–7.

Baer, T., Gore, J. C., Gracco, L. C., & Nye, P. W. (1991). Analysis of vocal tract shape and dimensions using magnetic resonance imaging—vowels. *Journal of the Acoustical Society of America, 90,* 799–828.

Baer, T., Löfqvist, A., McGarr, N. (1983a). Laryngeal vibrations: a comparison between high-speed filming and glottographic techniques. *Journal of the Acoustical Society of America, 73,* 1304–1308.

Baer, T., Löfqvist, A., McGarr, N. (1983b). Laryngeal vibrations: a comparison between high-speed filming and glottographic techniques. In *Status report on speech research* (pp. 283–291). New Haven, CT: Haskins Laboratories.

Baken, R. J. (1987). *Clinical measurement of speech and voice.* San Diego: College Hill Press.

Baker, A. B. (1958). *An outline of clinical neurology.* Dubuque, IA: William Brown & Co.

Balestrieri, F., & Watson, C. (1982). Intubation granuloma. *Otolaryngology Clinics of North America, 15,* 567–579.

Ball, J., & Lloyd, J. (1971). Myasthenia gravis as hysteria or the sounds of silence. *Medical Journal of Australia, 1,* 1018–1020.

Ballantyne, J. C., & Groves, J. (1978). *A synopsis of otolaryngology.* Bristol: John Wright and Sons Ltd.

Ballenger, J. J. (1985). Neurologic diseases of the larynx. In J. J. Ballenger (Ed.), *Diseases of the nose, throat, ear, head, and neck* (pp. 513–548). Philadelphia: Lea & Febiger.

Bamberger-Bozo, C. (1987). The Chiari II. In P. J. Vinken, G. W. Bruyn, H. L. Klawans, & N. C. Myrianthopoulos (Eds.), *Handbook of clinical neurology.* (pp. 403–412). Amsterdam: Elsevier.

Bannister, R., Gibson, W., Michaels, L., & Oppenheimer, D. R. (1981). Laryngeal abductor paralysis in multiple system atrophy. *Brain, 104,* 351–368.

Bannister, R., & Oppenheimer, D. R. (1972). Degenerative diseases of the nervous system associated with autonomic failure. *Brain, 95,* 457–474.

Barker, K. D., & Wilson, F. B. (1967). Comparative study of vocal utilization of children with hoarseness and normal voice. Paper presented at the convention of the American Speech-Language-Hearing Association, Chicago.

Barlow, S. M., Netsell, R., & Hunker, C. J. (1986). Phonatory disorders associated with CNS lesions. In C. Cummings, J. Fredrickson, L. Harker, C. Krause, & D. Schuller (Eds.), *Otolaryngology—Head and Neck Surgery* (pp. 2087–2093). St. Louis: CV Mosby.

Barry, H. C., & Eathorne, S. W. (1994). Exercise and aging. Issues for the practitioner [review]. *Medical Clinics of North America, 78,* 357–376.

Barton, R. T. (1979). Treatment of spastic dysphonia by recurrent laryngeal nerve section. *Laryngoscope, 89,* 244–249.

Basmajian, J. V. (1979). *Muscles alive: their functions revealed by electromyography.* Baltimore: Williams & Wilkins.

Bassich, C. J., & Ludlow, C. L. (1986). The use of perceptual methods by new clinicians for assessing voice quality. *Journal of Speech and Hearing Disorders, 51,* 125–133.

Bastian, R. W. (1985). Laryngeal biofeedback for voice modification. In V. Lawrence (Ed.), *Transcripts of the 14th symposium: care of the professional voice* (pp. 330–333). New York: Voice Foundation.

Bastian, R. W. (1986). Benign mucosal disorders, saccular disorders and neoplasms. In C. Cummings, J. Fredrickson, C. Krause, & D. Schuller (Eds.), *Otolaryngology—Head and Neck Surgery* (pp. 1965–1987). St. Louis: CV Mosby.

Bastian, R. W. (1987). Laryngeal image feedback for voice disorder patients. *Journal of Voice, 1,* 279–282.

Beasley, D. & Davis, G. (1981). *Aging communication processes and disorders.* New York: Grune & Stratton.

Beck, C., & Richstein, A. (1982). Medianverlagerung einer paretischen Stimmlippe durch partielle Schildknorpelimpression. *Laryngo-Rhino- Otologie (Stuttgart), 61,* 251.

Beckett, R. L., Thoelke, W., & Cowan, L. (1971). A normative study of air flow in children. *British Journal of Disorders of Communication, 6,* 13–17.

Behlau, M., & Pontes, P. (1990). *Princípios de reabilitaçào vocal nas disfonias* (2nd ed.). Sao Paulo, Brazil: Paulista Publicaçòes Medicas.

Benjamin, B. (1981). Frequency variability in the aged voice. *Journal of Gerontology, 36,* 722–726.

Benjamin, B. N., Gatenby, P. A., Kitchen, R., Harrison, H., & Cameron, K. (1988). Alpha-interferon (Wellferon) as an adjunct to standard surgical therapy in the management of recurrent respiratory papillomatosis. *Annals of Otology, Rhinology and Laryngology, 97,* 376–380.

Bennett, S., Bishop, S., & Lumpkin, S. (1987). Phonatory characteristics associated with bilateral diffuse polypoid degeneration. *Laryngoscope, 97,* 446–450.

Bernstein, L., & Bernstein, R. S. (1985). *Interviewing, a guide for health professionals.* East Norwalk, CT: Appleton-Lange.

Berry, R. J., Epstein, R., Fourcin, J., Freeman, M., & MacCurtain, F. (1982). An objective analysis of voice disorder: part one. *British Journal of Disorders of Communication, 17,* 67–76.

Berry, R. L., Epstein, R., Freeman, M., MacCurtain, F., & Noscoe, N. (1982). An objective analysis of voice disorders: part two. *British Journal of Disorders of Communication, 17,* 77–85.

Biever, D. M., & Bless, D. M. (1988). *Posterior glottal gap in normal young adult and geriatric women.* Unpublished manuscript.

Biever, D. M., & Bless, D. M. (1989). Vibratory characteristics of the vocal folds in young adult and geriatric women. *Journal of Voice, 3,* 120–131.

Bless, D., & Hirano, M. (1982). Verbal instructions: a critical variable in obtaining optimal performance for maximum phonation time. Paper presented at the convention of the American Speech-Language-Hearing Association, Toronto, Canada.

Bless, D., Hunker, C., & Weismer, G. (1981). Comparison of noninvasive methods to obtain chest-wall displacement and aerodynamic measures during speech. In V. Lawrence (Ed.), *Transcripts of the 10th symposium: care of the professional voice* (pp. 43–51). New York: Voice Foundation.

Bless, D. M., & Brandenburg, J. H. (1983). *Stroboscopic evaluation of "functional" voice disorders.* Paper presented at the middle section of the Triologic Society, Madison, WI.

Bless, D. M., Hirano, M., & Feder, R. (1987). Videostroboscopic evaluation of the larynx. *Ear, Nose, Throat Journal, 66,* 289–296.

Bless, D. M., Miller, J. (1972). Influence of mechanical and linguistic factors on lung volume effects during speech. Paper presented at the convention of the American Speech-Language-Hearing Association, San Francisco.

Bless, D. M., & Swift, E. (1995). Paradoxical vocal cord dysfunction: episodic laryngeal dyskinesia; one disorder, multiple causes? Paper presented at the convention of the American-Speech-Language-Hearing Association, Orlando, FL.

Blitzer, A., & Brin, M. F. (1991). Laryngeal dystonia: a series with botulinum toxin therapy. *Annals of Otology, Rhinology and Laryngology, 100,* 85–89.

Blitzer, A., & Brin, M. F. (1992). The dystonic larynx. *Journal of Voice, 6,* 294–297.

Blitzer, A., Brin, M. F., Fahn, S., & Lovelace, R. E. (1988). Clinical and laboratory characteristics of focal laryngeal dystonia: study of 110 cases. *Laryngoscope, 98,* 636–640.

Blitzer, A., Brin, M. F., Stewart, C., Aviv, J. E., & Fahn, S. (1992). Abductor laryngeal dystonia: a series treated with botulinum toxin. *Laryngoscope, 102,* 163–167.

Blitzer, A., Lovelace, R. E., Brin, M. F., Fahn, S., & Fink, M. E. (1985). Electromyographic findings in focal laryngeal dystonia (spastic dysphonia). *Annals of Otology, Rhinology and Laryngology, 94,* 591–594.

Block, P. (1965). Neuro-psychiatric aspects of spastic dysphonia. *Folia Phoniatrica, 17,* 301–364.

Blum, R. H. (1960). *The management of the doctor-patient relationship.* New York: McGraw-Hill.

Boone, D. R. (1977). *The voice and voice therapy.* Englewood Cliffs, NJ: Prentice-Hall.

Boone, D. R. (1983). *The voice and voice therapy* (2nd ed.). Englewood Cliffs, NJ: Prentice-Hall.

Boone, D. R. (1987). *Human communication and its disorders.* Englewood Cliffs, NJ: Prentice-Hall.

Boone, D. R., & McFarlane, S. C. (1988). *The voice and voice therapy* (4th ed). Englewood Cliffs, NJ: Prentice-Hall.

Borden, G. J., Baer, T., & Kenney, M. K. (1985). Onset of voice in stuttered and fluent utterances. *Journal of Speech and Hearing Research, 28,* 363–372.

Botez, M. I., & Barbeau, A. (1971). Role of subcortical structures and particularly of the thalamus in the mechanisms of speech and language. *International Journal of Neurology, 8,* 300–320.

Bouchayer, M., Cornut, G., Witzig, E., Loire, R., Roch, J., & Bastian R. (1985). Epidermoid cysts, sulci and mucosal bridges of the true vocal cord: a report of 157 cases. *Laryngoscope, 95,* 1087–1094.

Bralley, R. C., Bull, J. L., Gore, C. H., & Edgerton, M. T. (1978). Evaluation of vocal pitch in male transsexuals. *Journal of Communication Disorders, 11,* 443–449.

Brandt, J. F., Ruder, K. F., & Shipp, T. (1969). Vocal loudness and effort in continuous speech. *Journal of the Acoustical Society of America, 46,* 1543–1548.

Brantigan, C. O., Brantigan, T. A., & Joseph, N. (1982). Effects of beta blockade and beta stimulation on stage fright. *American Journal of Medicine, 72,* 88–94.

Brewer, D. W. (1975). Early diagnostic signs and symptoms of laryngeal disease. *Laryngoscope, 85,* 499–515.

Brewer, D. W., Brodnitz, F., Gould, W. J., Lawrence, V. L., Monaghan, J., Pratt, D., et al. (1979). Medical care for professional voice: panel discussion. In V. Lawrence (Ed.), *Transcripts of the 7th symposium: care of the professional voice* (pp. 8–38). New York: Voice Foundation.

Brewer, D. W., & Gould, L. V. (1974). Pyriform sinus: functional visualization. *Annals of Otology, Rhinology and Laryngology, 83,* 720–724.

Brewer, D. W., & McCall, G. N. (1974). Visible laryngeal changes during voice therapy. *Annals of Otology, Rhinology and Laryngology, 83,* 423–427.

Briant, T. D. R., Blair, R. L., Cole, P., & Singer, L. (1983). Laboratory investigation of abnormal voice. *Journal of Otolaryngology, 12,* 285–290.

Brin, M. F., Fahn, S., Blitzer, A., Ramig, L. O., & Stewart, C. (1992). Movement disorders of the larynx. In A. Blitzer, M. F. Brin, C. T. Sasaki, S. Fahn, & K. S. Harris (Eds.), *Neurologic disorders of the larynx* (pp. 248–278). New York: Thieme.

Broad, D. J. (1973). Phonation. In F. D. Minifie, T. J. Hixon, & W. Williams (Eds.), *Normal aspects of speech, hearing and language* (pp. 127–167). Englewood Cliffs, NJ: Prentice-Hall.

Brodie, K., Colton, R. H., & Swisher, L. (1988). *Reliability of inverse filtered and EGG measurements of vocal function.* Unpublished manuscript.

Brodnitz, F. (1976). Spastic dysphonia. *Annals of Otolaryngology, 85,* 210–214.

Brown, J. E., & Simonson, J. (1963). Organic voice tremor. *Neurology, 13,* 520–525.

Brown, J. R., Darley, F. L., & Aronson, A. E. (1970). Ataxic dysarthria. *International Journal of Neurology, 7,* 302–318.

Brown, W. S., Jr., Morris, R. J., Hollien, H., & Howell, E. (1991). Speaking fundamental frequency characteristics as a function of age and professional singing. *Journal of Voice, 5,* 310–315.

Brown, W. S., Jr., Morris, R., & Michel, J. (1989). Vocal jitter in young adult and aged female voices. *Journal of Voice, 3,* 113–119.

Browne, K., & Freeling, P. (1976). *The doctor-patient relationship.* New York: Churchill Livingstone.

Burch, P. R. (1981). Passive smoking and lung cancer. *British Medical Journal, 282,* 1393.

Canter, G. J. (1963). Speech characteristics of patients with Parkinson's disease. I. Intensity, pitch and duration. *Journal of Speech and Hearing Disorders, 28,* 221–229.

Canter, G. J. (1965). Speech characteristics of patients with Parkinson's disease. II: Physiological support for speech. *Journal of Speech and Hearing Disorders, 30,* 44–49.

Carpenter, R. J., McDonald, T. J., & Howard, F. M. (1979). The otolaryngologic presentation of myasthenia gravis. *Laryngoscope, 89,* 922–928.

Carpenter, R. J., McDonald, T. J., & Howard, F. M. (1988). The otolaryngologic presentation of amyotrophic lateral sclerosis. *Otolaryngology, 86,* 479–484.

Carrow, E., Mauldin, M., & Shamblin, L. (1974). Deviant speech characteristics in motor neuron disease. *Archives of Otolaryngology, 100,* 212–218.

Caruso, A., & Burton, E. K. (1987). Temporal acoustic measures of dysarthria associated with amyotrophic lateral sclerosis. *Journal of Speech and Hearing Research, 30,* 80–87.

Case, J. L. (1984). *Clinical management of voice disorders.* Rockville, MD: Aspen Systems.

Case, J. L. (1991). *Clinical management of voice disorders* (2nd ed). Austin: Pro-Ed.

Casper, J. K. (1983). *Frequency perturbation in normal speakers: a descriptive and methodological study.* Unpublished doctoral dissertation, Syracuse University, Syracuse, NY.

Casper, J. K. (1993). Objective methods for the evaluation of vocal function. In J. Stemple (Ed.), *Voice therapy: clinical methods* (pp. 39–45). St Louis: Mosby Yearbook.

Casper, J. K., Brewer, D. W., & Colton, R. H. (1987a). Variations in normal human laryngeal anatomy and physiology as viewed fiberscopically. *Journal of Voice, 1,* 180–185.

Casper, J. K., Brewer, D. W., & Colton, R. H. (1987b). Pitfalls and problems in flexible fiberoptic videolaryngoscopy. *Journal of Voice, 1,* 347–352.

Casper, J. K., Brewer, D. W., & Conture, E. G. (1981). Speech therapy patient evaluation techniques with the fiberscope. In V. Lawrence (Ed.), *Transcripts of the 10th symposium: care of the professional voice* (pp. 136–140). New York: Voice Foundation.

Casper, J. K., Colton, R. H., & Brewer, D. W. (1985). Selected Therapy Techniques and Laryngeal Physiological Changes in patients with vocal fold immobility. In V. Lawrence (Ed.), *Transcripts of the 14th symposium: care of the professional voice* (pp. 318–323). New York: Voice Foundation.

Casper, J. K., Colton, R. H., Brewer, D. W., Kelley, R., Woo, P., & Griffin, B. (1995). *Nodular diversity.* Unpublished manuscript.

Casper, J. K., Colton, R. H., Brewer, D. W., & Woo, P. (1989). Investigation of selected voice therapy techniques. Paper presented at the 18th symposium of the Voice Foundation, Care of the Professional Voice, New York.

Casper, J. K., Colton, R. H., Woo, P., & Brewer, D. (1992). Physiological characteristics of selected voice therapy techniques: a preliminary research note. *Voice, 1,* 131–141.

Charcot M. (1881). *Lectures on the diseases of the nervouse system.* London: The New Sydenham Society.

Cherry, J., & Margulies, S. I. (1968). Contact ulcer of the larynx. *Laryngoscope, 73,* 1937–1940.

Chevrie-Muller, C., Arabia-Guidet, C., & Pfauwadel, M. (1987). Can one recover from spasmodic dysphonia? *British Journal of Disorders of Communication, 22,* 117–128.

Chiari, H. (1896). Über Veränderungen des Kleinhirns, des Pons und Medulla oblongata in Folge von Kongenitaler Hydrocephalie des Grosshirns. *Dtsch Akad Wiss Wien, 63,* 71–116.

Childers, D. G., Alsaka, Y. A., Hicks, D. M., Moore, G. P. (1986). Vocal fold vibrations in dysphonia: model vs. measurement. *Journal of Phonetics, 14,* 429–434.

Childers, D. G., Moore, G. P., Naik, J. M., Larar, J. N., & Krishnamurthy, A. K. (1983). Assessment of laryngeal function by simultaneous synchronized measurement of speech, electroglottography and high-speed film. In V. Lawrence (Ed.), *Transcripts of the 11th symposium: care of the professional voice* (pp. 234–244). New York: Voice Foundation.

Childers, D. G., Naik, J. M., Larar, J. N., Krishnamurthy, A. K., & Moore, G. P. (1983). Electroglottography, speech, and ultra-high speed cinematography. In I. Titze

& R. Scherer (Eds.), *Vocal fold physiology biomechanics, acoustics and phonatory control* (pp. 202–220). Denver, CO: Denver Center for the Performing Arts.

Chipman, S. F., & Carey, S. (1975). Anatomy of a stimulus domain: the relation between multidimensional and unidimensional scaling of noise bands. *Perceptual Motor Skills, 17,* 417–424.

Chisnall, B. (1977). Increase in house fires. *Fire Protection, 4,* 119–121.

Chodosh, P. L. (1977). Gastro-esophageal-pharyngeal reflux. *Laryngoscope, 87,* 1418–1427.

Cisler, J. (1927). Sur les troubles du language articule et de la phonation au cours de l'encephalite epidemique. *Arch International Laryngol, 33,* 1054–1057.

Close, L. G., Catlin, F. I., & Cohn, A. M. (1980). Acute and chronic effects of ammonia burns on the respiratory tract. *Archives of Otolaryngology, 106,* 151–158.

Cohen, S. R., Geller, K. A., Birns, J. W., & Thompson, J. W. (1982). Laryngeal paralysis in children: a long term retrospective study. *Annals of Otology, Rhinology and Laryngology, 91,* 417–424.

Coleman, R. F., Mabis, J. H., & Hinson, J. K. (1977). Fundamental frequency-sound pressure level profiles of adult male and female voices. *Journal of Speech and Hearing Research, 20,* 197–204.

Coleman, R. F., & Wendahl, R. (1967). Vocal roughness and stimulus duration. *Speech Monographs, 34,* 85–92.

Coleman, R. O. (1971). Male and female voice quality and its relationship to vowel formant frequencies. *Journal of Speech and Hearing Research, 14,* 565–577.

Coleman, R. O. (1973). Speaker identification in the absence of inter-subject differences in glottal source characteristics. *Journal of the Acoustical Society of America, 53,* 1741–1743.

Coleman, R. O. (1976). A comparison of the contributions of two voice quality characteristics to the perception of maleness and femaleness in the voice. *Journal of Speech and Hearing Research, 19,* 168–180.

Colton, R. H. (1973). Vocal intensity in the modal and falsetto registers. *Journal of Speech and Hearing Research, 25,* 62–70.

Colton, R. H. (1987). The role of pitch in the discrimination of voice quality. *Journal of Voice, 1,* 240–245.

Colton, R. H. (1988). Physiological mechanisms of vocal frequency control: the role of tension. *Journal of Voice, 2,* 208–220.

Colton, R. H. (1989). Objective evaluation of voice dysfunction in the elderly. In J. C. Goldstein, H. K. Kashima, & C. F.

Koopmann, Jr. (Eds.), *Geriatric Otorhinolaryngology* (pp. 79–91). Toronto: BC Decker.

Colton, R. H. (1994). Physiology of phonation. In M. S. Benninger, B. H. Jacobson, & A. F. Johnson (Eds.), *Vocal arts medicine: the care and prevention of professional voice disorders* (pp. 30–60). New York: Thieme.

Colton, R. H., & Brewer, D. W. (1985). Fiberoptic/vibratory relationships in patients with voice disorders. In V. Lawrence (Ed.), *Transcripts of the 14th symposium: care of the professional voice* (pp. 271–275). New York: Voice Foundation.

Colton, R. H., Brewer, D., & Rothenberg, M. (1983). Evaluating vocal function. *Journal of Otolaryngology, 12,* 291–294.

Colton, R. H., & Brown, W. S. (1973). Some relationships between vocal effort and intraoral air pressure. *Journal of the Acoustical Society of America, 53,* 296A.

Colton, R. H., Casper, J. K., Brewer, D. W., & Conture, E. G. (1989). Digital processing of laryngeal images: a preliminary report. *Journal of Voice, 3,* 132–142.

Colton, R. H., & Estill, J. (1981). Elements of voice quality: perceptual, acoustic and physiologic aspects. In N. Lass (Ed.), *Speech and language: advances in basic research and practice* (pp. 311–403). New York: Academic Press.

Colton, R. H., & Hollien, H. (1972). Phonational range in the modal and falsetto registers. *Journal of Speech and Hearing Research, 15,* 708–713.

Colton, R. H., Reed, G., Sagerman, R., & Chung, C. (1982). An investigation of voice change after radiotherapy. In *Final Report, National Cancer Institute, NIH.* Bethesda, MD: National Institutes of Health.

Colton, R. H., Sagerman, R., Chung, C., Young, Y., & Reed, G. (1978). Voice change after radiotherapy. *Radiology, 127,* 821–824.

Colton, R. H., Woo, P., Brewer, D. W., Griffin, B., & Casper, J. K. (1995). Stroboscopic signs associated with benign lesions of the vocal folds. *Journal of Voice, 9,* 312–325.

Conture, E. G., Cudahy, E., Caruso, A., Schwartz, H., Brewer, D., & Casper, J. (1981). Computer assisted measures of video taped data: a description and case study. In V. Lawrence (Ed.), *Transcripts of the 10th symposium: care of the professional voice* (pp. 129–135). New York: Voice Foundation.

Conture, E. G., Schwartz, H., & Brewer, D. (1985). Laryngeal behavior during stuttering: a further study. *Journal of Speech and Hearing Research, 28,* 233–240.

Cooper, D., & Titze, I. (1985). Generation and dissipation of heat in vocal fold tissue. *Journal of Speech and Hearing Research, 28,* 207–215.

Cooper, M. (1973). *Modern techniques of vocal rehabilitation.* Springfield, IL: Charles C Thomas.

Cooper, M. (1984). Change your voice, change your life. New York: Macmillan.

Cooper, M., & Cooper, M. H. (1977). *Approaches to vocal rehabilitation.* Springfield, IL: Charles C Thomas.

Cotton, R. T., & Richardson, M. A. (1981). Congenital laryngeal anomalies. *Otolaryngology Clinics of North America, 14,* 203.

Countryman, S., Ramig, W., & Pawlas, A. A. (1994). Speech and voice deficits in Parkinsonian plus syndromes: Can they be treated? *Journal of Medical Speech Language Pathology, 2,* 211–225.

Crapo, R. O. (1981). Smoke inhalation injuries. *Journal of the American Medical Association, 246,* 1694–1696.

Critchley, M. (1949). Observations on essential (heredofamilial) tremor. *Brain, 72,* 9–139.

Crumley, R. L. (1983). Phrenic nerve graft for bilateral vocal cord paralysis. *Laryngoscope, 93,* 425–428.

Cudmore, R. E., & Vivori, E. (1981). Inhalation injury to the respiratory tract of children. *Progress in Pediatric Surgery, 14,* 173–188.

Cummings, C. W. (1986). Bilateral vocal cord paralysis/ankylosis. In C. Cummings, L. Harker, C. S. Krause, & D. Schuller (Eds.), *Otolaryngology—Head and Neck Surgery* (pp. 2181–2189). St. Louis: CV Mosby.

Damste, P. H. (1967). Voice change in adult women caused by virilizing agents. *Journal of Speech and Hearing Disorders, 32,* 126–132.

Damste, P. H. (1970). The phonetogram. *Practica Otology Rhinology Laryngology, 32,* 185–187.

Daniloff, R., Schuckers, G., & Feth, L. (1980). *The physiology of speech and hearing.* Englewood Cliffs, NJ: Prentice-Hall.

Darley, F. L., Aronson, A. E., & Brown, J. R. (1969a). Clusters of deviant speech dimensions in the dysarthrias. *Journal of Speech and Hearing Research, 12,* 462–496.

Darley, F. L., Aronson, A. E., & Brown, J. R. (1969b). Differential diagnostic patterns of dysarthria. *Journal of Speech and Hearing Disorders, 12,* 246–269.

Darley F. L., Aronson A. E., & Brown J. R. (1975). *Motor speech disorders.* Philadelphia: WB Saunders.

Darley, F. L., Brown, J. R., & Goldstein, N. P. (1972). Dysarthria in multiple sclerosis. *Journal of Speech and Hearing Research, 15,* 229–245.

Darley, F. L., & Spriesterbach, D. C. (1978). *Diagnostic methods in speech pathology* (2nd ed.). New York: Harper & Row.

Davis, P. J., Boone, D. R., Carroll, R. L., Darvenzia, P., & Harrison, G. A. (1988). Adductor spastic dysphonia: heterogeneity of physiologic and phonatory characteristics. *Annals of Otology, Rhinology and Laryngology, 97,* 179–185.

Davis, S. B. (1981). Acoustic characteristics of normal and pathological voices. In C. Ludlow & M. Hart (Eds.), *Proceedings of the conference on the assessment of vocal pathology* (pp. 97–115). Rockville, MD: American Speech-Language-Hearing Association.

Davis, P. J., & Zhang, S. P. (1991). What is the role of the midbrain periaqueductal gray in respiration and vocalization? In A. Depaulis & R. Bandler (Eds.), *Midbrain periaqueductal gray matter: functional, anatomical and immunohistochemical organization* (pp. 57–66). New York: Plenum Press.

Dedo, H. H. (1976). Recurrent laryngeal nerve section for spastic dysphonia. *Annals of Otology Rhinology and Laryngology, 85,* 451–459.

Dedo, H. H. (1988). Avoidance and treatment of complications of Teflon injection of the vocal cord. *Journal of Voice, 2,* 90–92.

Dedo, H. H. (1992). Injection and removal of Teflon for unilateral vocal cord paralysis. *Annals of Otology, Rhinology and Laryngology, 101,* 81–86.

Dedo, H. H., & Izdebski, K. (1981). Surgical treatment of spasmodic dysphonia. *Contemporary Surgery, 18,* 75–90.

Dedo, H. H., & Izdebski, K. (1983). Intermediate results of 306 recurrent laryngeal nerve sections for spastic dysphonia. *Annals of Otology, Rhinology and Laryngology, 92,* 9–15.

Dedo, H. H., Townsend, J., & Izdebski, K. (1978). Current evidence for the organic etiology of spastic dysphonia. *Otolaryngology, 86,* 875–880.

Dejonckere, P. H., Lebacq, J. (1985). Electroglottography and vocal nodules: an attempt to quantify the shape of the signal. *Folia Phoniatrica, 37,* 195–200.

Delahunty, J. E. (1972). Acid laryngitis. *Journal of Laryngology, 86,* 335–342.

Delahunty, J. E., & Cherry, J. (1968). Experimentally produced vocal cord granulomas. *Laryngoscope, 73,* 1941–1947.

Deveney, C. W., Benner, K., & Cohen, J. (1993). Gastroesophageal reflux and laryngeal disease. *Archives of Surgery, 128,* 1021–1027.

DeWeese, D. D., & Saunders, W. H. (1982). *Textbook of otolaryngology* (6th ed). St. Louis: CV Mosby.

Dickson, D. R., & Dickson, W. M. (1982). *Anatomical and physiological bases of speech.* Boston: Little, Brown.

Diehl, C. F. (1960). Voice and personality: an evaluation. In D.A. Barbara (Ed.), *Psychological and psychiatric aspects of speech and hearing* (pp. 171–203). Springfield IL: Charles C Thomas.

Dordain, M., & Dordain, G. (1972). L'epreuve du /a/ tenu au course des tremblements de la voix (tremblement idiopathique et dyskinesie volitionnelle, leurs rapports avec la dysphonie spasmodique). *Revue de Laryngologie, 93,* 167–182.

Dowling, P. C., Blumberg, B. M., & Cook, S. D. (1987). Guillain-Barre Syndrome. In P. J. Vinken, G. W. Bruyn, H. L. Klawans, & W. B. Matthews (Eds.), *Handbook of clinical neurology* (pp. 239–262). Amsterdam: Elsevier.

Dromey, C., Stathopoulos, E. T., Sapienza, C. M. (1992). Glottal airflow and electroglottographic measures of vocal function at multiple intensities. *Journal of Voice, 6,* 44–54.

Duvoisin, R. (1976). Parkinsonism. *Clinical Symposia, 28,* 1–29.

Dyer, R. F., & Esch, V. H. (1976). Polyvinyl chloride toxicity in fires. *Journal of the American Medical Association, 235,* 393–397.

Eccles, J. C. (1977). *The understanding of the brain.* New York: McGraw-Hill.

Eckel, F. C., & Boone, D. R. (1981). The s/z ratio as an indicator of laryngeal pathology. *Journal of Speech and Hearing Disorders, 46,* 147–149.

Emanuel, F., & Sansone, F. (1969). Some spectral features of normal "and simulated 'rough' vowels." *Folia Phoniatrica, 21,* 401–415.

Faaborg-Andersen, K. (1957). Electromyographic investigation of intrinsic muscles in humans: an investigation of subjects with normally movable vocal cords and patients with vocal cord paresis. *Acta Physiologica Scandinavica, 41 (suppl 140),* 1–148.

Faaborg-Andersen, K. (1964). The position of paretic vocal cords. *Acta Oto-laryngologica (Stockholm), 57,* 50–54.

Faaborg-Andersen, K., & Sonninen, A. (1960). The function of the extrinsic laryngeal muscles at different pitch. *Acta Oto-laryngologica (Stockholm), 51,* 89–93.

Faaborg-Andersen, K., & Vennard, W. (1964). Electromyography of extrinsic laryngeal muscles during phonation of different vowels. *Annals of Otology, Rhinology and Laryngology, 73,* 248–254.

Fairbanks, G. F. (1960). *Voice and articulation drillbook.* New York: Harper & Row.

Fairbanks, G., Herbert, E. L., & Hammond, J. M. (1949). An acoustical study of vocal pitch in seven and eight year old girls. *Child Development, 20,* 71–78.

Fairbanks, G. F., Wiley, J. H., & Lassman, F. M. (1949). An acoustical study of vocal pitch in 7 and 8 year old boys. *Child Development, 20,* 63–69.

Fant, G. (1970). *Acoustic theory of speech production.* The Hague: Mouton.

Farmakides, M. N., & Boone, D. R. (1960). Speech problems of patients with multiple sclerosis. *Journal of Speech and Hearing Disorders, 25,* 385–390.

Feder, R. (1986). On standardizing the laryngeal examination. *Archives of Otolaryngology—Head and Neck Surgery, 112,* 145.

Feder, R. J., & Michell, M. J. (1984). Hyperfunctional, hyperacidic and intubation granulomas. *Archives of Otolaryngology, 110,* 582–584.

Fex, S. (1970). Judging the movements of vocal cords in laryngeal paralysis. *Acta Oto-laryngologica Supplement (Stockholm), 263,* 82–83.

Finitzo-Hieber, T., Freeman, F. J., Gerling, I. J., Dobson, L., & Shaefer, S. D. (1982). Auditory brainstem response abnormalities in adductor spasmodic dysphonia. *American Journal of Otolaryngology, 3,* 26–30.

Finnegan, D. E. (1984). Maximum phonation time for children with normal voices. *Journal of Communication Disorders, 17,* 309–317.

Finnegan, D. E. (1985). Maximum phonation time for children with normal voices. *Folia Phoniatrica, 37,* 209–215.

Fitch, J. L., & Holbrook, A. (1970). Modal vocal fundamental frequency of young adults. *Archives of Otolaryngology, 92,* 379–382.

Fitz-Hugh, G. S., Smith, D. E., & Chiong, A. T. (1958). Pathology of three hundred clinically benign lesions of the vocal cords. *Laryngoscope, 68,* 855–875.

Flynn, P. T. (1983). Speech-language pathologists and primary prevention: from ideas to action. *Language Speech Hearing Services in Schools, 14,* 99–104.

Folkins, J. W. (1978). Lower lip displacement during voluntary activation of individual labial muscles. *Archives of Oral Biology, 23,* 189–193.

Ford, C. N., Bless, D. M., & Loftus, J. M. (1992). Role of injectable collagen in the treatment of glottic insufficiency: a study of 119 patients. *Annals of Otology, Rhinology and Laryngology, 101,* 237–247.

Ford, C. N., Bless, D. M., & Patel, N. Y. (1992). Botulinum toxin treatment of spasmodic dysphonia: techniques, indications, efficacy. *Journal of Voice, 6,* 370–376.

Ford, C. N., Martin, D. W., & Warner, T. F. (1984). Injectable collagen in laryngeal rehabilitation. *Laryngoscope, 94,* 513.

Freud, E. D. (1962). Functions and dysfunctions of the ventricular folds. *Journal of Speech and Hearing Disorders, 27,* 334–340.

Fritzell, B., & Fant, G. (1986). Voice acoustics and dysphonia. *Journal of Phonetics, 14 (Suppl),* 345–347.

Fritzell, B., Feuer, E., Haglund, S., Knutsson, E., & Schiratzki, H. (1982). Experiences with recurrent laryngeal nerve section for spastic dysphonia. *Folia Phoniatrica, 34,* 160–167.

Froeschels, E. (1952). Chewing method as therapy. *Archives of Otolaryngology, 56,* 427–434.

Fujimura, O. (1981). Body-cover theory of the vocal fold and its phonetic implications. In K. Stevens & M. Hirano (Eds.), *Vocal fold physiology* (pp. 271–288). Tokyo: University of Tokyo Press.

Fujiu, M., Hibi, S. R., & Hirano, M. (1988). An improved technique for measurement of the relative noise level using a sound spectrograph. *Folia Phoniatrica, 40,* 53–57.

Fulton, J., & Dow, R. (1937). The cerebellum: a summary of functional localization. *Yale Journal of Biology and Medicine, 10,* 89–119.

Furukawa, M. (1967). Studies on the mechanism of phonation in excised larynges. *Practica Otologica Kyoto, 60,* 145–181.

Garcia, M. (1855). Observations of the human voice. *Philosophical Mag J Science, 10,* 511–513.

Gardner, E. (1963). *Fundamentals of neurology.* Philadelphia: WB Saunders.

Garfinkle, T., & Kimmelman, C. (1982). Neurologic disorders: amyotrophic lateral sclerosis, myasthenia gravis, multiple sclerosis and poliomyelitis. *American Journal of Otolaryngology, 3,* 204–212.

Garrett, K., & Healey, E. (1987). An acoustic analysis of fluctuations in the voices of normal adult speakers across three times of day. *Journal of the Acoustical Society of America, 82,* 58–62.

Gates, G., & Montalbo, P. J. (1987). The effect of low-dose β-blockade on performance anxiety in singers. *Journal of Voice, 1,* 105–108.

Gates, G. A., Saegert, J., Wilson, N., Johnson, L., Shepard, A., & Hearne, E. A. (1985). The effect of beta blockage on singing performance. *Annals of Otology, Rhinology and Laryngology, 94,* 570–574.

Gaynor, E. B. (1991). Otolaryngologic manifestations of gastroesophageal reflux. *American Journal of Gastroenterology, 86,* 801–808.

Gerratt, B. R., Hanson, D. (1987). Glottographic measures of laryngeal function in individuals with abnormal motor control. In T. Baer, C. H. Sasaki, & K. Harris (Eds.), *Laryngeal function in phonation and respiration* (pp. 521–532). San Diego: College Hill Press.

Gerratt, B. R., Hanson, D. G., & Berke, G. S. (1988). Laryngeal configuration associated with glottography. *American Journal of Otolaryngology, 9,* 173–179.

Gerratt, B. R., Hanson, D. G., Berke, G. S., & Precoda, K. (1991). Photoglottography: a clinical synopsis. *Journal of Voice, 5,* 98–105.

Gerratt, B. R., Hanson, D. G., Hunt, S. M. J., & Karin, R. (1985). Glottographic measure-

ment of laryngeal paralysis. Paper presented at the convention of the American Speech-Language-Hearing Association, Washington, DC.

Golden, G. S. (1977). Tourette syndrome: the pediatric perspective. *American Journal of Disorders in Childhood, 131,* 531–534.

Gould, W. J. (1987). Surgery in professional singers. *Ear, Nose, Throat Journal, 66,* 327–332.

Gracco, C., & Kahane, J. C. (1989). Age-related changes in the vestibular folds of the human larynx: a histomorphometric study. *Journal of Voice, 3,* 204–212.

Gracco, C., Jones-Bryant, N., Fahey, J., DeStephens, R., & Naito, W. (1995). Videoendoscopic and cardiopulmonary measures of exercise induced upper airway dysfunction. Paper presented at the 24th symposium of the Voice Foundation, Care of the Professional Voice, Philadelphia.

Gray, S. D. (1991). Basement membrane zone injury in vocal nodules. In J. Gauffin & B. Hammarberg (Eds.), *Vocal fold physiology: acoustic, perceptual, and physiological aspects of voice mechanisms.* (pp. 21–28). San Diego: Singular Publishing Group.

Gray, S. D., Hirano, M., & Sato, K. (1993). Molecular and cellular structure of vocal fold tissue. In I. R. Titze (Ed.), *Vocal fold physiology: frontiers in basic science* (pp. 1–36). San Diego: Singular Publishing Group.

Gray, S. D., Pignatari, S. S., & Harding, P. (1994). Morphologic ultrastructure of anchoring fibers in normal vocal fold basement membrane zone. *Journal of Voice, 8,* 48–52.

Grob, D. (1961). Myasthenia gravis. *Archives of Internal Medicine, 108,* 615–638.

Guidi, A. M., Bannister, R., and Gibson, W. P. R. (1981). Laryngeal electromyography in multiple system atrophy with autonomic failure. *Journal of Neurology, Neurosurgery, and Psychiatry, 44,* 49–53.

Guillain-Barré Syndrome Study Group. (1985). Plasmapheresis and acute Guillain-Barré syndrome. *Neurology, 35,* 1096–1104.

Haji, T., Horiguchi, S., Baer T., & Gould, W. J. (1986). Perturbation analysis of electroglottograph during sustained phonation. *Folia Phoniatrica, 38,* 290A.

Hallewell, J., & Cole, T. B. (1970). Isolated head and neck symptoms due to hiatus hernia. *Archives of Otolaryngology, 92,* 499–501.

Hamlet, S. L. (1972). Vocal fold articulatory activity during whispered speech. *Archives of Otolaryngology, 95,* 211–312.

Hamlet, S. L. (1981). Ultrasound assessment of phonatory function. In C. Ludlow & M. Hart (Eds.), *Proceedings of the conference on the assessment of vocal pathology* (pp. 128–140).

Rockville, MD: American Speech-Language-Hearing Association.

Hammarberg, B., Fritzell, B., Gauffin, J., & Sundberg, J. (1986). Acoustic and perceptual analysis of vocal dysfunction. *Journal of Phonetics, 14,* 533–548.

Hammarberg, B., Fritzell, B., & Schiratzki, H. (1984). Teflon injection in 16 patients with paralytic dysphonia: perceptual and acoustic evaluations. *Journal of Speech and Hearing Disorders, 49,* 72–82.

Hammond, E. C. (1966). Smoking in relation to the death rate of 1 million men and women. *National Cancer Institute Monograph, 19,* 127–204.

Hanson, D. G., Gerratt, B. R., Karin, R. R., & Berke, G. S. (1988). Glottographic measures of vocal fold vibration: an examination of laryngeal paralysis. *Laryngoscope, 98,* 541–549.

Hanson, D. G., Gerratt, B. R., & Ward, P. H. (1983). Glottographic measurement of vocal dysfunction: a preliminary report. *Annals of Otology, Rhinology and Laryngology, 92,* 413–420.

Hanson, D. G., Gerratt, B. R., & Ward, P. H. (1984). Cineradiographic observations of laryngeal function in Parkinson's disease. *Laryngoscope, 94,* 348–353.

Hanson, D. G., Ludlow, C., & Bassich, C. (1983). Vocal fold paresis in Shy-Drager syndrome. *Annals of Otology, Rhinology and Laryngology, 92,* 85–90.

Hanson, D. G., Ward, P. H., Gerratt, B. R., Berci, G., & Berke, G. S. (1989). Diagnosis of neuromuscular impairment. In J. C. Goldstein, H. K. Kashima, & C. F. Koopman (Eds.), *Geriatric otorhinolaryngology* (pp. 71–78). Toronto: BC Decker.

Hanson, W., & Emanuel, F. W. (1979). Spectral noise and vocal roughness relationships in adults with laryngeal pathology. *Journal of Communication Disorders, 12,* 113–124.

Hanson, W. R., & Metter, E. J. (1980). DAF as instrumental treatment for dysarthria in progressive supranuclear palsy. *Journal of Speech and Hearing Disorders, 45,* 268–276.

Harris, T. M. (1992). The pharmacological treatment of voice disorders. *Folia Phoniatrica, 44,* 143–154.

Harrison, G. A., Davis, P. J., Troughear, R. H., & Winkworth, A. L. (1992). Inspiratory speech as a management option for spastic dysphonia—case study. *Annals of Otology, Rhinology and Laryngology, 101,* 375–382.

Hartman, D. E., Abbs, J. H., & Vishwanat, B. (1988). Clinical investigations of adductor spastic dysphonia. *Annals of Otology, Rhinology and Laryngology, 97,* 247–252.

Hartman, D. E., & Aronson, A. E. (1981). Clinical investigations of intermittent breathy dysphonia. *Journal of Speech and Hearing Disorders, 46,* 428–432.

Heaver, L. (1959). Spastic dysphonia: II. Psychiatric considerations. *Logos, 2,* 15–24.

Hecker, M. H., & Kreul, E. J. (1971). Descriptions of the speech of patients with cancer of the vocal folds. Part I: Measures of fundamental frequency. *Journal of the Acoustical Society of America, 49,* 1275–1282.

Henschen, T. L., & Burton, N. G. (1978). Treatment of spastic dysphonia by EMG biofeedback. *Biofeedback and Self Regulation, 3,* 91–96.

Hersen, M., & Turner, S. M. (1985). *Diagnostic interviewing.* New York: Plenum.

Hibi, S. R., Bless, D. M., Hirano, M., & Yoshida, T. (1988). Distortions of videofiberscopy imaging: reconstruction and correction. *Journal of Voice, 2,* 168–175.

Hicks, D. M., Larar, J. N., Moore, G. P., & Childers, D. G. (1985). Electroglottography for assessing laryngeal function. *Institute for Advanced Study of the Communication Processes Bulletin, 1,* 41–50.

Higgins, M. B., & Saxman, J. H. (1993). Inverse-filtered air flow and EGG measures for sustained vowels and syllables. *Journal of Voice, 7,* 47–53.

Hill, A. V. (1938). The heat of shortening and the dynamic constants of muscle. *Proceedings of the Royal Society, 126,* 136–195.

Hillman, R. E., & Weinberg, B. (1981). A new procedure for venting a reflectionless tube. *Journal of the Acoustical Society of America, 69,* 1449–1451.

Hirano, M. (1974). Morphological structure of the vocal cord as a vibrator and its variations. *Folia Phoniatrica, 26,* 89–94.

Hirano, M. (1975). Phonosurgery: basic and clinical applications. *Otologia (Fukuoka), 21,* 239–242.

Hirano, M. (1981a). Structure of the vocal fold in normal and disease states: anatomical and physical studies. In C. Ludlow & M. Hart (Eds.), *Proceedings of the conference on the assessment of vocal pathology.* (pp. 11–30). Rockville, MD: American Speech-Language-Hearing Association.

Hirano, M. (1981b). *Clinical examination of voice.* Vienna: Springer-Verlag.

Hirano, M. (1983). Epithelial hyperplasia of the larynx. In M. Hirano (Ed.), *Illustrated handbook of clinical otolaryngology* (pp. 100–101). Tokyo: Medical View.

Hirano, M., & Bless, D. M. (1993). *Videostroboscopic examination of the larynx.* San Diego: Singular Publishing Group.

Hirano, M., Feder, R., & Bless, D. M. (1983). Clinical evaluation of patients with voice disorders: stroboscopic evaluation. Paper presented at the convention of the American

Speech-Language-Hearing Association, Cincinnati, OH.

Hirano, M., Kakita, Y., Kawasaki, H., Gould, W. J., & Lambiase, A. (1981). Data from high-speed motion picture studies. In K. N. Stevens & M. Hirano (Eds.), *Vocal fold physiology* (pp. 85–91). Tokyo: University of Tokyo Press.

Hirano, M., Kakita, Y., Kawasaki, H., & Matsushita, H. (1977). *Vocal cord vibration: behavior of the layer-structured vibrator in normal and pathological conditions.* [16 mm film, also available on videotape]. New York: Voice Foundation.

Hirano, M., Koike, Y., & von Leden, H. (1968). Maximum phonation time and air usage during phonation. *Folia Phoniatrica, 20*, 185–201.

Hirano, M., Kurita, S., Kyokawa, K., & Sato, K. (1986). Posterior glottis: morphological study in excised human larynges. *Annals of Otology, Rhinology and Laryngology, 95*, 576–581.

Hirano, M., Kurita, S., Matsuo, K., & Nagata, K. (1980). Laryngeal tissue reaction to stress. In V. Lawrence (Ed.), *Transcripts of the 9th symposium: care of the professional voice* (pp. 10–20). New York: Voice Foundation.

Hirano, M., Kurita, S., & Nakashima, T. (1983). Growth, development and aging of human vocal folds. In D. M. Bless & J. H. Abbs (Eds.), *Vocal fold physiology: contemporary research and clinical issues* (pp. 22–43). San Diego: College Hill Press.

Hirano, M., Yoshida, Y., & Matsushita, H. (1974). An apparatus for ultra-high-speed cinematography of vocal folds. *Annals of Otology, Rhinology and Laryngology, 83*, 12–18.

Hirose, H. (1988). High speed digital imaging of vocal fold vibration. *Acta Oto-laryngologica (Stockholm), 458*(Suppl.), 151–158.

Hirose, H., Kiritani, S., & Imagawa, H. (1987). High speed digital image analysis of laryngeal behavior in running speech. *Annual Bulletin RILP, 21*, 25–40.

Hirose, H., Kiritani, S., & Imagawa, H. (1988). High speed digital image analysis of laryngeal behavior in running speech. In O. Fujimura (Ed.), *Vocal fold physiology: voice production, mechanisms and function* (pp. 335–345.). New York: Raven Press.

Hirose, H., Kiritani, S., & Imagawa, H. (1991a). High-speed digital imaging of vocal fold vibration and its application for analysis of hoarseness. In J. A. Cooper (Ed.), *Assessment of speech and voice production: research and clinical applications* (pp. 146–149). Bethesda, MD: U.S. Department of Health and Human Services.

Hirose, H., Kiritani, S., & Imagawa, H. (1991b). Clinical application of high-speed digital imaging of vocal fold vibration. In J. Gauffin

& B. Hammarberg (Eds.), *Vocal fold physiology: acoustic, perceptual, and physiological aspects of voice mechanisms.* (pp. 213–216). San Diego: Singular Publishing Group.

Hiroto, I. (1976). Surgical voice improvement for unilateral recurrent laryngeal nerve paralysis. *Otologia (Fukuoka), 22*, 473–474.

Hiroto, I., Hirano, M., & Tomita, H. (1968). Electromyographic investigation of human vocal cord paralysis. *Annals of Otology, Rhinology and Laryngology, 77*, 296–304.

Hixon, T. (1987). *Respiratory function in speech and song.* Boston: Little, Brown & Co.

Hixon, T. J., & Smitheran, J. R. (1982). A reply to Rothenberg. *Journal of Speech and Hearing Disorders, 47*, 220–223.

Hoehn, M. M., & Yahr, M. D. (1967). Parkinsonism: onset, progression and mortality. *Neurology, 17*, 427–442.

Holbrook, A., Rolnick, M. I., & Bailey, C. W. (1974). Treatment of vocal abuse disorders using a vocal intensity controller. *Journal of Speech and Hearing Disorders, 39*, 298–303.

Hollien, H. (1975). On vocal registers. *Journal of Phonetics, 2*, 125–143.

Hollien, H. (1987). 'Old Voices': what do we really know about them. *Journal of Voice, 1*, 2–17.

Hollien, H., Dew, D., & Phillips, P. (1971). Phonational frequency ranges of adults. *Journal of Speech and Hearing Research, 14*, 755–760.

Hollien, H., & Jackson, B. (1973). Normative data on the speaking fundamental frequency characteristics of young adult males. *Journal of Phonetics, 19*, 117–120.

Hollien, H., Michel, J., & Doherty, E. T. (1973). A method of analyzing vocal jitter in sustained phonation. *Journal of Phonetics, 1*, 85–91.

Hollien, H., & Moore, G. P. (1960). Measurements of the vocal folds during changes in pitch. *Journal of Speech and Hearing Research, 3*, 157–165.

Hollien, H., & Shipp, T. (1972). Speaking fundamental frequency and chronologic age in males. *Journal of Speech and Hearing Research, 15*, 155–159.

Hollinger, P., & Brown, W. T. (1967). Congenital webs, cysts, laryngoceles, and other anomalies of the larynx. *Annals of Otology, Rhinology and Laryngology, 76*, 744–752.

Holmberg, E. B., Hillman, R. E., & Perkell, J. S. (1988). Glottal airflow and transglottal air pressure measurements for male and female speakers in soft, normal and loud voice. *Journal of the Acoustical Society of America, 84*, 511–529.

Honjo, I., & Isshiki, N. (1980). Laryngoscopic and voice characteristics of aged persons. *Archives of Otolaryngology, 106*, 149–150.

Horii, Y. (1979). Fundamental frequency perturbation observed in sustained phonation. *Journal of Speech and Hearing Research, 22,* 5–19.

Horii, Y. (1980). Vocal shimmer in sustained phonation. *Journal of Speech and Hearing Research, 23,* 202–209.

Horii, Y. (1982). Jitter and shimmer differences among sustained vowels. *Journal of Speech and Hearing Research, 25,* 12–14.

Horii, Y. (1983). Some acoustic characteristics of oral reading by ten-to twelve year-old children. *Journal of Communication Disorders, 16,* 257–267.

Horii, Y., & Cooke, P. A. (1978). Some airflow, volume and duration characteristics of oral reading. *Journal of Speech and Hearing Research, 21,* 470–481.

Houben, G. B., Buekers, R., & Kingma, H. (1992). Characterization of the electroglottographic waveform: a primary study to investigate vocal fold functioning. *Folia Phoniatrica, 44,* 269–281.

House, A. S. (1959). Note on optimal vocal frequency. *Journal of Speech and Hearing Research, 2,* 55–60.

House, E. L., & Pansky, B. (1967). *A functional approach to neuroanatomy.* New York: Mc-Graw-Hill.

Hufnagle, J., & Hufnagle, K. (1988). S/Z ratio in dysphonic children with and without vocal cord nodules. *Language Speech Hearing Services in Schools, 19,* 418–422.

Hunt, J. L., Agee, R. N., & Pruitt, B. A. (1975). Fiberoptic bronchoscopy in acute inhalation injury. *Journal of Trauma, 15,* 641–648.

Irwin, R. J., & Mills, A. W. (1965). Matching loudness and vocal level: an experiment requiring no apparatus. *British Journal of Psychology, 56,* 143–146.

Isshiki, N. (1964). Regulatory mechanism of voice intensity regulation. *Journal of Speech and Hearing Research, 7,* 17–29.

Isshiki, N. (1965). Vocal intensity and air flow rate. *Folia Phoniatrica, 17,* 92–104.

Isshiki, N. (1977). *Functional surgery of the larynx with special reference to percutaneous tension of the vocal cords.* Kyoto: Maeda Press.

Isshiki, N., & Ishikawa, T. (1976). Diagnostic value of tomography in unilateral vocal cord paralysis. *Laryngoscope, 86,* 1573–1578.

Isshiki, N., Kitajima, K., Kojima, M., & Harita, Y. (1978). Turbulent noise in dysphonia. *Folia Phoniatrica, 30,* 214–224.

Isshiki, N., Morita, H., Okamura, H., & Hiramoto, M. (1974). Thyroplasty as a new phono-surgical technique. *Acta Oto-laryngologica (Stockholm), 78,* 451–457.

Isshiki, N., Okamura, H., & Ishikawa, T. (1975). Thyroplasty type I (lateral compression) for dysphonia due to vocal cord paralysis or atrophy. *Acta Oto-laryngologica (Stockholm), 80,* 465–473.

Isshiki, N., Tanabe, M., Ishizaka, K., & Board, C. (1977). Clinical significance of asymmetrical tension of the vocal cords. *Annals of Otology, Rhinology and Laryngology, 86,* 1–9.

Isshiki, N., & von Leden, H. S. (1964). Hoarseness: aerodynamic studies. *Archives of Otolaryngology, 80,* 206–213.

Ivers, R. R., & Goldstein, N. P. (1963). Multiple sclerosis: a current appraisal of symptoms and signs. *Proceedings of the Staff Meetings of the Mayo Clinic, 38,* 457–466.

Iwata, S., Esaki, T., Iwami, K., & Mimura, Y. (1976). Air flow studies in the patients with laryngeal diseases during phonation. *Journal of the Nagoya Cy University Medical Association, 26,* 398–406.

Iwata, S., von Leden, H. S., & Williams, D. (1972). Air flow measurement during phonation. *Journal of Communication Disorders, 5,* 67–79.

Izdebski, K. (1981). Magnetic sound recording in laryngology. *American Journal of Otolaryngology, 2,* 48–53.

Izdebski, K. (1983). Practical techniques of office voice recording. *Otolaryngology and Head and Neck Surgery, 91,* 638–642.

Izdebski, K. (1984). Overpressure and breathiness in spastic dysphonia. *Acta Oto-laryngologica (Stockholm), 97,* 373–378.

Izdebski, K. (1992). Symptomatology of adductor spasmodic dysphonia: a physiologic model. *Journal of Voice, 6,* 306–319.

Izdebski, K., & Dedo, H. H. (1979). Characteristics of vocal tremor in spastic dysphonia: a preliminary study. In V. Lawrence (Ed.), *Transcripts of the 8th symposium: care of the professional voice* (pp. 17–23). New York: Voice Foundation.

Izdebski, K., Dedo, H. H., & Shipp, T. (1981). Postoperative and follow-up studies of spastic dysphonia patients treated by recurrent nerve section. *Otolaryngology and Head and Neck Surgery, 89,* 96–101.

Jackson, C. L. (1941). Vocal nodules. *Transactions of the American Laryngological Association, 63,* 185–193.

Jacobson, E. (1938). *Progressive relaxation* (2nd ed.). Chicago: University of Chicago Press.

Jako, J. G. (1972). Laser surgery of the vocal cords: an experimental study with carbon dioxide lasers on dogs. *Laryngoscope, 82,* 2204–2216.

James, I. M., Pearson, R. M., Griffith, D. N. M., & Newburg, P. (1977). Effect of oxprenolol on stage fright in musicians. *Lancet, 2,* 952–954.

Janzen, V. D., Rae, R. E., & Hudson, A. J. (1988). Otolaryngologic manifestations of amyotrophic lateral sclerosis. *Journal of Oto-laryngology, 17,* 41–42.

Jarema, A. D., Kennedy, J. L., & Shoulson, I. (1985). Acoustic and aerodynamic measurements of hyperkinetic dysarthria in Huntington's disease. Paper presented at the convention of the American-Speech-Language-Hearing Association, Washington, DC.

Javkin, H. R., Antonanzas-Barros, H., & Maddieson, I. (1987). Digital inverse filtering for linguistic research. *Journal of Speech and Hearing Research, 30,* 122–129.

Jensen, J. R. (1960). *A study of certain motor-speech aspects of the speech of multiple sclerotic patients.* Unpublished doctoral dissertation, University of Wisconsin, Madison.

Jentzsch, H., Sasama, R., & Unger, E. (1978). Elektroglottographische Untersuchungen zur Problematik des Stimmeinsatzes bei zu sammenhangenden Sprechen. *Folia Phoniatrica, 30,* 59–66.

Jiang, J. J., Titze, I. R., Wexler, D. B., & Gray, S. D. (1994). Fundamental frequency and amplitude perturbation in reconstructed canine vocal folds. *Annals of Otology, Rhinology and Laryngology, 103,* 145–148.

Johns, M. E., & Rood, S. R. (1987). *Vocal cord paralysis: diagnosis and management.* Washington, DC: American Academy of Otolaryngology.

Johnson, J. A., & Pring, T. R. (1990). Speech therapy and Parkinson's disease: a review and further data. *British Journal of Disorders of Communication, 25,* 183–194.

Johnson, T. S. (1983). Treatment of vocal abuse in children. In Perkins, W. H. (Ed.), *Current therapy of communication disorders: voice disorders* (pp. 3–11). New York: Thieme.

Johnson, T. S. (1985). Voice disorders: the measurement of clinical progress. In Costello, J. (Ed.), *Speech disorders in adults: recent advances* (pp. 127–154). San Diego: College Hill Press.

Jürgens, U., & Pratt, R. (1979). Role of the periaqueductal grey in vocal expression of emotion. *Brain Research, 167,* 367–378.

Kahane, J., & Mayo, R. (1989). The need for aggressive pursuit of healthy childhood voices. *Language Speech Hearing Services in Schools, 20,* 102–107.

Kahane, J. C. (1981a). Anatomic and physiologic changes in the aging peripheral speech mechanism. In D. Beasley & G. Davis (Eds.), *Aging communication processes and disorders* (pp. 22–45). New York: Grune & Stratton.

Kahane, J. C. (1981b). A survey of age-related changes in the connective tissues of the human adult larynx. In D. M. Bless & J. H. Abbs (Eds.), *Vocal fold physiology: contemporary research and clinical issues* (pp. 44–49). San Diego: College Hill Press.

Kahane, J. C. (1982). Growth of the human prepubertal and pubertal larynx. *Journal of Speech and Hearing Research, 25,* 446–455.

Kahane, J. C. (1987). Connective tissue changes in the larynx and their effects on voice. *Journal of Voice, 1,* 27–30.

Kahn, H. A. (1966). The Dorn study of smoking and mortality among US veterans: A report of 8½ years of observation. *National Cancer Institute Monograph, 19,* 1–125.

Kakita, Y., Hirano, M., & Okmaru, K. (1981). Physical properities of the vocal fold tissue: measurement on excised larynges. In K. N. Stevens & M. Hirano (Eds.), *Vocal fold physiology* (pp. 377–397). Tokyo: University of Tokyo Press.

Kallen, L. A. (1932). Laryngostroboscopy in the practice of otolaryngology. *Archives of Otolaryngology, 16,* 791–807.

Kammermeier, M. A. (1969). A comparison of phonatory phenomena among groups of neurologically impaired speakers. Unpublished doctoral dissertation, University of Minnesota.

Karnell, M. P., Li, L., & Panje, W. R. (1991). Glottal opening in patients with vocal fold tissue changes. *Journal of Voice, 5,* 239–246.

Kaszniak, A. W., Garron, D. C., Fox, J. H., Bergen, D., & Huckman, M. (1979). Cerebral atrophy, EEG slowing, age, education, and cognitive functioning in suspected dementia. *Neurology, 29,* 1273–1279.

Kasuya, H., Ogawa, S., Mashima, K., & Ebihara, S. (1986). Normalized noise energy as an acoustic measure to evaluate pathologic voice. *Journal of the Acoustical Society of America, 80,* 1329–1334.

Keaton, A. L. (1983). The physiology of imagery. In V. Lawrence (Ed.), *Transcripts of the 12th symposium: care of the professional voice* (Part II, pp. 281–283). New York: Voice Foundation.

Kellman, R. M., & Leopold, D. A. (1982). Paradoxical vocal cord motion: an important cause of stridor. *Laryngoscope, 92,* 58–60.

Kelly, A. H., Beaton, L. E., & Magoun, H. W. (1946). A midbrain mechanism for facio-vocal activity. *Journal of Neurophysiology, 9,* 181–189.

Kempster, G. B. (1984). *A multidimensional analysis of vocal quality in two dysphonic groups.* Unpublished doctoral dissertation, Northwestern University, Evanston, IL.

Kent, R. D., Kent, J., & Rosenbek, J. (1987). Maximum performance tests of speech production. *Journal of Speech and Hearing Research, 52,* 367–387.

Kent, R. D., Kim, H., Weismer, G., Kent, J. F., Rosenbek, J. C., Brooks, B. R., & Workinger, M. (1994). Laryngeal dysfunction in neurological disease: amyotrophic lateral sclerosis, parkinson disease, and stroke. *Journal of Medical Speech Language Pathology, 2*, 157–175.

Kent, R. D., & Netsell, R. (1975). A case study of an ataxic dysarthric cineradiographic and spectrographic observations. *Journal of Speech and Hearing Disorders, 40*, 115–134.

Kent, R. D., Netsell, R., & Abbs, J. H. (1979). Acoustic characteristics of dysarthria associated with cerebellar disease. *Journal of Speech and Hearing Research, 22*, 627–648.

Kent, R. D., Sufit, R. L., Rosenbek, J. C., Kent, J. F., Weismer, G., Martin, R. E., & Brooks, B. R. (1991). Speech deterioration in amyotrophic lateral sclerosis: a case study. *Journal of Speech and Hearing Research, 34*, 1269–1275.

Kim, K. M., Kakita, Y., & Hirano, M. (1982). Sound spectrographic analysis of the voice of patients with recurrent laryngeal nerve paralysis. *Folia Phoniatrica, 34*, 124–133.

King, J. B., Ramig, L. O., Lemke, J. H., & Horii, Y. (1994). Parkinson's disease: Longitudinal changes in acoustic parameters of phonation. *Journal of Medical Speech Language Pathology, 2*, 29–42.

Kinney, J. P., Kado, R. T., & Royner, L. D. (1972). A simple encoder for labelling events recorded on analogue tape. *Medical and Biological Engineering, 10*, 431–432.

Kiritani, S., Imagawa, H., & Hirose, H. (1986). Simultaneous high-speed digital recording of vocal fold vibration, speech and EGG. *Annual Bulletin RILP, 20*, 11–15.

Kitajima, K. (1981). Quantitative evaluation of the noise level in the pathologic voice. *Folia Phoniatrica, 33*, 115–124.

Kitzing, P. (1985). Stroboscopy—a pertinent laryngological examination. *Journal of Otolaryngology, 14*, 151–157.

Kitzing, P., & Löfqvist, A. (1978). *Clinical application of combined electro- and photoglottography.* Paper presented at the 17th Congress of Logopedics and Phoniatrics, Copenhagen, Denmark.

Kleinsasser, O. (1987). *Surgery in unilateral vocal cord paralysis.* Paper presented at the International Symposium on Phonosurgery. Cairo, Egypt.

Klingholz, F., & Martin, F. (1985). Quantitative spectral evaluation of shimmer and jitter. *Journal of Speech and Hearing Research, 28*, 169–174.

Koike, Y. (1967a). Experimental studies on vocal attack. *Practica Otologica Kyoto, 60*, 663–688.

Koike, Y. (1967b). Applications of some acoustic measures for the evaluation of laryngeal dysfunction. *Journal of the Acoustical Society of America, 42*, 1209.

Koike, Y., & Hirano, M. (1968). Significance of the vocal velocity index. *Folia Phoniatrica, 20*, 285–296.

Kojima, H., Gould, W. J., & Lambiase, A. (1979). Computer analysis of hoarseness. *Journal of the Acoustical Society of America, 65*, S67.

Kojima, H., Gould, W. J., Lambiase, A., & Isshiki, N. (1980). Computer analysis of hoarseness. *Acta Oto-laryngologica (Stockholm), 89*, 547–554.

Koller, W. C., Busenbark, K., & Miner, K. (1994). The relationship of essential tremor to other movement disorders: report on 678 patients. *Annals of Neurology, 35*, 717–723.

Komiyama, S., Watanabe, H., & Ryu, S. (1984). Phonetographic relationship between pitch and intensity of the human voice. *Folia Phoniatrica, 36*, 1–7.

Kooper, R., & Sullivan, C. A. (1986). Professional liability: management and prevention. In KG Butler (Ed.), *Prospering in private practice* (pp. 59–80). Rockville, MD: Aspen Systems.

Kornhuber, H. H. (1977). A reconsideration of the cortical and subcortical mechanisms involved in speech and aphasia. In J. E. Desmedt (Ed.), *Progress in clinical neurophysiology* (pp. 28–35). Basel: S Karger.

Kotby, M. N., & Haugen, L. K. (1970). The mechanics of laryngeal function. *Acta Otolaryngologica (Stockholm), 70*, 203–211.

Koufman, J. A. (1986). Laryngoplasty for vocal cord medialization: an alternative to teflon. *Laryngoscope, 96*, 726–731.

Koufman, J. A. (1991). The otolaryngologic manifestations of gastroesophageal reflux disease (GERD): a clinical investigation of 225 patients using ambulatory 24-hour pH monitoring and an experimental investigation of the role of acid and pepsin in the development of laryngeal injury. *Laryngoscope, 101*, 1–78.

Koufman, J. A. (1995). Gastroesophageal reflux and voice disorders. In J. S. Rubin, R. T. Sataloff, G. Korovin, & W. J. Gould (Eds.), *Diagnosis and treatment of voice disorders* (pp. 161–175). New York: Igaku-Shoin.

Koufman, J. A., Wiener, G. J., Wu, W. C., & Castell, D. O. (1988). Reflux laryngitis and its sequelae: the diagnostic role of ambulatory 24-hour pH monitoring. *Journal of Voice, 2*, 78–89.

Kreindler, A., & Pruskauer-Apostol, B. (1971). Neurologic and psychopathologic aspects of compulsive crying and laughter in pseudobulbar palsy patients. *Revue Roumaine de Neurologie, 8*, 125–139.

Kunze, L. H. (1964). Evaluation of methods of estimating sub-glottal air pressure. *Journal of Speech and Hearing Research, 7*, 151–164.

Kurita, S. (1980). Layer structure of the human vocal fold: morphological investigation. *Otologia (Fukuoka), 26*, 973–997.

Kuroki, K. (1969). Subglottic pressure of normal and pathological larynges. *Otologia (Fukuoka), 15,* 54–74.

Kurtzke, J. F., Beebe, G. W., Nagler, B., Auth, T. L., & Kurland, L. T. (1972). Studies on the natural history of multiple sclerosis. *Acta Neurologica Scandinavia, 48,* 19–46.

Ladefoged, P., & McKinney, N. P. (1963). Loudness, sound pressure and subglottal pressure in speech. *Journal of the Acoustical Society of America, 35,* 454–460.

Lane, H. L., Catania, A. C., & Stevens, S. S. (1961). Voice level: autophonic scale, perceived loudness and effects of sidetone. *Journal of the Acoustical Society of America, 33,* 160–167.

Lang, A. E., & Marsden, C. D. (1983). Spasmodic dysphonia in Gilles de la Tourette's disease. *Archives of Neurology, 40,* 51–52.

Langworthy, O. R., & Hesser, F. H. (1940). Syndrome of pseudobulbar palsy: an anatomic and physiologic analysis. *Archives of Internal Medicine, 65,* 106–121.

Larson, C. (1985). The midbrain periaqueductal gray: a brainstem structure involved in vocalization. *Journal of Speech and Hearing Research, 28,* 241–249.

Larson, C. R. (1988). Brain mechanisms involved in the control of vocalization. *Journal of Voice, 2,* 301–311.

Larson, C. R., & Kistler, M. K. (1986). The relationship of periaqueductal gray neurons to vocalization and laryngeal EMG in the behaving monkey. *Experimental Brain Research, 63,* 596–606.

Larson, C. R., Sutton, D., & Lindeman, R. C. (1978). Cerebellar regulation of phonation in rhesus monkey (Macaca mulatta). *Experimental Brain Research, 33,* 1.

Larson, K. K., Ramig, L. O., & Scherer, R. C. (1994). Acoustic and glottographic voice analysis during drug-related fluctuations in Parkinson disease. *Journal of Medical Speech Language Pathology, 2,* 227–239.

Larsson, T., & Sjogren, T. (1960). Essential tremor. A clinical and genetic population study. *Acta Psychiatry Neurology (Scand), 36 (Suppl 144),* 1–176.

Lawrence, V. L. (1987). Common medications with laryngeal effects. *Ear Nose and Throat Journal, 66,* 318–322.

Leanderson, R., Meyerson, B. A., & Persson, A. (1972). Lip muscle function in Parkinsonian dysarthria. *Acta Oto-laryngologica (Stockholm), 74,* 350–357.

Leboldus, G. M., Savoury, L. W., Carr, T. J., & Nicholson, R. L. (1986). Magnetic resonance imaging: a review of basic principles and potential use in otolaryngology. *Journal of Otolaryngology, 15,* 273–278.

Lebrun, Y., Devreux, F., Rousseau, J., & Darimont, P. (1982). Tremulous speech. *Folia Phoniatrica, 34,* 134–142.

Lechtenberg, R., & Gilman, S. (1978). Speech disorders in cerebellar disease. *Annals of Neurology, 3,* 285–290.

Lee, K. J. (1973). *The otolaryngology boards.* New York: Medical Exam Publishing.

Lehmann, Q. H. (1965). Reverse phonation: a new maneuver for examining the larynx. *Radiology, 84,* 215–222.

LeJeune, F. E., Guice, C. E., & Samuels, P. M. (1983). Early experiences with vocal ligament tightening. *Annals of Otology, Rhinology and Laryngology, 92,* 475–477.

Leonard, R. J., & Ringel, R. L. (1979). Vocal shadowing under conditions of normal and altered laryngeal sensation. *Journal of Speech and Hearing Research, 22,* 794–817.

Lessac, A. (1987). *The use and training of the human voice: a practical approach to speech and voice dynamics.* New York: Drama Book Publishers.

Lester, B. M. (1985). Introduction: there's more to crying than meets the ear. In B. M. Lester & C. F. Boukydis (Eds.), *Infant crying: theoretical and research perspectives* (pp. 1–28). New York: Plenum.

Levine, L., Hatlali, J. M., & Zaggy, M. (1985). Myasthenia gravis presenting as intermittent laryngeal paralysis. In V. Lawrence (Ed.), *Transcripts of the 14th symposium: care of the professional voice* (pp. 348–351). New York: Voice Foundation.

Lewis, K., Casteel, R., & McMahon, J. (1982). Duration of sustained /a/ related to number of trials. *Folia Phoniatrica, 34,* 41–48.

Lewy, R. B. (1993). Teflon injection: pointers and pitfalls. *Annals of Otology, Rhinology and Laryngology, 102,* 283–284.

Liden, S., & Gottfries, C. (1974). Beta-blocking agents in the treatment of catecholamine-induced symptoms in musicians. *Lancet, 2,* 529.

Lieberman, P. (1963). Some acoustic measures of the fundamental periodicity of normal and pathologic larynges. *Journal of the Acoustical Society of America, 35,* 344–353.

Lieberman, P. (1968). Vocal cord motion in man. *Annals of the New York Academy of Sciences, 155,* 28–38.

Lindestad, P., & Persson, A. (1994). Quantitative analysis of EMG interference patterns in patients with laryngeal paresis. *Acta Oto-laryngologica (Stockholm), 114,* 91–97.

Linebaugh, C. (1979). The dysarthrias of Shy-Drager syndrome. *Journal of Speech and Hearing Disorders, 44,* 55–60.

Linville, S. E. (1987a). Acoustic-perceptual studies of aging voice in women. *Journal of Voice, 1,* 44–48.

Linville, S. E. (1987b). Maximum phonational frequency range capabilities of women's voices with advancing age. *Folia Phoniatrica, 39,* 297–301.

Linville, S. E. (1992). Glottal gap configurations in two age groups of women. *Journal of Speech and Hearing Research, 35,* 1209–1215.

Linville, S. E., & Fisher, H. (1985). Acoustic characteristics of women's voices with advancing age. *Journal of Gerontology, 40,* 324–330.

Löfqvist, A. (1993). Aerodynamic measurements of vocal function. In A. Blitzer, M. F. Brin, C. T. Sasaki, S. Fahn, & K. S. Harris (Eds.), *Neurologic disorders of the larynx* (pp. 98–107). New York: Thieme.

Logemann, J. A., Fisher, H. B., Boshes, B., & Blonsky, E. R. (1978). Frequency and cooccurrence of vocal tract dysfunctions in the speech of a large sample of Parkinson patients. *Journal of Speech and Hearing Disorders, 42,* 47–57.

Longridge, N. S. (1987). Bilateral vocal cord paralysis in Shy-Drager syndrome. *Journal of Otolaryngology, 16,* 146–148.

Lou, J. S., & Jankovic, J. (1991). Essential tremor: clinical correlates in 350 patients. *Neurology, 41,* 234–238.

Lowenthal, D. T., Kirschner, D. A., Scarpace, N. T., Pollock, M., & Graves, J. (1994). Effects of exercise on age and disease [review]. *Southern Medical Journal, 87,* S5–12.

Lowenthal, G. (1958). The treatment of polypoid laryngitis. *Laryngoscope, 68,* 1095–1104.

Luchsinger, R., & Arnold, G. E. (1965). *Voice speech language clinical communicology: its physiology and pathology.* Belmont, CA: Wadsworth.

Ludlow, C. (1981). Research needs for the assessment of phonatory function. In C. Ludlow & M. Hart (Eds.), *Proceedings of the conference on vocal assessment of vocal pathology* (pp. 3–8). Rockville, MD: American Speech-Language-Hearing Association.

Ludlow, C. L. (1990). Treatment of speech and voice disorders with botulinum toxin. *Journal of the American Medical Association, 264,* 2671–2675.

Ludlow, C. L. (1995). Management of the spasmodic dysphonias. In J. S. Rubin, R. T. Sataloff, G. Korovin, & W. J. Gould (Eds.), *Diagnosis and treatment of voice disorders* (pp. 436–454). New York: Igaku-Shoin.

Ludlow, C. L., Bassich, C. J., Connor, N. P., & Coulter, D. C. (1986). Phonatory characteristics of vocal fold tremor. *Journal of Phonetics, 14,* 509–516.

Ludlow, C. L., Connor, N. P., & Coulter, D. (1984). A preliminary investigation into the validity of an optimum frequency for phonatory functioning in patients with laryngeal pathology. In V. Lawrence (Ed.), *Transcripts of the 12th symposium: care of the professional voice* (pp. 155–168). New York: Voice Foundation.

Ludlow, C. L., Coulter, D., & Gentges, F. (1983). Differential sensitivity of frequency perturbation to laryngeal neoplasms and neuropathologies. In D. M. Bless & J. H. Abbs (Eds.), *Vocal fold physiology: contemporary research and clinical issues* (pp. 381–392). San Diego: College Hill Press.

Ludlow, C. L., Naunton, R. F., Terada, S., Anderson, B. J. (1991). Successful treatment of selected cases of abductor spasmodic dysphonia using botulinum toxin *injection. Archives of Otolaryngology—Head and Neck Surgery, 104,* 849–855.

Ludlow, C. L., Schulz, G. M., & Naunton, R. F. (1988). The effects of Diazepam on intrinsic laryngeal muscle activation during respiration and speech. *Journal of Voice, 2,* 70–77.

Lufkin, R. B., & Hanafee, W. N. (1985). Application of surface coils to MR anatomy of the larynx. *American Journal of Nuclear Resonance, 6,* 491–497.

MacCurtain, F., & Fourcin, A. J. (1982). Applications of the electroglottograph wave form display. In V. Lawrence (Ed.), *Transcripts of the 10th symposium: care of the professional voice* (pp. 51–57). New York: Voice Foundation.

Marge, M. (1984). The prevention of communication disorders. *ASHA, 26,* 29–37.

Markel, N. N., Bern, M. F., & Philis, J. A. (1973). The relationship between words and tone of voice. *Language and Speech, 16,* 15–21.

Markel, N. N., Meisels, M., & Houck, J. (1964). Judging personality from voice quality. *Journal of Abnormal Social Psychology, 69,* 458–463.

Martin, F. G. (1983). Drugs and the voice. In V. Lawrence (Ed.), *Transcripts of the 12th symposium: care of the professional voice* (pp. 124–132). New York: Voice Foundation.

Martin, F. G. (1984). The influence of drugs on voice. In V. Lawrence (Ed.), *Transcripts of the 13th symposium: care of the professional voice* (pp. 191–201). New York: Voice Foundation.

Martin, F.G. (1988). Tutorial: drugs and vocal function. *Journal of Voice, 2,* 338–344.

Martin, R., Blager, F., Gay, M., & Wood, R. (1987). Paradoxic vocal cord motion in presumed asthmatics. *Seminars in Respiratory Medicine, 9,* 332–337.

Martínez-Martín, P., & Bermejo-Pareja, F. (1988). Rating scales in Parkinson's disease. In J. Jankovic & E. Tolosa (Eds.), *Parkinson's disease and movement disorders* (pp. 235–240). Baltimore: Urban & Schwarzenberg.

Maxwell, S., & Locke, J. (1969). Voice in myasthenia gravis. *Laryngoscope, 79,* 1902–1906.

McClean, M. D. (1987). Surface EMG recordings of the perioral reflexes: preliminary observations on stutterers and non stutterers. *Journal of Speech and Hearing Research, 30,* 283–287.

McClean, M. D. (1988). Neuromotor aspects of speech production and dysarthria. In K. M. Yorkston, D. R. T. Beukelman, & K. R. Bell (Eds.), *Clinical management of dysarthric speakers* (pp. 19–58). Boston: College Hill Press.

McFarlane, S. C., Fujiki, M., & Brinton, B. (1984). *Coping with communicative handicaps: resources for the practicing clinician.* San Diego: College Hill Press.

McGlone, R. E., & Hollien, H. (1963). Vocal pitch characteristics of aged women. *Journal of Speech and Hearing Research, 6,* 164–170.

McGlone, R. E., Richmond, W. H., & Bosma, J. F. (1966). A physiological model for investigation of the fundamental frequency of phonation. *Folia Phoniatrica, 18,* 109–116.

McGowan, R. S. (1992). Tongue-tip trills and vocal-tract wall compliance. *Journal of the Acoustical Society of America, 91,* 2903–2910.

Merritt, H. H. (1975). *A textbook of neurology* (5th ed.). Philadelphia: Lea & Febiger.

Merritt, H. H. (1979). *A textbook of neurology* (6th ed.). Philadelphia: Lea & Febiger.

Merson, R. M., & Ginsberg, A. P. (1979). Spasmodic dysphonia: abductor type. A clinical report of acoustic aerodynamic and perceptual characteristics. *Laryngoscope, 89,* 129–139.

Metz, D. E., Whitehead, R. L., Peterson, D. H. (1980). An optical illumination system for high speed laryngeal cinematography. *Journal of the Acoustical Society of America, 67,* 719–720.

Meurman, R. (1952). Operative mediofixation of the vocal cord in complete unilateral paralysis. *Archives of Otolaryngology, 55,* 544.

Miehlke, V. A., Arnold, R. (1982). Chirurgie des Nervus recurrense-ein Ausblick. In J. Berendes, R. Link, & F. Zollner (Eds.), *Hals-Nasen-Ohren-Heilkunde in Praxis and Klinik (Band 4 Teil 1)* (pp. 1–24). Stuttgart: Thieme Verlag.

Millar, J. H. D. (1971). *Multiple sclerosis: a disease acquired in childhood.* Springfield: Charles C Thomas.

Miller, J. E., & Mathews, M. V. (1963). Investigation of the glottal waveshape by automatic inverse filtering. *Journal of the Acoustical Society of America, 35,* 1876.

Miller, R. P., Gray, S. D., Cotton, R. T., & Myer, C. M. (1988). Airway reconstruction following laryngotracheal thermal trauma. *Laryngoscope, 98,* 826–829.

Minifie, F. D. (1984). Against the clinical use of optimal pitch. In V. Lawrence (Ed.), *Transcripts of the 12th symposium: care of the professional voice* (Part II, pp. 148–154). New York: Voice Foundation.

Mitchell, G. (1993). Update on multiple sclerosis therapy [review]. *Medical Clinics of North America, 77,* 231–249.

Moll, K. L., & Peterson, G. E. (1969). Speaker and listener judgments of vowel levels. *Phonetica, 19,* 104–117.

Monday, L. A. (1983). Clinical evaluation of functional dysphonia. *Journal of Otolaryngology, 12,* 307–310.

Monoson, P., & Zemlin, W. R. (1984). Quantitative study of whisper. *Folia Phoniatrica, 36,* 53–65.

Moore, G. P. (1937). A short history of laryngeal investigation. *Quarterly Journal of Speech, 23,* 531–564.

Moore, G. P. (1975). Ultra high speed photography in laryngeal research. *Canadian Journal of Otolaryngology, 4,* 793–799.

Moore, G. P. (1977). Have the major issues in voice disorders been answered by research in speech science? A 50–year retrospective. *Journal of Speech and Hearing Disorders, 42,* 152–160.

Moore, G. P. (1986). Voice disorders. In G. H. Shames & E. H. Wiig (Eds.), *Human communication disorders an introduction* (pp. 183–241). Columbus, OH: Charles E. Merrill.

Moore, G. P., & Childers, D. G. (1984). Glottal area (real size) related to voice production. In V. Lawrence (Ed.), *Transcripts of the 12th symposium: care of the professional voice* (pp. 92–96). New York: Voice Foundation.

Moore, G. P, Hicks, D. M., & Abbott, T. B. (1985). Defects of speech and language. In J. J. Ballenger (Ed.), *Diseases of the nose, throat, ear, head, and neck* (pp. 692–731). Philadelphia: Lea & Febiger.

Moore, G. P., & von Leden, H. S. (1958). Dynamic variations of the vibratory pattern in the normal larynx. *Folia Phoniatrica, 10,* 205–238.

Moore, G. P., White, F., & von Leden, H. S. (1962). Ultra high speed photography in laryngeal physiology. *Journal of Speech and Hearing Disorders, 27,* 165–171.

Morris, R. J., & Brown, W. S., Jr. (1994). Age-related differences in speech intensity among adult females. *Folia Phoniatrica et Logopedica, 46,* 64–69.

Morrison, M., & Rammage, L. (1994). *The management of voice disorders.* San Diego: Singular Publishing Group.

Morrison, M. D., Rammage, L. A., Belisle, G. M., Pullan, C. B., & Nichol, H. (1983). Muscular tension dysphonia. *Journal of Otolaryngology, 12,* 302–306.

Mueller, P. B., Larson, G. W., & Summers, P. A. (1993). Additional data on s/z ratios in kindergarten children. *Language Speech Hearing Services in Schools, 24,* 177–178.

Mueller, P. B., Sweeney, R. J., & Baribeau, L. J. (1984). Acoustic and morphologic study of the senescent voice. *Ear, Nose, and Throat Journal, 63,* 292–295.

Murry, T. (1971). Subglottal pressure and airflow measures during vocal fry phonation. *Journal of Speech and Hearing Research, 14,* 544–551.

Murry, T. (1978). Speaking fundamental frequency characteristics associated with voice pathologies. *Journal of Speech and Hearing Disorders, 43,* 374–379.

Murry, T., Bone, R., & von Essen, C. (1974). Changes in voice production during radiotherapy for laryngeal cancer. *Journal of Speech and Hearing Disorders, 39,* 194–201.

Murry, T., & Woodson, G. E. (1995). Combined-modality treatment of adductor spasmodic dysphonia with Botulinum toxin and voice therapy. *Journal of Voice, 9,* 460–465.

Mysak, E. D. (1959). Pitch and duration characteristics of older males. *Journal of Speech and Hearing Research, 2,* 46–54.

Mysak, E., & Hanley, T. (1959). Vocal aging. *Geriatrics, 14,* 652–656.

Nagler, W. (1987). *Dr. Nagler's body maintenance and repair book.* New York: Simon and Schuster.

Neiman, G. S., & Edeson, B. (1981). Procedural aspects of eliciting maximum phonation time. *Folia Phoniatrica, 33,* 285–293.

Newman, R. A., & Emanuel, F. W. (1991). Pitch effects on vowel roughness and spectral noise for subjects in four musical voice classifications. *Journal of Speech and Hearing Research, 34,* 753–760.

Nielsen, V. M., Hojslet, P. E., & Karlsmose, M. (1986). Surgical treatment of Reinke's oedema (long-term results). *Journal of Laryngology and Otology, 100,* 187–190.

Nilson, H., & Schneiderman, C. R. (1983). Classroom program for the prevention of vocal abuse in elementary school children. *Language Speech Hearing Services in Schools, 14,* 172–178.

Noffsinger, D., Olsen, W. O., Carhart, R., Hart, C. W., & Sahgal, V. (1972). Auditory and vestibular aberrations in multiple sclerosis. *Acta Oto-laryngologica (Stockholm), Suppl 303,* 1–63.

Olson, N. R. (1991). Laryngopharyngeal manifestations of gastroesophageal reflux disease. *Otolaryngology Clinics of North America, 24,* 1201–1213.

Orlikoff, R. F. (1990). The relationship of age and cardiovascular health to certain acoustic characteristics of male voices. *Journal of Speech and Hearing Research, 33,* 450–457.

Ortega, J. D., DeRosier, E., Park, S., & Larson, C. (1988). Brainstem mechanisms of laryngeal control as revealed by microstimulation studies. In O. Fujimura (Ed.), *Vocal fold physiology: voice production, mechanisms and function* (pp. 19–28). New York: Raven Press.

Osserman, K. E. (1958). *Myasthenia gravis.* New York: Grune & Stratton.

Oxtoby M. (1982). *Parkinson's disease patients and their social needs.* London: Parkinson's Disease Society.

Padberg, G. W., & Bruyn, G. W. (1986). Chorea—differential diagnosis. In P. J. Vinken, G. W. Bruyn, & H. L. Klawans (Eds.), *Handbook of clinical neurology* (pp. 549–564). Amsterdam: Elsevier.

Pahn, J. (1966). Zur entwicklung und behandlung funktioneller singstimmerkrankugen. *Folia Phoniatrica, 18,* 117–130.

Painter, C. (1986). The laryngeal vestibule and voice quality. *Archives of Otolaryngology, 243,* 329–337.

Painter, C. (1988). Electroglottogram waveform types. *Archives of Otolaryngology, 245,* 116–121.

Painter, C. (1991). The laryngeal vestibule, voice quality and paralinguistic markers. *European Archives of Oto-rhino-laryngology, 248,* 452–458.

Papp, P. (1983). *The process of change.* New York: Guilford Press.

Parnes, S. M. (1988). Laryngeal electromyography. *ENTechnology,* 48–51.

Parnes, S. M., Lavarato, A. B., & Myers, E. N. (1978). Study of spastic dysphonia using videofiberoptic laryngoscopy. *Annals of Otology, Rhinology and Laryngology, 87,* 322–326.

Parnes, S. M., & Satya-Murti, S. (1985). Predictive value of laryngeal electromyography in patients with vocal cord paralysis of neurogenic origin. *Laryngoscope, 95,* 1323–1326.

Peacher, G. (1947). Contact ulcer of the larynx I. History. *Journal of Speech and Hearing Disorders, 12,* 67.

Penfield, W., & Roberts, L. (1959). *Speech and brain mechanisms.* Princeton, NJ: Princeton University Press.

Perez, K. S., Ramig, L. O., Smith, M. E., & Dromey, C. (1994). The Parkinson larynx: tremor and videostroboscopic findings. *NCVS Status and Progress Report, 7,* 33–39.

Perkins, W. (1971). *Speech pathology: an applied behavioral science.* St Louis: CV Mosby.

Perkins, W. H. (1983). Quantification of vocal behavior: a foundation for clinical management of voice. In D. M. Bless & J. H. Abbs (Eds.), *Vocal fold physiology: contemporary research and clinical issues* (pp. 425–431). San Diego: College Hill Press.

Perkins, W. H. (1985). Assessment and treatment of voice disorders: state of the art. In Costello, J. (Ed.), *Speech disorders in adults:*

*recent advances* (pp. 79–112). San Diego: College Hill Press.

Perlman, A. L., & Titze, I. R. (1988). Development of an in vitro technique for measuring elastic proper ties of vocal fold tissue. *Journal of Speech and Hearing Research, 31,* 288–298.

Perlman, A. L., Titze, I. R., & Cooper, D. S. (1984). Elasticity of canine vocal fold tissue. *Journal of Speech and Hearing Research, 27,* 212–219.

Pinto, N. B., & Titze, I. R. (1990). Unification of perturbation measures in speech signals. *Journal of the Acoustical Society of America, 87,* 1278–1289.

Plomp, R. (1976). *Aspects of tone sensation.* New York: Academic Press.

Pontes, P., & Behlau, M. (1993). Treatment of sulcus vocalis: auditory perceptual and acoustical analysis of the slicing mucosa surgical technique. *Journal of Voice, 7,* 365–376.

Pontes, P., Mara, B., & Oscar, T. (1989). Computer acoustical analysis of the treatment of sulcus vocalis. *Folia Phoniatrica, 41,* 204–205.

Prater, R. J., & Swift, R. W. (1984). *Manual of voice therapy.* Boston: Little, Brown.

Pressman, J. J. (1942). Physiology of vocal cords in phonation and respiration. *Archives of Otolaryngology, 35,* 355–398.

Pressman, J. J., & Kelemen, G. (1955). Physiology of the larynx. *Physiological Reviews, 35,* 506–554.

Prosek, R. A., Montgomery, A., Walden, B., & Schwartz, D. (1978). EMG feedback in the treatment of hyperfunctional voice disorders. *Journal of Speech and Hearing Disorders, 43,* 282–294.

Ptacek, P. H., Sander, E., Maloney, W., & Jackson, C. C. (1966). Phonatory and related changes with advanced age. *Journal of Speech and Hearing Research, 9,* 353–360.

Rabuzzi, D., & McCall, G. N. (1972). Spasmodic dysphonia: a clinical perspective. *Transactions of the American Academy of Ophthalmology and Otolaryngology, 76,* 724–728.

Ramig, L. A. (1986). Acoustic analysis of phonation in patients with Huntington's disease. *Annals of Otology, Rhinology and Laryngology, 95,* 288–293.

Ramig, L. A., & Gould, W. J. (1986). Speech characteristics in Parkinson's disease. *Neurologic Consultant, 4,* 1–8.

Ramig, L. A., & Ringel, R. (1983). Effects of physiological aging on selected acoustic characteristics of voice. *Journal of Speech and Hearing Research, 26,* 22–30.

Ramig, L. A., Scherer, R. C., Klasner, E. R., Titze, I. R., & Horii, Y. (1990). Acoustic analysis of voice in amyotrophic lateral sclerosis: a longitudinal case study. *Journal of Speech and Hearing Disorders, 55,* 2–14.

Ramig, L. A., Scherer, R. C., Titze, I. R., & Ringel, S. P. (1988). Acoustic analysis of voices of patients with neurologic disease: rationale and preliminary data. *Annals of Otology, Rhinology and Laryngology, 97,* 164–172.

Ramig, L. O. (1995). Speech therapy for patients with Parkinson's disease. In W. C. Koller & G. Paulson (Eds.), *Therapy of Parkinson's disease.* (pp. 539–550). New York: Marcel Dekker.

Ramig, L. O., Bonitati, C. M., Lemke, J. H., & Horii, Y. (1994). Voice treatment for patients with Parkinson disease: development of an approach and preliminary efficacy data. *Journal of Medical Speech Language Pathology, 2,* 191–209.

Ramig, L. O., Mead, C., Scherer, R., Horii, Y., Larson, K., & Kohler, D. (1988). Voice therapy and Parkinson's disease: a longitudinal study of efficacy. Paper presented at the Clinical Dysarthria Conference, San Diego.

Ramig, L. O., & Scherer, R. C. (1992). Speech therapy for neurologic disorders of the larynx. In A. Blitzer, M. F. Brin, C. T. Sasaki, S. Fahn, & K. S. Harris (Eds.), *Neurologic disorders of the larynx* (pp. 163–181). New York: Thieme.

Randall, W. L. (1964). The behavior of cats (Felis catus) with lesions in the caudal midbrain region. *Behavior, 23,* 107–139.

Raphael, B. N., & Scherer, R. (1987). Voice modifications of stage actors: acoustic analyses. *Journal of Voice, 1,* 83–87.

Rasinger, G. A., Neuwirth-Riedi, K., & Kment, G. (1986) Erst ergebnisse digitaler Videobildanalyseverfahren zur Auswertung von endoskopischen. *Laryngo- Rhino- Otologie (Stuttgart), 65,* 333–335.

Rastatter, M. P., & Hyman, M. (1982). Maximum phoneme duration of /s/ and /z/ by children with vocal nodules. *Language Speech Hearing Services in Schools, 13,* 197–199.

Ravits, J. (1988). Myasthenia gravis. A well-understood neuromuscular disorder. *Postgraduate Medicine, 83,* 219–223.

Reed, C. G. (1980). Voice therapy: a need for research. *Journal of Speech and Hearing Disorders, 45,* 157–169.

Reich, A. R., & Lerman, J. W. (1978). Teflon laryngoplasty: an acoustical and perceptual study. *Journal of Speech and Hearing Disorders, 43,* 496–505.

Reich, A. R., Mason, J. A., & Polen, S. B. (1986). Task administration variables affecting phonation time measures in 3rd grade girls with normal voice quality. *Language Speech Hearing Services in Schools, 17,* 262–269.

Reik, T. (1948). *Listening with the third ear.* New York: Farrar, Strauss & Giroux.

Reiser, D. E., & Schroder, A. K. (1980). *Patient interviewing, the human dimension.* Baltimore: Williams & Wilkins.

Riklan, M., & Levita, E. (1969). *Subcortical correlates of human behavior.* Baltimore: Williams & Wilkins.

Ringel, R. L., & Chodzko-Zajko, W. (1987). Vocal indices of biological age. *Journal of Voice, 1,* 31–37.

Robe, E., Brumlik, J., & Moore, G. P. (1960). A study of spastic dysphonia. *Laryngoscope, 70,* 219–245.

Robertson, S., & Thompson, F. (1984). Speech therapy in Parkinson's disease: a study of the efficacy and long-term effect in intensive treatment. *British Journal of Disorders of Communication, 19,* 213–224.

Rogers, J. H., & Stell, P. M. (1978). Paradoxical movement of the vocal cords as a cause of stridor. *Journal of Laryngology and Otology, 92,* 157–158.

Rontal, E., & Rontal, M. (1986). The immobile cord. In C. Cummings, L. Harker, C. S. Krause, & D. Schuller (Eds.), *Otolaryngology—Head and Neck Surgery* (pp. 2055–2071). St. Louis: CV Mosby.

Rontal, M., Rontal, E., Leuchter, W., & Rolnick, M. (1978). Voice spectrography in the evaluation of myasthenia gravis of the larynx. *Archives of Otolaryngology, 87,* 722–728.

Rontal, M., Rontal, E., Rolnick, M., Merson, R., Silverman, B., & Truong, D. D. (1991). A method for the treatment of abductor spasmodic dysphonia with botulinum toxin injections: a preliminary report. *Laryngoscope, 101,* 911–914.

Rosenfield, D. B. (1987). Neurolaryngology. *Ear, Nose, and Throat Journal, 66,* 323–326.

Rosenthal, R. S. (1978). Malpractice: cause and its prevention. *Laryngoscope, 88,* 1–11.

Rothenberg, M. (1968). The breath stream dynamics of simple-released plosive production. *Bibliotheca Phonetica, 6,* (whole volume).

Rothenberg, M. (1973). A new inverse filtering technique for deriving the glottal air flow during voicing. *Journal of the Acoustical Society of America, 53,* 1632–1645.

Rothenberg, M. (1977). Measurement of air flow during speech. *Journal of Speech and Hearing Research, 2,* 155–176.

Rothenberg, M. (1981). Some relations between glottal air flow and vocal fold contact area. In C. Ludlow & M. Hart (Eds.), *Proceeding of the conference on the assessment of vocal pathology.* Rockville, MD: American Speech-Language-Hearing Association.

Rothenberg, M. (1982). Interpolating subglottal pressure from oral pressure. *Journal of Speech and Hearing Disorders, 47,* 218–224.

Rothenberg, M., & Mahshie, J. J. (1988). Monitoring vocal fold abduction through vocal fold contact area. *Journal of Speech and Hearing Research, 31,* 338–351.

Roy, N. (1994). Manual tension reduction: an alternative with functional voice disorders. Paper presented at the convention of the American Speech-Language-Hearing Association, New Orleans, LA.

Roy, N., & Leeper, H. A. (1993). Effects of the manual laryngeal musculoskeletal tension reduction technique as a treatment for functional voice disorders: perceptual and acoustic measures. *Journal of Voice, 7,* 242–249.

Roy, N., Tasko, S. M., & Harvey, S. (1995). Treatment results using the manual laryngeal musculoskeletal tension reduction procedure. Paper presented at the convention of the American Speech-Language-Hearing Association, New Orleans, LA.

Rubin, H. J. (1965). Pitfalls in treatment of dysphonias by intracordal injection of synthetics. *Laryngoscope, 75,* 381–395.

Rubin, H. J., & Hirt, C. (1960). The falsetto: A high speed cinematographic study. *Laryngoscope, 70,* 1305–1324.

Rubin, H. J., & LeCover, M. (1960). Technique of high speed photography of the larynx. *Annals of Otology, Rhinology and Laryngology, 69,* 1072–1082.

Rullan, A. (1991). Associated laryngeal paralysis. *Archives of Otolaryngology, 64,* 207–212.

Rutala, D. R., Rutala, W. A., Weber, D. J., & Thomann, C. A. (1991). Infection risks associated with spirometry. *Infection Control and Hospital Epidemiology, 12,* 89–92.

Rutala, W. A. (1990). APIC guideline for selection and use of disinfectants. *American Journal of Infection Control, 18,* 99–117.

Rutala, W. A., Clontz, E. P., Weber, D. J., & Hoffmann, K. K. (1991). Disinfection practices for endoscopes and other semicritical items. *Infection Control and Hospital Epidemiology, 12,* 282–288.

Ryan, E. B., & Capadano, H. L. (1978). Age perceptions and evaluative reactions toward adult speakers. *Journal of Gerontology, 33,* 98–102.

Ryan, S., & Gelfer, M. P. (1993). *Normative data for vocal intensity.* Paper presented at the convention of the American Speech-Language-Hearing Association, Anaheim, CA.

Ryan, W. J. (1972). Acoustic aspects of the aging voice. *Journal of Gerontology, 27,* 265–268.

Sackner, M. A. (1980). Monitoring of ventilation without physical connection to the airway. In M. A. Sackner (Ed.), *Diagnostic techniques in pulmonary disease.* (pp. 503–537). New York: Marcel Dekker.

Saito, S. (1977). Phonosurgery: basic study of the mechanism of phonation and endolaryngeal microsurgery. *Otologia (Fukuoka), 23,* 171–384.

Saito, S., Ogino, M., Ishikura, M., Niino, Y., & Fukuda, H. (1966). Endolaryngeal microsurgery. *Journal of the Japanese Bronchoesophagology Society, 17*, 253–266.

Salam, M. Z., & Adams, R. D. (1978). The Arnold-Chiari malformation. In P. J. Vinken, G. W. Bruyn, & N. C. Myrianthopoulos (Eds.), *Handbook of clinical neurology* (pp. 99–110). Amsterdam: North Holland.

Salamy, J. N., & Sessions, R. B. (1980). Spastic dysphonia. *Journal of Fluency Disorders, 5*, 281–290.

Sander, E. K. (1989). Arguments against the aggressive pursuit of voice treatment for children. *Language Speech Hearing Services in Schools, 20*, 94–101.

Sanders, D. B., & Scoppetta, C. (1994). The treatment of patients with myasthenia gravis [review]. *Neurologic Clinics, 12*, 343–368.

Sataloff, R. T. (1981). Professional singers: the science and art of clinical care. *American Journal of Otolaryngology, 2*, 251–266.

Sataloff, R. T. (1986). The professional voice. In C. Cummings, L. Harker, C. S. Krause, & D. Schuller (Eds.), *Otolaryngology—Head and Neck Surgery* (pp. 2029–2053). St. Louis: CV Mosby.

Sataloff, R. T. (1987a). Clinical evaluation of the professional singer. *Ear, Nose, and Throat Journal, 66*, 267–277.

Sataloff, R.T. (1987b). The professional voice: Part II. Physical examination. *Journal of Voice, 1*, 191–201.

Sataloff, R. T. (1987c). The professional voice: Part III. Common diagnoses and treatments. *Journal of Voice, 1*, 283–292.

Sataloff, R. T., Spiegel, J., Carroll, L., Darby, K., & Rulnik, R. (1987). Objective measures of voice function. *Ear, Nose, and Throat Journal, 66*, 307–312.

Sawashima, M. (1966). Measurements of the phonation time. *Japanese Journal of Logopedics and Phoniatrics, 7*, 23–29.

Sawashima, M., & Hirose, H. (1981). Abduction-adduction of the glottis in speech and voice production. In K. N. Stevens & M. Hirano (Eds.), *Vocal fold physiology* (pp. 329–346). Tokyo: University of Tokyo Press.

Sawashima, M., Sato, M., Funasaka, S., & Totsuk, G. (1958). Electromyographic study of the human larynx and its clinical application. *Journal of Otolaryngology of Japan, 61*, 1357–1364.

Sawashima, M., Totsuka, G., Kobayashi, T., & Hirose, M. (1968). Reconstructive surgery for hoarseness due to unilateral vocal cord paralysis. *Archives of Otolaryngology, 87*, 289.

Saxman, J., & Burk, K. W. (1967). Speaking fundamental frequency characteristics of middle aged women. *Folia Phoniatrica, 19*, 167–172.

Scherer, R. C., & Titze, I. R. (1987). The abduction quotient related to vocal quality. *Journal of Voice, 1*, 246–251.

Schiffman, S. S., Reynolds, M. L., & Young, F. W. (1981). *Introduction to multidimensional scaling: theory, methods, application.* New York: Academic Press.

Schilling, R. (1925). Experimentell-phonetische Untersuchunger bei Erkrankunger des extrapyramidalen Systems. *Archives Psychiatrica Nevenkr, 75*, 419–471.

Schutte, H. K. (1980). *The efficiency of voice production.* Groningen: Kemper.

Scott, S., & Cairn, F. L. (1983). Speech therapy for Parkinson's disease. *Journal of Neurology, Neurosurgery and Psychiatry, 46*, 140–144.

Segre, R. (1971). Senescence of the voice. *Ear Nose and Throat Monthly, 50*, 223–233.

Senturia, B. H., & Wilson, F. B. (1968). Otorhinolaryngologic findings in children with voice deviations. *Annals of Otology, Rhinology and Laryngology, 77*, 1027–1042.

Sercarz, J. A., Berke, G. S., Ming, Y., Gerratt, B. R., & Natividad, M. (1992). Videostroboscopy of human vocal fold paralysis. *Annals of Otology, Rhinology and Laryngology, 101*, 567–577.

Sessions, R. B., Miller, S. D., Martin, G. F., Solomon, B. I., Harrison, L. B., & Stackpole, S. (1989). Videolaryngostroboscopic analysis of minimal glottic cancer. *Transactions American Laryngological Association, 110*, 56–59.

Shaefer, S. D. (1983). Neuropathology of spasmodic dysphonia. *Laryngoscope, 93*, 1183–1202.

Shaefer, S. D., Freeman, F., Finitzo, T., Close, L., & Cannito, M. (1985). Magnetic resonance imaging findings and correlations in spasmodic dysphonia patients. *Annals of Otology, Rhinology and Laryngology, 94*, 595–601.

Shaefer, S. D., Roark, R. M., Watson, B. C., Kondraske, G. V., Freeman, F. J., Butsch, R. W., & Pohl, J. (1992). Multichannel electromyographic observations in spasmodic dysphonia patients and normal control subjects. *Annals of Otology, Rhinology and Laryngology, 101*, 67–75.

Sharbrough, F. W., Stockard, J. J., & Aronson, A. E. (1975). Brainstem auditory evoked responses in spastic dysphonia. *Transactions of the American Neurological Association, 103*, 198–201.

Shearer, W. (1983). s/z ratio for detection of vocal nodules. *Folia Phoniatrica, 35*, 172.

Shigemori, Y. (1977). Some tests related to the air usage during phonation: clinical investigations. *Otologia (Fukuoka), 23*, 138–166.

Shindo, M. L., & Hanson, D. G. (1990). Geriatric voice and laryngeal dysfunction [review]. *Otolaryngologic Clinics of North America, 23*, 1035–1044.

Shipp, T. (1975). Vertical laryngeal position during continuous and discrete vocal frequency change. *Journal of Speech and Hearing Research, 18*, 707–718.

Shipp, T. (1987). Vertical laryngeal position: research findings and application for singers. *Journal of Voice, 1*, 217–219.

Shipp, T., Guinn, L., Sundberg, J., & Titze, I. R. (1987). Vertical laryngeal position—research findings and their relationship to singing. *Journal of Voice*, 220–222.

Shipp, T., & Hollien H. (1969). Perception of the aging male voice. *Journal of Speech and Hearing Research, 12*, 703–710.

Shipp, T., & Huntington, D. (1965). Some acoustic and perceptual factors in acute-laryngitic hoarseness. *Journal of Speech and Hearing Disorders, 30*, 350–359.

Shipp, T., & Izdebski, K. (1975). Vocal frequency and vertical larynx positioning by singers and nonsingers. *Journal of the Acoustical Society of America, 58*, 1104–1106.

Shipp, T., Izdebski, K., Schutte, H. K., & Morrissey, P. (1988). Subglottal air pressure in spastic dysphonia speech. *Folia Phoniatrica, 40*, 105–110.

Shipp, T., & McGlone, R. (1971). Laryngeal dynamics associated with voice frequency change. *Journal of Speech and Hearing Research, 14*, 761–768.

Shipp, T., Mueller, P., & Zwitman, D. (1980). Intermittent abductory dysphonia. *Journal of Speech and Hearing Disorders, 45*, 283.

Shy, G. M., & Drager, G. (1960). A neurological syndrome associated with orthostatic hypotension. *AMA Arch Neurology, 2*, 511–527.

Simkin, B. (1964). Corticosteroids in clinical practice. *Eye, Ear, Nose and Throat Monthly, 43* (3), 47–54.

Singh, W., & Ainsworth, W. A. (1992). Computerised measurement of fundamental frequency in Scottish neoglottal patients. *Folia Phoniatrica, 44*, 231–237.

Siribodhi, C., Sundmaker, W., Atkins, J. P., & Bonner, F. L. (1963). Electromyographic studies of laryngeal paralysis and regeneration of laryngeal motor nerve in dogs. *Laryngoscope, 73*, 148–164.

Smith, M. E., Ramig, L. O., Dromey, C., Perez, K. S., & Samandari, R. (1994). Intensive voice treatment in Parkinson's disease: Laryngostroboscopic findings. *NCVS Status and Progress Report, 6*, 127–133.

Smitheran, J. R., & Hixon, T. J. (1981). A clinical method for estimating air way resistance during vowel production. *Journal of Speech and Hearing Disorders, 46*, 138–146.

Snidecor, J. C. (1943). A comparative study of the pitch and duration characteristics of impromptu speaking and oral reading. *Speech Monographs, 10*, 50–57.

Snow, J. B., Hirano, M., & Balough, K. (1966). Postintubation granuloma of the larynx. *Anesthesia and Analgesia, 45*, 425.

Södersten, M., & Lindestad, P. A. (1990). Glottal closure and perceived breathiness during phonation in normally speaking subjects. *Journal of Speech and Hearing Research, 33*, 601–611.

Solomon, N. P., McCall, G. N., Trosset, M. W., Gray, W. C. (1989). Laryngeal configuration and constriction during two types of whispering. *Journal of Speech and Hearing Research, 32*, 161–174.

Sondi, M. M. (1975). Measurement of the glottal waveform. *Journal of the Acoustical Society of America, 57*, 228–232.

Sonnesson, B. (1959). A method for studying the vibratory movements of the vocal cords. *Journal of Laryngology and Otology, 73*, 732–737.

Sorensen, D., & Parker, P. (1993). Response to Mueller, Larson and Summers. *Language Speech Hearing Services in Schools, 24*, 178–179.

Sorin, R., McClean, M. D., Ezerzer, F., & Meissner-Fishbein, B. (1987). Electroglottographic evaluation of the swallow. *Archives of Physical Medicine and Rehabilitation, 68*, 232–235.

Spector, G. J., & Ogura, J. H. (1985). Tumors of the larynx and laryngopharynx. In J. J. Ballenger (Ed.), *Diseases of the nose, throat, ear, head, and neck* (pp. 549–602). Philadelphia: Lea & Febiger.

Stark, D. D., Moss, A. A., Gamsu, G., Clark, O. H., & Gooding, G. A. (1984). Magnetic resonance imaging of the neck. Part I: Normal anatomy. *Radiology, 150*, 447–454.

Stathopoulos, E. T., & Sapienza, C. (1993). Respiratory and laryngeal function of women and men during vocal intensity variation. *Journal of Speech and Hearing Research, 36*, 64–75.

Stemple, J., Weider, E., Whitehead, W., & Komray, R. (1980). Electromyographic biofeedback training with patients exhibiting a hyperfunctional voice disorder. *Laryngoscope, 90*, 471–475.

Stemple, J. C., Glaze, L., & Gerdeman, B. (1995). *Clinical voice pathology: theory and management* (2nd ed.). San Diego: Singular Publishing Group.

Stevens, K. N., & House, A. (1961). An acoustical theory of vowel production and some of its implications. *Journal of Speech and Hearing Research, 4*, 303–320.

Stoicheff, M. (1981). Speaking fundamental frequency characteristics of nonsmoking female adults. *Journal of Speech and Hearing Research, 24*, 437–441.

Stoicheff, M., Giampi, A., Passi, J., & Fredrickson, J. (1983). The irradiated larynx and voice: a perceptual study. *Journal of Speech and Hearing Research, 26,* 482–485.

Stone, R. E., Jr. (1983). Issues in clinical assessment of laryngeal function: Contraindications for subscribing to maximum phonation time and optimum fundamental frequency. In D. M. Bless & J. H. Abbs (Eds.), *Vocal fold physiology: contemporary research and clinical issues* (pp. 410–424). San Diego: College Hill Press.

Strand, E. A., Buder, E. H., Yorkston, K. M., & Ramig, L. O. (1993). Differential phonatory characteristics of women with amyotrophic lateral sclerosis. *NCVS Status and Progress Report, 4,* 151–167.

Streifler, M., & Hofman, S. (1984). Disorders of verbal expression in Parkinsonism. *Advances in Neurology, 40,* 385–393.

Strong, M. S., & Jako, G. J. (1972). Laser surgery in the larynx: early clinical experience with continous $CO_2$ laser. *Annals of Otolaryngology, 81,* 791–798.

Stuart, W. D. (1965). The otolaryngologic aspects of myasthenia gravis. *Laryngoscope, 75,* 112–121.

Sundberg, J. (1974). Articulatory interpretation of the 'singing formant'. *Journal of the Acoustical Society of America, 55:* 838–844.

Sundberg, J. (1987). *The science of the singing voice.* DeKalb, IL: Northern Illinois University Press.

Sundberg, J., & Askenfelt, A. (1983). Larynx height and voice source: a relationship. In D. M. Bless & J. H. Abbs (Eds.), *Vocal fold physiology: contemporary research and clinical issues* (pp. 307–316). San Diego: College Hill Press.

Sundberg, J., Titze, I., & Scherer, R. (1993). Phonatory control in male singing: a study of the effects of subglottal pressure, fundamental frequency, and mode of phonation on the voice source. *Journal of Voice, 7,* 15–29.

Swenson, M. R., Zwirner, P., Murry, T., & Woodson, G. E. (1992). Medical evaluation of patients with spasmodic dysphonia. *Journal of Voice, 6,* 320–324.

Taft, J. M. (1988). Acute inflammatory demyelinating polyradiculoneuropathy: The Landry, Guillain-Barré, Strol syndrome. *American Academy of Physician Assistants, 1,* 219–223.

Tait, N. A., Michel, J. F., & Carpenter, M. A. (1980). Maximum duration of sustained /s/ and /z/ in children. *Journal of Speech and Hearing Disorders, 45,* 239–246.

Takahashi, H., & Koike, Y. (1975). Some perceptual dimensions and acoustical correlates of pathologic voices. *Acta Oto-laryngologica (Stockholm), 338,* 1–24.

Tanaka, S., & Gould, W. (1985). Vocal efficiency and aerodynamic aspects in voice disorders. *Annals of Otology and Laryngology, 94,* 29–33.

Tasko, S. M., Roy, N., & Harvey, S. (1994). Using manual laryngeal tension reduction techniques with benign mucosal disorders. Paper presented at the convention of the American Speech-Language-Hearing Association, New Orleans, LA.

Terris, D. J., Arnstein, D. P., & Nguyen, H. H. (1992). Contemporary evaluation of unilateral vocal cord paralysis [review]. *Otolaryngology-Head and Neck Surgery, 107,* 84–90.

Teter, D. L. (1976). Voice disorders. In English, G. M. (Ed.), *Otolaryngology: a textbook* (pp. 584–599). New York: Harper & Row.

Thomas, J. E., & Schirger, A. (1970). Idiopathic orthostatic hypotension. A study of its natural history in 57 neurologically affected patients. *Archives of Neurology, 22,* 289–293.

Thompson, A. R. (1995). Medications and the voice. In J. S. Rubin, R. T. Sataloff, G. S. Korovin, & W. J. Gould (Eds.), *Diagnosis and treatment of voice problems* (pp. 237–246). New York: Igaku-Shoin.

Thurman, W. L. (1958). Frequency-intensity relationships and optimum pitch level. *Journal of Speech and Hearing Research, 1,* 117–123.

Timcke, R., von Leden, H. S., & Moore, G. P. (1958). Laryngeal vibrations: measurements of the glottic wave Part I: The normal vibratory cycle. *Archives of Otolaryngology, 68,* 1–19.

Timcke, R., von Leden, H. S., & Moore, G. P. (1959). Laryngeal vibrations: measurements of the glottic wave Part II: Physiologic variations. *Archives of Otolaryngology, 69,* 438–444.

Titze, I. R. (1981). Heat generation in the vocal folds and its possible effect on vocal endurance. In V. Lawrence (Ed.), *Transcripts of the 10th symposium: care of the professional voice* (pp. 52–59). New York: Voice Foundation.

Titze, I. R. (1984). Parameterization of the glottal area, glottal flow and vocal fold contact area. *Journal of the Acoustical Society of America, 75,* 570–580.

Titze, I. R. (1990). Interpretation of the electroglottographic signal. *J Voice 4:1-9.*

Titze, I. R. (1992a). Vocal efficiency. *Journal of Voice, 6,* 135–138.

Titze, I. R. (1992b). Phonation threshold pressure—A missing link in glottal aerodynamics. *Journal of the Acoustical Society of America, 91,* 2926–2935.

Titze, I. R. (1994). *Principles of voice production.* Englewood Cliffs, NJ: Prentice-Hall.

Titze, I. R. (1995). Workshop on *Acoustic Voice Analysis—Summary Statement.* Iowa City: National Center for Voice and Speech.

Titze, I. R., & Sundberg, J. (1992). Vocal intensity in speakers and singers. *Journal of the Acoustical Society of America, 91,* 2936–2946.

Titze, I. R., Talkin, D. (1981). Simulation and interpretation of glottographic waveforms.

In C. Ludlow & M. Hart (Eds.), *Proceedings of the conference on the assessment of vocal pathology* (pp. 48–55). Rockville, MD: American Speech-Language-Hearing Association.

Toohill, R. J. (1975). The psychosomatic aspects of children with nodules. *Archives of Otolaryngology, 101,* 591–595.

Trapp, T. K., & Berke, G. S. (1988). Photoelectric measurement of laryngeal paralyses correlated with videostroboscopy. *Laryngoscope, 98,* 486–492.

Tucker, H. M. (1978). Human laryngeal reinnervation: long term experience with the nerve-muscle pedicle technique. *Laryngoscope, 88,* 598–604.

Tucker, H. M. (1980). Vocal cord paralysis-etiology and management. *Laryngoscope, 90,* 585–590.

Tucker, H. M. (1985). Anterior commissure laryngoplasty for adjustment of vocal fold tension. *Annals of Otology, Rhinology and Laryngology, 94,* 547–549.

Tucker, H. M., & Lavertu, P. (1992). Paralysis and paresis of the vocal folds. In A. Blitzer, M. F. Brin, C. T. Sasaki, S. Fahn, & K. S. Harris (Eds.), *Neurologic disorders of the larynx* (pp. 182–189). New York: Thieme.

Tucker, H. M., & Rusnov, M. (1981). Laryngeal reinnervation for unilateral vocal cord paralysis: long term results. *Annals of Otology, Rhinology and Laryngology, 90,* 457–459.

Ungerleider, S. (1986). Athletes in motion: training for the Olympic games with mind and body: two case studies. Paper presented at International Conference on Mental Health and Technology, Winnipeg, Canada.

U.S. Department of Health and Human Services. (1985). *The health consequences of smoking: Cancer and chronic diseases in the workplace; a report of the Surgeon General.* Washington, DC: U.S. Government Printing Office.

U.S. Department of Health and Human Services. (1986). *The health consequences of smoking: a public health service review, 1967–1985.* Washington, DC: U. S. Government Printing Office.

Vallancien, B., Gautheron, B., Pasternak, L., Guisez, D., & Paley, B. (1971). Comparaison des signaux microphoniques, diaphanographiques et glottographiques avec application au laryngographe. *Folia Phoniatrica, 23,* 371–380.

van den Berg, J. W. (1956). Physiology and physics of voice production. *Acta Physiologica et Pharmacologica Neerl, 5,* 40–55.

van den Berg, J. W. (1958). Myoelastic-aerodynamic theory of voice production. *Journal of Speech and Hearing Research, 1,* 227–244.

van den Berg, J. W., & Tan, T. S. (1959). Results of experiments with human larynges. *Practica Otology Rhinology Laryngology, 21,* 425–450.

Vaughan, C. W. (1982). Diagnosis and treatment of organic voice disorders. *New England Journal of Medicine, 307,* 863–866.

Verdolini, K., & Titze, I. R. (1994). The application of laboratory formulas to clinical voice management. In Titze, I. R. (Ed.), *NCVS status and progress report* (pp. 197–205). Iowa City, IA: National Center for Voice and Speech.

Verdolini, K., & Titze, I. R. (1995). The application of laboratory formulas to clinical voice management. *American Journal of Speech Language Pathology, 4,* 62–69.

Verdolini-Marston, K., Burke, M. K., Lessac, A., Glaze, L., & Caldwell, E. (1995). Preliminary study of two methods of treatment for laryngeal nodules. *Journal of Voice, 9,* 74–85.

Verdolini-Marston, K., Titze, I. R., & Druker, D. G. (1990). Changes in phonation threshold pressure with induced conditions of hydration. *Journal of Voice, 4,* 142–151.

von Euler, C. (1986). Brain stem mechanisms for generation and control of breathing pattern. In N. S. Cherniack & J. G. Widdicombe (Eds.), *Handbook of physiology. Section 3. The respiratory system* (pp. 1–67). Bethesda, MD: American Physiological Society.

von Leden, H., & Isshiki, N. (1965). An analysis of cough at the level of the larynx. *Archives of Otolaryngology, 81,* 616–625.

von Leden, H. S., LeCover, M., Ringel, R. L., & Isshiki, N. (1966). Improvements in laryngeal cinematography. *Archives of Otolaryngology—Head and Neck Surgery, 83,* 482–487.

von Leden, H., & Moore, G. P. (1960). Contact ulcer of the larynx: experimental observations. *Archives of Otolaryngology, 72,* 746–752.

von Leden, H., & Moore, G. P. (1961). The mechanics of the cricoarytenoid joint. *Archives of Otolaryngology, 73,* 541–550.

von Leden, H., Moore, P., & Timcke, R. (1960). Laryngeal vibrations: measurements of the glottic wave. Part III. The pathologic larynx. *Archives of Otolaryngology, 71,* 26–45.

von Leden, H., Poyle, P. J., Goff, W. F., & Miller, A. L. (1969). Symposium on surgery for the improvement of voice. *Transactions of the Pacific Coast Oto-Ophthalmology Society, 50,* 351–362.

von Leden, H., Yanagihara, N., & Werner-Kukuk, E. (1967). Teflon in unilateral vocal cord paralysis: preoperative and postoperative function studies. *Archives of Otolaryngology, 85,* 666–674.

Ward, D. (1990). Voice-onset time and electroglottographic dynamics in stutterers' speech: implications for a differential diagnosis.

*British Journal of Disorders of Communication,* *25,* 93–104.

Ward, P. H., & Berci, G. (1982a). Observations on so-called idiopathic vocal cord paralysis. *Annals of Otology, Rhinology and Laryngology, 91,* 558–563.

Ward, P. H., & Berci, G. (1982b). Observations on the pathogenesis of chronic non-specific pharyngitis and laryngitis. *Laryngoscope, 92,* 1377–1382.

Ward, P. H., Cannon, D., & Lindsay, J. R. (1965). The vestibular system in multiple sclerosis. *Laryngoscope, 75,* 1031–1046.

Ward, P. H., Hanson, D., & Berci, G. (1981). Observations on central neurologic etiology for laryngeal dysfunction. *Annals of Otolaryngology, 90,* 430–441.

Ward, P. H., Zwitman, D., Hanson, D., & Berci, G. (1980). Contact ulcers and granulomas of the larynx: new insights into their etiology as a basis for a more rational treatment. *Archives of Otolaryngology-Head Neck Surgery, 88,* 262–269.

Warr-Leeper, G. A., McShea, R. S., & Leeper, H. (1979). The incidence of voice and speech deviations in a middle school population. *Language Speech Hearing Services in Schools, 10,* 14–20.

Warren, R. M. (1962). Are 'autophonic' judgments based on loudness? *American Journal of Psychology, 75,* 452–456.

Warren, W. R., Gutmann, L., & Cody, R. (1977). Stapedius reflex decay in myasthenia gravis. *Archives of Neurology, 34,* 496–497.

Watkin, K. L., & Ewanowski, S. J. (1979). The effects of Triamcinolone Acetonide on the voice. *Journal of Speech and Hearing Research, 22,* 446–455.

Watson, H. (1979). The technology of respiratory inductive plethysmography. Paper presented at the 3rd International Symposium on Ambulatory Monitoring, Middlesex, United Kingdom.

Watson, P. J., Hixon, T. J., & Maher, M. Z. (1987). To breathe or not to breathe—That is the question: an investigation of speech breathing kinematics in world class Shakespearean actors. *Journal of Voice, 1,* 269–272.

Watterson, T., Hensen-Magorian, H. J., & McFarlane, S. C. (1988). A demographic description of laryngeal contact ulcers. Paper given at the convention of American Speech-Language-Hearing Association, Boston.

Wechsler, E. (1976). A laryngographic study of voice disorders. *British Journal of Disorders of Communication, 12,* 9–22.

Weinberg, B., Bosma, J. F., Shanks, J. C., & DeMyer, W. (1968). Myotonic dystrophy initially manifested by speech disability. *Journal of Speech and Hearing Disorders, 33,* 51–59.

Wendahl, R. W. (1963). Laryngeal analog synthesis of harsh voice quality. *Folia Phoniatrica, 15,* 241–250.

Wendahl, R. (1966). Some parameters of auditory roughness. *Folia Phoniatrica, 18,* 26–32.

Wendahl, R. W., & Coleman, R. F. (1967). Vocal cord spectra derived from glottal-area waveforms and subglottal photocell monitoring. *Journal of the Acoustical Society of America, 41,* 1613A.

Wendler, J., & Köppen, K. (1988). Schwingungsmessunger der Stimmlippen: Zur klinischen relevantz der Stroboskopie. *Folia Phoniatrica, 40,* 297–302.

Wendler, J., Rauhut, A., & Kruger, H. (1986). Classification of voice qualities. *Journal of Phonetics, 14,* 483–488.

Weymuller, E. A. (1988). Laryngeal injury from prolonged endotracheal intubation. *Laryngoscope, 98,* 1–15.

Wexler, D. B., Jiang, J., Gray, S. D., & Titze, I. R. (1989). Phonosurgical studies: fat-graft reconstruction of injured canine vocal cords. *Annals of Otology, Rhinology and Laryngology, 98,* 668–673.

Williams, A. J., Baghat, M. S., DeStableforth, C. R. M., Shenoi, P. M., & Skinner, C. (1983). Dysphonia caused by inhaled steroids: recognition of a characteristic laryngeal abnormality. *Thorax, 38,* 813–821.

Williams, A. J., Hanson, D., & Calne, D. B. (1979). Vocal cord paralysis in the Shy-Drager syndrome. *Journal of Neurology, Neurosurgery and Psychiatry, 42,* 151–153.

Williams, R. T., Farquharson, I. M., & Anthony, J. (1975). Fiberoptic laryngoscopy in the assessment of laryngeal disorder. *Journal of Laryngology and Otology, 89,* 299–306.

Wilson, D. K. (1987). *Voice problems of children* (3rd ed). Baltimore: Williams & Wilkins.

Wilson, F. B., & Lamb, M. M. (1973). Comparison of personality characteristics of children with and without vocal nodules on Rorschach protocol interpretation. Paper presented at the convention of the American Speech-Language-Hearing Association, Atlanta, GA.

Wilson, F. B., Oldring, D. J., & Mueller, K. (1980). Recurrent laryngeal nerve dissection: a case report involving return of spastic dysphonia after initial surgery. *Journal of Speech and Hearing Disorders, 45,* 112–118.

Wilson, F. B., & Rice, M. A. (1977). *A programmed approach to voice therapy.* Austin, TX: Learning Concepts.

Wilson, F. B., Wellen, C. J., & Kimbarow, M. L. (1983). Perception of the fundamental frequencies of children's voices by trained and untrained listeners. *Journal of Otolaryngology, 12,* 341–344.

Wilson, J., Pryde, A., Cecilia, A., & MacIntyre, C. (1989). Normal pharyngoesophageal motility.

A study of 50 healthy subjects. *Digestive Diseases and Sciences, 34*, 1590–1599.

Wirz, S., Anthony, J. (1979). The use of the Voiscope in improving the speech of profoundly deaf children. *British Journal of Disorders of Communication, 14*, 137–152.

Wolfe, V. I., & Bacon, M. (1976). Spectrographic comparison of two types of spastic dysphonia. *Journal of Speech and Hearing Disorders, 41*, 325–332.

Wolfe, V. I., & Ratusnik, D. L. (1988). Acoustic and perceptual measurements of roughness influencing judgments of pitch. *Journal of Speech and Hearing Disorders, 53*, 15–22.

Wolfe, V. I., & Steinfatt, T. (1987). Prediction of vocal severity within and across voice types. *Journal of Speech and Hearing Research, 30*, 230–240.

Wolski, W. (1967). Hypernasality as the presenting symptom of myasthenia gravis. *Journal of Speech and Hearing Research, 32*, 36–38.

Woo, P., Casper, J., Brewer, D., & Colton, R. H. (in press). Long-term voice complications after prolonged intubation. *Archives of Otolaryngology—Head and Neck Surgery.*

Woo, P., Casper, J., Colton, R., & Brewer, D. (1992). Dysphonia in the aging: physiology versus disease. *Laryngoscope, 102*, 139–144.

Woo, P., Casper, J., Griffin, B., Colton, R. H., & Brewer, D. (1995). Endoscopic microsuture repair of vocal fold defects. *Journal of Voice, 9*, 332–339.

Woo, P., Colton, R., Brewer, D., & Casper, J. (1991). Functional staging for vocal cord paralysis. *Otolaryngology—Head and Neck Surgery, 105*, 440–448.

Woo, P., Colton, R. H., Casper, J. K., & Brewer, D. W. (1991). Diagnostic value of stroboscopic examination in hoarse patients. *Journal of Voice, 5*, 231–238.

Woo, P., Colton, R. H., Casper, J. K., & Brewer, D. W. (1992). Analysis of spasmodic dysphonia by aerodynamic and laryngostroboscopic measurements. *Journal of Voice, 6*, 344–351.

Woo, P., Colton, R. H., & Shangold, L. (1987). Phonatory airflow analysis in patients with laryngeal disease. *Annals of Otology, Rhinology and Laryngology, 96*, 549–555.

Wright, H. N., & Colton, R. H. (1972a). Some parameters of vocal effort. *Journal of the Acoustical Society of America, 51*, 141A.

Wright, H. N., & Colton, R. H. (1972b). Some parameters of autophonic level. Paper presented at the convention of the American Speech-Language-Hearing Association, San Francisco.

Wyke, B. (1967). Recent advances in the neurology of phonation: phonatory reflex mechanisms in the larynx. *British Journal of Disorders of Communication, 2*, 2–14.

Wyke, B. (1969). Deus ex machina vocis: an analysis of the laryngeal reflex mechanisms of speech. *British Journal of Disorders of Communication, 4*, 3–25.

Wynder, E. L., Covey, L. S., Mabuchi, K., & Muchinski, M. (1976). Environmental factors in cancer of the larynx: a second look. *Cancer, 38*, 1591–1601.

Wynder, E. L., & Stellman, S. D. (1977). Comparative epidemiology of tobacco-related cancers. *Cancer, 37*, 4608–4622.

Yajima, Y., Hayashi, Y., & Yoshii, N. (1982). Ambiguus motoneurons discharging closely associated with ultrasonic vocalization in rats. *Brain Research, 238*, 445–450.

Yamaguchi, H., Yotsukura, Y., Sata, H., Watanabe, Y., Hirose, H., & Kobayashi, N. (1993). Pushing exercise program to correct glottal incompetence. *Journal of Voice, 7*, 250–256.

Yanagihara, N. (1967a). Hoarseness: investigation of the physiological mechanisms. *Annals of Otology, Rhinology and Laryngology, 76*, 472–488.

Yanagihara, N. (1967b). Significance of harmonic changes and noise components in hoarseness. *Journal of Speech and Hearing Research, 10*, 531–541.

Yanagihara, N., & von Leden, H. (1967). Respiration and phonation. *Folia Phoniatrica, 19*, 153–166.

Yoshida, Y., Mitsumasu, T., Hirano, M., Morimoto, M., & Kanaseki, T. (1987). Afferent connections to the nucleus ambiguus in the brainstem of the cat—an HRP study. In T. Baer, C. Sasaki, & K. Harris (Eds.), *Laryngeal function in phonation and respiration* (pp. 45–61). San Diego: College Hill Press.

Young, M. A., Bless, D. M., McNeil, M. R., & Braun, S. R. (1983). Relation of physical condition to age-related voice changes. *Folia Phoniatrica, 35*, 185.

Young, R. R. (1986). Essential-familial tremor. In P. J. Vinken, G. W. Bruyn, & H. L. Klawans (Eds.), *Handbook of clinical neurology* (pp. 565–582). Amsterdam: Elsevier.

Yumoto, E. (1987). Quantitative assessment of the degree of hoarseness. *Journal of Voice, 1*, 310–313.

Yumoto, E., Gould, W. J., & Baer, T. (1982). Harmonics-to-noise ratio as an index of the degree of hoarseness. *Journal of the Acoustical Society of America, 71*, 1544–1550.

Yumoto, E., Sasaki, Y., & Okamura, H. (1984). Harmonics-to-noise ratio and psychological measurement of the degrees of hoarseness. *Journal of Speech and Hearing Research, 27*, 2–6.

Zemlin, W. R. (1962). A comparison of the periodic function of vocal fold vibration in a multiple sclerosis and a normal population.

Unpublished doctoral dissertation, University of Minnesota.

Zemlin, W. R. (1988). *Speech and hearing science: anatomy and physiology.* Englewood Cliffs, NJ: Prentice-Hall.

Zhang, S. P., Davis, P. J., Bandler, R., & Carrive, P. (1994). Brain stem integration of vocalization: role of the midbrain periaqueductal gray. *Journal of Neurophysiology, 72,* 1337–1356.

Zhang, S. P., Davis, P. J., Carrive, P., & Bandler, R. (1992). Vocalization and marked pressor effect evoked from the region of the nucleus retroambigualis in the caudal ventrolateral medulla of the cat. *Neuroscience Letters, 140,* 103–107.

Zwirner, P., Murry, T., Swenson, M., & Woodson, G. E. (1991). Acoustic changes in spasmodic dysphonia after Botulinum Toxin injection. *Journal of Voice, 5,* 78–84.

Zwirner, P., Murry, T., & Woodson, G. E. (1991). Phonatory function of neurologically impaired patients. *Journal of Communication Disorders, 24,* 287–300.

Zwitman, D. (1979). Bilateral cord dysfunctions: abductor type spastic dysphonia. *Journal of Speech and Hearing Disorders, 44,* 373–378.

# Figure and Table Credits

## Figures

**Figure 2.4.** Coleman, R. F., Mabis, J. H., & Hinson, J. K. (1977). Fundamental frequency-sound pressure level profiles of adult male and female voices. *Journal of Speech and Hearing Research, 20,* 197–204.

**Figure 3.2.** Gray, S. D., Hirano, M., & Sato, K. (1993). Molecular and cellular structure of vocal fold tissue. In I. R. Titze (Ed.), *Vocal fold physiology: frontiers in basic science* (pp. 1–36). San Diego: Singular Publishing Group.

**Figure 3.7. A,** Hirano, M. (1981). Structure of the vocal fold in normal and disease states: anatomical and physical studies. In C. Ludlow & M. Hart (Eds.), *Proceedings of the conference on the assessment of vocal pathology* (pp. 11–30). Rockville, MD: American Speech-Language-Hearing Association.

**Figure 3.8.** Kurita, S. (1980). Layer structure of the human vocal fold: morphological investigation. *Otologia (Fukuoka), 26,* 973–997.

**Figure 3.9. B,** Hirano, M. (1981). Structure of the vocal fold in normal and disease states: anatomical and physical studies. In C. Ludlow & M. Hart (Eds.), *Proceedings of the conference on the assessment of vocal pathology* (pp. 11–30). Rockville, MD: American Speech-Language-Hearing Association.

**Figures 3.10–3.11.** Hirano, M., Kurita, S., & Nakashima, T. (1983). Growth, development and aging of human vocal folds. In D. M. Bless & J. H. Abbs (Eds.), *Vocal fold physiology: contemporary research and clinical issues* (pp. 22–43). San Diego: College Hill Press.

**Figure 3.12.** Hirano, M. (1983). Epithelial hyperplasia of the larynx. In M. Hirano (Ed.), *Illustrated handbook of clinical otolaryngology* (pp. 100–101). Tokyo: Medical View.

**Figure 3.13.** Hirano, M. (1981). Structure of the vocal fold in normal and disease states: anatomical and physical studies. In C. Ludlow & M. Hart (Eds.), *Proceedings of the conference on the assessment of vocal pathology* (pp. 11–30). Rockville, MD: American Speech-Language-Hearing Association.

**Figure 3.15. A,** Hirano, M. (1981). *Clinical examination of voice.* Vienna: Springer-Verlag. **B,** Hirano, M. (1975). Phonosurgery: basic and clinical applications. *Otologia (Fukuoka), 21,* 239–242.

**Figures 3.16-3.17.** Hirano, M. (1981). Structure of the vocal fold in normal and disease states: anatomical and physical studies. In C. Ludlow & M. Hart (Eds.), *Proceedings of the conference on the assessment of vocal pathology* (pp. 11–30). Rockville, MD: American Speech-Language-Hearing Association.

**Figure 3.19.** Hirano, M., Kurita, S., Kyokawa, K., & Sato, K. (1986). Posterior glottis: morphological study in excised human larynges. *Annals of Otology, Rhinology and Laryngology, 95,* 576–581.

**Figure 3.21.** Hirano, M. (1975). Phonosurgery: basic and clinical applications. *Otologia (Fukuoka), 21,* 239–242.

**Figure 3.22. A,** Hirano, M. (1981). Structure of the vocal fold in normal and disease states: anatomical and physical studies. In C. Ludlow & M. Hart (Eds.), *Proceedings of the conference on the assessment of vocal pathology* (pp. 11–30). Rockville, MD: American Speech-Language-Hearing Association.

**Figure 3.23.** Hirano, M. (1975). Phonosurgery: basic and clinical applications. *Otologia (Fukuoka), 21,* 239–242.

**Figures 4.1–4.6.** Color photographs by Eiji Yanagisawa, M.D.

**Figure 4.7.** Bouchayer, M., Cornut, G., Witzig, E., Loire, R., Roch, J., & Bastian R. (1985). Epidermoid cysts, sulci and mucosal bridges of the true vocal cord: a report of 157 cases. *Laryngoscope, 95,* 1087–1094.

**Figure 5.1.** Darley F. L., Aronson A. E., & Brown J. R. (1975). *Motor speech disorders.* Philadelphia: WB Saunders, p. 50.

**Figures 5.2–5.3.** Aronson, A. E., Brown, J. R., Litin, E. M., & Pearson, J. S. (1968). Spastic dysphonia II. Comparison with essential (voice) tremor and other neurologic and psychogenic dysphonias. *Journal of Speech and Hearing Disorders, 33,* 219–231.

**Figure 5.4.** Smith, M. E., Ramig, L. O., Dromey, C., Perez, K. S., & Samandari, R. (1994). Intensive voice treatment in Parkinson's disease: Laryngostroboscopic findings. *NCVS Status and Progress Report, 6,* 127–133.

**Figures 5.5–5.6.** Perez, K. S., Ramig, L. O., Smith, M. E., & Dromey, C. (1994). The Parkinson larynx: tremor and videostroboscopic findings. *NCVS Status and Progress Report, 7,* 33–39.

**Figure 5.7.** Hanson, D. G., Ludlow, C., & Bassich, C. (1983). Vocal fold paresis in Shy-Drager syndrome. *Annals of Otology, Rhinology and Laryngology, 92,* 85–90.

**Figures 5.8–5.10.** Aronson, A. E., Brown, J. R., Litin, E. M., & Pearson, J. S. (1968). Spastic dysphonia II. Comparison with essential (voice) tremor and other neurologic and psychogenic dysphonias. *Journal of Speech and Hearing Disorders, 33,* 219–231.

**Figure 5.11.** Aronson, A. E., Brown, J. R., Litin, E. M., & Pearson, J. S. (1968). Spastic dysphonia.

I. Voice, neurologic, and psychiatric aspects. *Journal of Speech and Hearing Disorders, 33*, 203–218.

**Figure 5.12.** Izdebski, K. (1984). Overpressure and breathiness in spastic dysphonia. *Acta Otolaryngologica (Stockholm), 97*, 373–378.

**Figure 5.13.** Wolfe, V. I., & Bacon, M. (1976). Spectrographic comparison of two types of spastic dysphonia. *Journal of Speech and Hearing Disorders, 41*, 325–332.

**Figure 5.14.** Aronson, A. E., Brown, J. R., Litin, E. M., & Pearson, J. S. (1968). Spastic dysphonia II. Comparison with essential (voice) tremor and other neurologic and psychogenic dysphonias. *Journal of Speech and Hearing Disorders, 33*, 219–231.

**Figure 5.15.** Colton, R. H., & Brewer, D. W. (1985). Fiberoptic/vibratory relationships in patients with voice disorders. In V. Lawrence (Ed.), *Transcripts of the 14th symposium: care of the professional voice* (pp. 271–275). New York: Voice Foundation.

**Figure 5.16. A,** Terris, D. J., Arnstein, D. P., & Nguyen, H. H. (1992). Contemporary evaluation of unilateral vocal cord paralysis [review]. *Otolaryngology—Head and Neck Surgery, 107*, 84–90. **B,** Tucker, H. M. (1980). Vocal cord paralysis-etiology and management. *Laryngoscope, 90*, 585–590.

**Figure 5.17.** Cohen, S. R., Geller, K. A., Birns, J. W., & Thompson, J. W. (1982). Laryngeal paralysis in children: a long term retrospective study. *Annals of Otology, Rhinology and Laryngology, 91*, 417–424.

**Figures 5.18-5.19.** Hanson, D. G., Gerratt, B. R., Karin, R. R., & Berke, G. S. (1988). Glottographic measures of vocal fold vibration: an examination of laryngeal paralysis. *Laryngoscope, 98*, 541–549.

**Figure 5.20.** Casper, J. K., Colton, R. H., & Brewer, D. W. (1985). Selected Therapy Techniques and Laryngeal Physiological Changes in patients with vocal fold immobility. In V. Lawrence (Ed.), *Transcripts of the 14th symposium: care of the professional voice* (pp. 318–323). New York: Voice Foundation.

**Figures 6.1.–6.7.** Color photographs by Eiji Yanagisawa, M.D.

**Figures 6.8–6.10.** Colton, R. H., Reed, G., Sagerman, R., & Chung, C. (1982). An investigation of voice change after radiotherapy. In *Final Report, National Cancer Institute*, NIH. Bethesda, MD: National Institutes of Health.

**Figure 7.1.** Conture, E. G., Schwartz, H., & Brewer, D. (1985). Laryngeal behavior during stuttering: a further study. *Journal of Speech and Hearing Research, 28*, 233–240.

**Figures 7.2-7.3.** Color photographs by Eiji Yanagisawa, M.D.

**Figure 7.4.** Redrawn from Kitzing, P. (1985). Stroboscopy—a pertinent laryngological examination. *Journal of Otolaryngology, 14*, 151–157.

**Figure 7.5.** Hirano, M., & Bless, D. M. (1993). *Videostroboscopic examination of the larynx.* San Diego: Singular Publishing Group.

**Figure 7.6.** Metz, D. E., Whitehead, R. L., Peterson, D. H. (1980). An optical illumination system for high speed laryngeal cinematography. *Journal of the Acoustical Society of America, 67*, 719–720.

**Figures 7.8–7.9.** Drawn from data of Colton, R. H., Reed, G., Sagerman, R., & Chung, C. (1982). An investigation of voice change after radiotherapy. In *Final Report, National Cancer Institute, NIH.* Bethesda, MD: National Institutes of Health.

**Figure 7.11.** *Application notes: acoustic measurement of vocal function.* Courtesy of Kay Elemetrics Co., Pine Brook, NJ.

**Figure 7.17.** Data drawn from Tait, N. A., Michel, J. F., & Carpenter, M. A. (1980). Maximum duration of sustained /s/ and /z/ in children. *Journal of Speech and Hearing Disorders, 45*, 239–246.

**Figure 7.18.** Based on data reported by Wright, H. N., & Colton, R. H. (1972a). Some parameters of vocal effort. *Journal of the Acoustical Society of America, 51*, 141A.

**Figures 8.1–8.8.** Hirano, M. (1988). Endolaryngeal microsurgery. In G. M. English (Ed.), *Otolaryngology* (Vol. 3, pp. 1–22). Philadelphia: JB Lippincott.

**Figures 8.13-8.17.** Reproduced by permission from Hirano, M. (1989). Surgical alteration of voice quality. In C. W. Cummings, J. M. Fredrickson, L. A. Harker, C. J. Krause, D. E. Schuller (Eds.), *Otolaryngology—Head and Neck Surgery, Update I.* St. Louis: CV Mosby.

**Figure 8.24.** Pontes, P., & Behlau, M. (1993). Treatment of sulcus vocalis: auditory perceptual and acoustical analysis of the slicing mucosa surgical technique. *Journal of Voice, 7*, 365–376.

**Figure 9.1.** Hixon, T. J. (1973). Respiratory function in speech. In F. D. Minifie, T. J. Hixon, & W. Williams (Eds.), *Normal aspects of speech, hearing and language* (p. 107). Englewood Cliffs, NJ: Prentice-Hall.

**Figure 9.3.** Data obtained from Holmberg, E. B., Hillman, R. E., & Perkell, J. S. (1988). Glottal airflow and transglottal air pressure measurements for male and female speakers in soft, normal and loud voice. *Journal of the Acoustical Society of America, 84*, 511–529.

**Figure 10.5.** Hirano, M. (1981). *Clinical examination of voice.* Vienna: Springer-Verlag.

**Figure 10.6.** Dickson, D. R., & Dickson, W. M. (1982). *Anatomical and physiological bases of speech.* Boston: Little, Brown.

**Figure 11.2.** Titze, I. R. (1994). *Principles of voice production.* Englewood Cliffs, NJ: Prentice-Hall, p. 101.

**Figure 11.3.** Based on data from Hollien, H., & Moore, G. P. (1960). Measurements of the vocal folds during changes in pitch. *Journal of Speech and Hearing Research, 3,* 157–165.

**Figure 11.4.** Based on data from Hollien, H., & Colton, R.H. (1969). Four laminagraphic studies of vocal fold thickness. *Folia Phoniatrica, 21,* 179–198.

**Figure 11.5.** Based on data from van den Berg, J. W., & Tan, T. S. (1959). Results of experiments with human larynges. *Practica Otology Rhinology Laryngology, 21,* 425–450.

**Figures 11.6–11.7.** Data obtained from Holmberg, E. B., Hillman, R. E., & Perkell, J. S. (1988). Glottal airflow and transglottal air pressure measurements for male and female speakers in soft, normal and loud voice. *Journal of the Acoustical Society of America, 84,* 511–529 (Tables AI–AVI).

**Figure 11.9.** Based on data from Colton, R. H., Estill, J., & Gerstman, L. (1981). *Identification of four selected voice qualities by spectral analysis.* Paper presented at the Vocal Fold Physiology Conference, Madison, WI.

**Figure 12.1.** McClean, M. D. (1988). Neuromotor aspects of speech production and dysarthria. In K. M. Yorkston, D. R. T. Beukelman, & K. R. Bell (Eds.), *Clinical management of dysarthric speakers* (pp. 19–58). Boston: College Hill Press.

**Figure 12.2.** Based on data from Penfield, W., & Roberts, L. (1959). *Speech and brain mechanisms.* Princeton, NJ: Princeton University Press.

**Figures 12.3–12.4.** Riklan, M., & Levita, E. (1969). *Subcortical correlates of human behavior.* Baltimore: Williams & Wilkins.

**Figure 12.5.** Based on data from Penfield, W., & Roberts, L. (1959). *Speech and brain mechanisms.* Princeton, NJ: Princeton University Press.

**Figures 12.6-12.7.** Eccles, J. C. (1977). *The understanding of the brain.* New York: McGraw-Hill.

**Figure 12.8.** House, E. L., & Pansky, B. (1967). *A functional approach to neuroanatomy.* New York: McGraw-Hill.

## Tables

**Table 5.1.** Adapted from Hoehn, M. M., & Yahr, M. D. (1967). Parkinsonism: onset, progression and mortality. *Neurology, 17,* 427–442.

**Table 5.3.** Adapted from Carpenter, R. J., McDonald, T. J., & Howard, F. M. (1988). The otolaryngologic presentation of amyotrophic lateral sclerosis. *Otolaryngology, 86,* 479–484.

**Table 5.4.** Adapted from Carrow, E., Mauldin, M., & Shamblin, L. (1974). Deviant speech characteristics in motor neuron disease. *Archives of Otolaryngology, 100,* 212–218.

**Table 5.6.** Adapted from Jarema, A. D., Kennedy, J. L., & Shoulson, I. (1985). Acoustic and aerodynamic measurements of hyperkinetic dysarthria in Huntington's disease. Paper presented at the convention of the American-Speech-Language-Hearing Association, Washington, DC.

**Table 5.7.** Adapted from Ballenger, J. J. (1985). Neurologic diseases of the larynx. In J. J. Ballenger (Ed.), *Diseases of the nose, throat, ear, head, and neck* (pp. 513–548). Philadelphia: Lea & Febiger.

**Tables 5.8-5.9.** Adapted from Darley, F. L., Brown, J. R., & Goldstein, N. P. (1972). Dysarthria in multiple sclerosis. *Journal of Speech and Hearing Research, 15,* 229–245.

**Table 5.10.** Adapted from Ballenger, J. J. (1985). Neurologic diseases of the larynx. In J. J. Ballenger (Ed.), *Diseases of the nose, throat, ear, head, and neck* (pp. 513–548). Philadelphia: Lea & Febiger.

**Table 5.11.** Adapted from Hirano, M., Feder, R., & Bless, D. M. (1983). Clinical evaluation of patients with voice disorders: stroboscopic evaluation. Paper presented at the convention of the American Speech-Language-Hearing Association, Cincinnati, OH.

**Table 6.1.** Based on American Joint Committee for Cancer Staging and End Results Reporting. (1983). Philadelphia: JB Lippincott.

**Table 13.2.** Data from Brown, W. S., Jr., Morris, R. J., Hollien, H., & Howell, E. (1991). Speaking fundamental frequency characteristics as a function of age and professional singing. *Journal of Voice, 5,* 310–315.

**Table 13.3.** Data from Casper, J. K. (1983). *Frequency perturbation in normal speakers: a descriptive and methodological study.* Unpublished doctoral dissertation, Syracuse University, Syracuse, NY.

**Table 13.6.** Adapted from Baken, R. J. (1987). *Clinical measurement of speech and voice.* San Diego: College Hill Press, p. 117.

**Table 13.9.** Adapted from Table 2 in Kent, R. D., Kent, J., & Rosenbek, J. (1987). Maximum performance tests of speech production. *Journal of Speech and Hearing Research, 52,* 367–387.

# Index

Page numbers followed by "t" or "f" denote tables or figures respectively.